# Secrets of Cooking for Long Life

# Secrets of Cooking for Long Life

## Sandra Woodruff, RD

AVERY PUBLISHING GROUP

*Garden City Park • New York*

The information in this book is intended for general purposes only. While this information can be used to help prevent and treat a wide variety of health problems, realize that certain medical problems and the use of certain medications may require very specific dietary guidelines. Therefore, the recommendations presented in this book should never replace the sound medical advice of a qualified medical professional who is familiar with your health history and your special health-care needs.

Text Illustrator: John Wincek
Interior Color Photographs: Victor Giordano
Photo Food Styling: BC Giordano
Front Cover Photograph: Victor Giordano
Back Cover Photographs: Victor Giordano
Cover Design: Eric Macaluso
Typesetting: Helen Contoudis and Gary Rosenberg
In-House Editor: Joanne Abrams

**Avery Publishing Group**
120 Old Broadway
Garden City Park, NY 11040
1–800–548–5757
www.averypublishing.com

**Library of Congress Cataloging-in-Publication Data**
Woodruff, Sandra L.
    Secrets of cooking for long life : over 200 delicious dishes that
maximize health and longevity / Sandra Woodruff.
        p. cm.
    Includes bibliographical references and index.
    ISBN 0–89529–861–9
    1. Cookery. 2. Low-fat diet—Recipes. I. Title.
TX714.W657 1999                                            98-37567
641.5′63—dc21                                                CIP

Printed in the United States of America

10   9   8   7   6   5   4   3   2   1

# Contents

*This book is dedicated
to my favorite taste testers,
Wiley, C.D., and Belle.*

# Acknowledgments

I am very grateful to have had the opportunity to do work that I love *and* to work with great people while doing it. It has been a tremendous pleasure to produce this book with the talented and dedicated professionals at Avery Publishing Group, who lend their support and creativity at every stage of production. Special thanks go to Rudy Shur and Ken Rajman for providing the opportunity to publish this book, and to my editor, Joanne Abrams, whose hard work, diligent attention to detail, and endless patience have added so much.

Thanks also go to my husband, Tom, and to my dear friends and family members for their long-term support and encouragement. And last but not least, I would like to express my gratitude to my clients and coworkers, whose many questions, ideas, and suggestions keep me learning and experimenting with new things.

# Preface

The relationship between a nutrient-rich low-fat diet, optimal health, and longevity is becoming more apparent every day. And as researchers explore the causes of aging, it has become abundantly clear that excessive intakes of fat and calories—combined with deficiencies of antioxidant nutrients, vitamins, minerals, and other substances—hasten the aging process. This is good news, because these dietary shortcomings are easily corrected. Even better news is that what has long been thought of as "normal" aging can be substantially delayed and even partially reversed by proper nutrition and exercise.

As millions of Americans approach middle age and beyond, they are becoming aware of the need to improve the quality of their diets, but many simply don't know where to start. How do you know which foods are the best choices? Unless you're a nutritionist, it's hard to be sure. Certainly, the flood of often contradictory information about nutrition can be overwhelming. This is why *Secrets of Cooking for Long Life* was written.

Part I of *Secrets* explores the relationship between what you eat—and what you don't eat—and longevity. You will discover how you can use the vast array of powerful nutrients in foods to maximize your body's potential, bolster your defenses against disease, and prevent premature aging. You will also learn about the many healthful ingredients that will allow you to create delicious meals that can help maintain optimal health, enabling you to get the most from life.

Following this important information, each of the first nine chapters of Part II focuses on a specific meal of the day or a specific type of dish, each of which offers a virtual food pharmacy of nutrients and protective substances. Looking for breakfast foods that are not only tempting enough to lure you out of bed, but also nutritious enough to keep you going strong until lunch time? Chapter 4, "Breakfasts for Champions," presents a wide selection of breakfast dishes, from Cinnamon-Vanilla French Toast to Sausage and Potato Strata. Or perhaps you want to serve hors d'oeuvres and appetizers that will make your buffet table the life of the party without adding an unhealthy dose of fat and calories. "Hors D'Oeuvres With a Difference" will lead the way with a sumptuous selection of treats that take the fat out of celebrations and get-togethers. Still other chapters will show you how to make warming soups like Roasted Onion Soup; refreshing salads like Mediterranean Chef's Salad; bountiful breads like Buttermilk Cornbread; savory pasta dishes like Lasagna Siciliana; hearty home-style entrées like Dilled Salmon Burgers; meatless main dishes like Black Bean Burritos; and wholesome side dishes like Southwestern Roasted Sweet Potatoes. And because for some of us, the meal just isn't complete until we've enjoyed dessert, there's a delightful selection of cakes, cobblers, crisps, puddings, pies, and other treats designed to provide a sweet but nutritious conclusion to your meal.

Finally, Chapter 14, "Menus for a Longer Life," pulls principles and practice together. In this chapter, you will find sample menus that guide you in the prevention and treatment of health problems through wise meal planning. I think you'll be delighted to discover that healthy eating does not have to mean deprivation. In fact, by modeling your own food choices after these sample menus, you may find your diet more varied and satisfying than ever before!

All of the recipes in *Secrets of Cooking for Long Life* have been designed to be as nutrient-dense as possible. This means that you get maximum amounts of vitamins, minerals, fiber, antioxidants, and other anti-aging sub-

stances, but not unhealthy amounts of sugar, salt, harmful fats, or calories. How has this been accomplished? These recipes start with plenty of nutrient-packed vegetables, fruits, whole grains, and other foods with proven health benefits. They then limit the use of overly processed, refined foods—foods that accelerate the aging process. Ultra-lean meats, legumes, wholesome meat alternatives, and low-fat dairy products are used to supply protein, calcium, and other essential nutrients, while keeping fat and cholesterol to a minimum. Finally, creative cooking techniques keep fat, calories, sugar, and sodium in check while keeping recipes high in flavor.

Through your food choices, you have a tremendous power to determine your health. The information presented in this book can be instrumental in helping you make the right choices. It is my hope that *Secrets of Cooking for Long Life* will prove to you that healthful, nutritious, and delicious foods can both enhance the quantity of your life and help you enjoy each and every day to the fullest.

# Introduction

Who doesn't want to live a longer, more productive, and more energetic life? Billions of dollars are spent each year on potions, pills, and other concoctions that promise to add years to your life and life to your years. Yet the single most powerful tool you have to promote health and longevity is inexpensive, easy to implement, and too often ignored. What is this tool? Food. Scientists have long known that what you eat—as well as what you don't eat—can have a profound effect on your susceptibility to disease and premature aging. In fact, just after smoking, diet is the second leading cause of premature death!

The role of a healthful low-fat diet in promoting health and vitality is becoming more apparent every day. Scientists are offering an abundance of evidence that poor nutrition—including subclinical deficiencies of vitamins and minerals, nutritional imbalances, and nutritional excesses—are responsible for much of what has long been considered "normal" aging. Researchers have also offered scientific proof that healthful low-fat diets can actually help reverse atherosclerosis and other life-threatening health problems that have always been thought to be a normal consequence of aging. And as millions of Americans reach middle age and beyond, they are taking this information to heart.

Unfortunately, the typical American diet does not even come close to supporting optimal health or longevity. The reason? For decades, fat has played a central role in the American diet. Butter, margarine, oil, mayonnaise, and fatty meats and cheeses have long been considered an essential part of good eating. To make matters worse, excessive amounts of sugar and salt are frequently added to foods during processing. And whole grains have taken a back seat to nutrient-poor refined grains like white rice and white flour. The fact is that the typical American diet may actually be shortening our lives, or at the very least keeping us from achieving our maximum potential.

*Secrets of Cooking for Long Life* was written to help you use the power of food to get the most from life. Although this book emphasizes the importance of low-fat eating, it goes beyond fat, because if you want optimal health, you must also go for optimal nutrition. And the plethora of nutrient-poor fat-free foods that has entered the market has created a whole new set of problems for the unaware consumer. *Secrets* alerts you to these problems, shows you how to balance your diet, and helps you avoid the common pitfalls of low-fat eating.

Within these pages, you will also discover that eating for health and longevity does not have to mean dieting and deprivation. The

1

recipes in this book bring you the best of traditional home cooking, as well as a wealth of ideas from other cuisines and cultures. The result? A whole new world of flavors that are never bland or boring, and over 200 recipes that are as delicious as they are nutritious. But perhaps best of all, most of the recipes in this book are surprisingly simple to make from readily available ingredients. Every effort has been made to keep the number of ingredients to a minimum, and to use as few bowls, pots, and pans as possible.

As you will see, what you have become conditioned to think of as normal aging is really premature aging brought on largely by nutritionally poor diets and inactivity. And there is plenty that you can do to slow down and even reverse the aging process. While no one will live forever, you can, through positive lifestyle choices, greatly extend both the quality and quantity of your life. I wish you the best of luck and health in all your eating adventures!

# Part I

# Understanding
# the Power of Food

# 1.

# Maximizing Your Body's Potential

So much has been written about the optimal diet for health and longevity, it's no wonder that people are confused about what they should be eating. Mediterranean diets, Asian diets, macrobiotic diets, and vegetarian diets have each been touted as the best way to lengthen life. Which of these claims is true? They all are, in a sense. You see, all of these diets have a common thread—they are low in saturated fat and animal products; rich in vegetables, fruits, and grains; low in sugar; and low in refined and processed foods. This is the essence of eating for health and vitality, and these are the principles upon which this book is based.

Scientists have generated volumes of research on the relationship between diet, health, and longevity, and it is now abundantly clear that there is much you can do to extend both the quantity and the quality of your life. Your food choices *do* directly influence your body chemistry and, thus, your risk of suffering from certain diseases and disorders. For instance, certain foods make your blood "sticky," and more likely to form dangerous clots that cause heart attacks and strokes. Other foods, however, have the opposite effect. What you eat—or don't eat—also influences the ability of your immune system to defend your body against cancer and other diseases, and the rate at which free radicals promote the aging process.

In this chapter, you will discover how you can use the power of food to change your body chemistry into an environment that promotes optimal health and longevity, instead of one that promotes poor health and a decreased life span. The chapter begins by explaining how fat, calories, carbohydrates, proteins, and a variety of other nutrients affect the rate at which you age. You will learn why a low-fat, high-fiber eating plan that is rich in vitamins and minerals can help you live longer and better. Finally, you will learn the simple guidelines for good eating that can help you put these healthy principles into practice in your everyday life.

## THE BUILDING BLOCKS OF A LONGER LIFE

We all know someone who appears and acts much younger than their years. And we all know someone who appears and acts much older than their years. What makes these two people so very different? Except for the fortunate few who are genetically programmed to live long, healthy lives no matter what they do, lifestyle—including diet, exercise habits, stress, and smoking—decides how fast and how well we age. This is good news, because these are all things that can be controlled.

This section will provide you with the rationale and strategies you need to take charge of your diet, and will familiarize you with the nutrients that are the building blocks of a healthier body. First, you will learn about the major nutrients—fat, protein, carbohydrates, and water. Then, you will learn about vitamins and minerals, which are often referred to as *micronutrients* because they're needed in only small amounts. In each case, you'll see how these nutrients either can enhance your health and promote longevity, or—if eaten in the wrong amount or the wrong form—can actually lead to chronic, life-shortening disorders.

## The Role of Fat

Nearly everyone now knows about the health dangers posed by a high-fat diet. In fact, excess fat has long been one of the biggest dietary problems in America. What you may not have considered is that dietary fat is one of the key determinants of how fast you age, and that each specific type of fat presents its own problems or benefits. Let's see how fat can affect your health. First, we'll look at the different categories of fat. You'll find that while some types are harmful, others are actually necessary for life. Then you'll learn how fat can be budgeted into your diet for maximum health.

### Knowing Your Fats

Most people have heard about the three main types of fat—polyunsaturated fat, saturated fat, and monounsaturated fat. However, when you seek to maximize health and longevity, it is important to familiarize yourself with certain subcategories of fats, too. Each of these fats affects your health in different ways.

*Polyunsaturated Fats.* Polyunsaturated fats were once highly recommended as the solution to heart disease, so it may surprise you to learn that these fats are now one of the biggest factors implicated in premature aging and dis-

ease. Why? When eaten in excess, polyunsaturated fats are now known to be powerful generators of free radicals. And free radicals are at the very heart of the aging process because they damage cells and promote disease. (To learn more about free radicals and antioxidants, see the inset "Free Radicals and Aging" on page 7.)

Where are polyunsaturated fats found? Nuts, seeds, and vegetable oils like safflower, sunflower, and corn oils—as well as margarine, mayonnaise, salad dressings, and other products made from these oils—are rich in polyunsaturated fats. Once eaten, these fats are incorporated into cells, where they are readily attacked by free radicals. To make matters worse, during processing, polyunsaturated vegetable oils are stripped of much of their vitamin E—an antioxidant that helps squelch free radicals. In fact, up to 40 percent of an oil's vitamin E may be lost during processing. If you fry foods in these oils, you lose even more of this important nutrient.

Considering the problems caused by polyunsaturated fats, you may think it would be best to completely eliminate them from your diet. But the fact is that two different polyunsaturated fats are essential for life. The first type of essential fat, *linoleic acid*, belongs to a family of fats known as omega-6 fats, and is naturally abundant in nuts and seeds. The average adult needs at least 3 to 6 grams of linoleic acid per day—the amount present in about two teaspoons of polyunsaturated vegetable oil (such as corn, safflower, and sunflower) or about two tablespoons of nuts or seeds (such as walnuts or sunflower seeds). The other essential fat, *linolenic acid*, belongs to the omega-3 family of fats. This fat is present mainly in fish and leafy green plant foods. Flaxseeds are also a rich source of linolenic acid, and walnuts and soy products provide some, as well. How much omega-3 fat do you need? As of yet, no formal recommendation

# Free Radicals and Aging

By now, most people have heard that free radicals pose a threat to their health. But what exactly are free radicals, and how are they related to disease and to the aging process? To understand this, it's helpful to learn a little about some of the chemical reactions that are constantly occurring in your body.

The cells of the body are made up of atoms, small particles that, in turn, contain electrons—even smaller particles. Electrons usually occur in pairs, forming a chemically stable arrangement. A free radical is an atom or group of atoms (a molecule) that has at least one unpaired electron. This makes the free radical highly unstable, causing it to roam around, looking for an electron that it can snatch from other parts of the cell. This leads to a chain reaction of electron snatching, as each affected electron tries to restabilize itself by stealing another electron—a process known as oxidation. As the process of oxidation continues, the cells experience a type of damage known as oxidative stress. This damage has been associated with a range of disorders, including arthritis, cardiovascular disease, mental decline, and visual disorders such as cataracts. It has also been linked to premature aging.

There is no way to prevent free radicals from forming in the body. These molecules are continuously formed as a normal part of body processes. You are also exposed to free radicals from external sources such as smoking, air pollution, and radiation. However, you can protect yourself from free radicals. How? The body uses a variety of antioxidants to defend itself against these destructive molecules. Vitamin E, vitamin C, and beta-carotene are the most well-known antioxidants. The body also uses a variety of enzymes such as superoxide dismutase and glutathione peroxidase to quench free radicals. Researchers have also discovered many substances in vegetables, fruits, and legumes—substances such as lycopene in tomatoes—that function as powerful antioxidants.

The relationship between free radicals and antioxidants is easy to understand if you think of your body as a battlefield where war is constantly being waged between two opposing forces. The polyunsaturated fats located in cell membranes as well as the cell's reproductive material—the DNA—are favorite targets of free radicals. If the body's antioxidant defense system is inadequate to neutralize these free radicals, these destructive molecules will alter the structure and function of cells, setting the stage for disease and premature aging. LDL cholesterol particles that circulate in the blood are another prime target for free radicals. When these particles become oxidized by free radicals, they more readily form plaques on artery walls, and promote premature cardiovascular disease.

It's clear that one of your best strategies for longevity is a means of protection against free radical damage. How can you establish such a defense? The answer is two-fold. First, feed your body's antioxidant defense system by making sure that your diet contains plenty of vegetables, fruits, whole grains, and legumes. These foods are rich in antioxidant vitamins, minerals, and other protective substances. Second, avoid exposing yourself to the foods and pollutants that cause free radicals to be generated. For instance, stay away from foods that contain large amounts of polyunsaturated vegetable oils, avoid chemical additives and pesticides in foods, don't smoke, and limit your exposure to environmental pollutants. This will keep the good forces in your body—the antioxidants—strong enough to repel the free radical forces.

---

exists in the United States, but researchers believe we need about a fourth as much linolenic acid as we do linoleic acid.

Omega-6 and omega-3 fats are important because they are the raw material for *eicosan*oids—hormone-like substances that control many aspects of metabolism, including blood clotting, blood pressure regulation, inflammation, and immune system function. There is still much to be learned about omega-6 and

# Getting the Right Balance of Essential Fats

*Two kinds of essential fats are needed in the diet every day. The first is an omega-6 fat known as linoleic acid, and the other is an omega-3 fat known as linolenic acid. These two types of fat exert very powerful—and very different—effects on the body. Most people eat far too much omega-6 fat and too little omega-3 fat—and the health implications of doing so include an increased risk of blood clots, high blood pressure, cancer, and various inflammatory diseases. Most foods provide a mixture of these two fats, and a food is usually higher in one type of fatty acid than another. Clearly, it makes sense to choose an overall diet that provides the most healthy balance of these fats.*

*The following table lists the omega-6 and omega-3 content of selected foods, along with the ratio of omega-6 to omega-3 fats. When evaluating this table, keep two things in mind. First, you need only small amounts of these fats in your diet. About 3 to 6 grams of linoleic acid and 1.1 to 1.5 grams of linolenic acid are the minimum suggested daily amounts. Most Americans eat at least ten times as much omega-6 fats as they do omega-3 fats. Researchers estimate that some people may be eating*

*up to twenty times more omega-6 fats than omega-3 fats. And while no one knows exactly what the optimal ratio of these fats is, it is thought that a diet that provides only four times as much omega-6 as omega-3 would greatly reduce the risk of many common diseases.*

*By examining this table, you will see how a diet overly rich in mayonnaise, margarine, oily dressings, and other foods made with corn, sunflower, and safflower oil can contribute to an overdose of omega-6 fat. You will also understand how foods like vegetables, fruits, and fish contribute to a favorable balance of fats. You will notice that meats like venison have the most favorable ratio of omega-6 to omega-3 fats. Why? Wild game feeds mostly on green plants, which provide the animals with omega-3 fat. On the other hand, domestic livestock consume more grains, which make their meat higher not only in total fat, but also in omega-6 fats.*

*Don't get caught up trying to calculate your ratio of omega-6 to omega-3 fats. If you follow the Guidelines for Good Eating presented on page 21, you will automatically consume a healthful balance of these essential nutrients.*

omega-3 fatty acids, but many researchers believe that humans evolved on a diet that provided about equal amounts of these fats. This began to change rapidly around the turn of the century, when industry developed ways to mass produce vegetable oils rich in omega-6 fats. At the same time, farmers began feeding their livestock grains, which made the animals fatter—and higher in omega-6 fats. As people began eating more fatty meats, as well as more vegetable oils, the ratio of omega-6 to omega-3 fats in the diet rose from about 1 to 1, to as high as 20 to 1. And, while the eicosanoids made from omega-6 fats are vital—they enable blood to clot, maintain normal blood pressure and immune function, and perform many other

essential functions—when omega-6 fats are consumed in excess, the resulting overabundance of eicosanoids favors the development of blood clots, high blood pressure, cancerous tumors, and inflammatory diseases.

At the same time that many people are overdosing on omega-6 fat, they are getting too little omega-3 fat. Why? Most people eat very little fish and not nearly enough vegetables. Another problem is that omega-6 fat competes with omega-3 fat for processing by the body. So when people eat large amounts of omega-6 fat, it blocks the metabolism of what little omega-3 fat they do eat, making matters worse. Why do you need omega-3 fats? Like omega-6 fats, omega-3 fats are made into eicosanoids, but

| Essential Fatty Acid Content of Selected Foods | | | |
|---|---|---|---|
| Food | Omega-6 Fats | Omega-3 Fats | Ratio of Omega-6 to Omega-3 |
| Spinach, raw (2 cups) | 0.02 g | 0.13 g | 0.2 to 1 |
| Salmon, poached (4 ounces) | 0.49 g | 1.78 g | 0.3 to 1 |
| Flaxseeds (2 tbsp) | 1.06 g | 3.23 g | 0.3 to 1 |
| Strawberries (2 cups) | 0.36 g | 0.26 g | 1.4 to 1 |
| Canola oil (1 tbsp) | 2.77 g | 1.27 g | 2.2 to 1 |
| Walnuts (2 tbsp) | 4.8 g | 1.02 g | 4.7 to 1 |
| Venison, roasted (4 ounces) | 0.6 g | 0.1 g | 6 to 1 |
| Soybean oil (1 tbsp) | 6.95 g | 0.93 g | 7.5 to 1 |
| Tofu (4 ounces) | 2.7 g | 0.36 g | 7.5 to 1 |
| Skinless chicken breast, roasted (4 ounces) | 0.74 g | 0.07 g | 10.6 to 1 |
| Olive oil (1 tbsp) | 1.07 g | 0.08 g | 13.3 to 1 |
| Beef rib eye steak, broiled and trimmed (4 ounces) | 0.35 g | 0.02 g | 17.5 to 1 |
| Pork chop, broiled and trimmed (4 ounces) | 0.61 g | 0.02 g | 30 to 1 |
| Corn oil (1 tbsp) | 7.9 g | 0.10 g | 79 to 1 |
| Sunflower oil (1 tbsp) | 8.95 g | 0.05 g | 179 to 1 |
| Safflower oil (1 tbsp) | 10.1 g | 0.05 g | 202 to 1 |

omega-3 eicosanoids alter body chemistry in a very different way. They "thin" the blood, preventing deadly blood clots from forming. They also help to lower blood pressure, reduce blood triglycerides, inhibit tumor formation, and protect against inflammatory diseases like rheumatoid arthritis.

It has become obvious that too much omega-6 fat and too little omega-3 fat plays an important role in promoting a number of diseases. How can you restore the right balance of fat to your diet? Reduce the amount of omega-6 fat in your diet to a healthy level by minimizing the use of vegetable oils, shortenings, full-fat margarine, and full-fat mayonnaise. Instead, eat a diet rich in vegetables, fruits, and whole grains; include fish several times a week, along with small amounts of nuts and seeds; and choose lean meats and low-fat dairy products. The inset "Getting the Right Balance of Essential Fats," found on page 8, provides more information on omega-6 and omega-3 fats.

*Saturated Fats.* While you may have been surprised to learn of the perils of polyunsaturated fats, you are probably well aware of the dangers posed by another type of fat—saturated fat. Found in fatty meats, butter, and high-fat dairy products, saturated fat very powerfully raises blood cholesterol levels, leading to atherosclerosis, a condition in which blood vessels throughout the body become clogged with plaque. As plaques get larger and larger over the years, they begin to harden arteries and reduce blood flow to the heart, brain, kidneys, and many other parts of the body, contributing to high blood pressure, mental decline, impotence, and many other problems.

Fortunately, with the wide variety of fat-free dairy products, ultra-lean meats, and meat alternatives that are available, it is a simple matter to keep saturated fat under control. The recipes in this book will show you how to do so easily and deliciously.

*Hydrogenated Fats.* Hydrogenated vegetable oil is yet another type of fat that should be avoided. This fat is different from the others being discussed in that, while the others occur naturally in food, this one is manmade—manufactured through the addition of hydrogen to liquid vegetable oils. Why do this? Hydrogenation transforms liquid oils into solid margarines and shortenings, giving these products a butter-like consistency, improving the oils' cooking and baking qualities, and extending their shelf life. But it does one other thing, as well—it creates undesirable by-products known as *trans-fatty acids* or *trans fats*. Unfortunately, trans fats act much like saturated fat to raise blood cholesterol levels. Many researchers believe that trans fats may be linked to some kinds of cancer and to other health problems, as well.

*Monounsaturated Fats.* If polyunsaturated fats must be limited, and saturated and hydrogenated fats should be avoided, are there any fats that are safe to eat? Yes. Monounsaturated fats—found in olive oil, canola oil, avocados, almonds, cashews, peanuts, and macadamia nuts—have no known harmful effects other than being a concentrated source of calories, like all fats. This makes monounsaturated fats a good fat choice as long as you stay within your fat budget. (More about this later in the chapter.)

## Budgeting Your Fat

You now understand why it's so important to limit your intake of fat. Just how much fat should you eat? It depends on how many calories you need each day to maintain a healthy body weight. Health experts recommend that fat calories constitute no more than 30 percent of your daily calorie intake, and, in fact, 20 to 25 percent would be even better in most cases. So the first step in determining your fat budget is to know your calorie needs. Since calorie needs depend on weight, age, gender, activity level, and metabolic rate, these needs vary greatly among people. Most adults, though, must consume 13 to 15 calories per pound to maintain their weight. Of course, some people require even fewer calories, while very physically active people need more.

Suppose you are a moderately active person who weighs 150 pounds. You will probably need about 15 calories per pound to maintain your weight, or about 2,250 per day. To limit your fat intake to 20 percent of your calorie intake, you can eat no more than 450 calories derived from fat per day (2,250 x .20 = 450). To convert this into grams of fat, divide by 9, as one gram of fat has 9 calories. Therefore, you should limit yourself to 50 grams of fat per day (450 ÷ 9 = 50). The table on page 11 shows two maximum daily fat gram budgets—one based on 20 percent of calorie intake, and one based on 25 percent of calorie intake. If you are overweight or underweight, go by the weight you would like to be. And keep in mind that although you shouldn't become obsessed with counting fat grams, it is important to have a sense of how much fat is healthy for you. This "budget" will help you make wise decisions when purchasing and preparing food. Finally, if you are watching your weight, realize that the limitation of fat by itself will not guarantee weight loss. You must also make sure that you are not overshooting your calorie budget. The discussion on page 13 explains more about the role of calories in weight control.

# Filling Up With Fiber

*Wholesome whole grains, legumes, vegetables, and fruits should be staples in the diet of anyone who wants to live long and well—and not only because they are loaded with vitamins, minerals, and phytochemicals. You see, all of these foods are rich in health-promoting fiber. Why is fiber so important? Fiber helps maintain blood sugar levels, controls cholesterol, and keeps the intestinal tract healthy, thus protecting against a wide range of health problems and disorders. In addition, fiber provides a feeling of fullness and prevents the overeating that can lead to obesity.*

*To optimize your health, aim for 25 to 35 grams of fiber per day—about twice the amount that most Americans consume. You'll find it easy to meet this*

*goal if you choose whole grains and whole grain breads and cereals instead of their refined counterparts, eat at least five servings of fruits and vegetables per day, and regularly include legumes in your diet.*

*If you are not used to eating high-fiber foods, be sure to add them to your diet gradually. Why? Some people experience bloating and gas when they begin a high-fiber regimen—although this usually passes in a few weeks, as the body becomes accustomed to eating whole natural foods. When following a high-fiber diet, it is also important to drink at least six to eight cups of water per day. Fiber needs to absorb water in order to move smoothly through the digestive system and exert its beneficial effects.*

## Recommended Daily Calorie and Fat Intakes

| Weight | Recommended Daily Cal. Intake | Daily Fat Gram Intake | Daily Fat Gram Intake |
|--------|-------------------------------|------------------------|------------------------|
| (Pounds) | (13–15 Calories per pound) | (20% of Calorie Intake) | (25% of Calorie Intake) |
| 100 | 1,300–1,500 | 29–33 | 36–42 |
| 110 | 1,430–1,650 | 32–37 | 40–46 |
| 120 | 1,560–1,800 | 34–40 | 43–50 |
| 130 | 1,690–1,950 | 38–43 | 47–54 |
| 140 | 1,820–2,100 | 40–46 | 51–58 |
| 150 | 1,950–2,250 | 43–50 | 54–62 |
| 160 | 2,080–2,400 | 46–53 | 58–67 |
| 170 | 2,210–2,550 | 49–57 | 61–71 |
| 180 | 2,340–2,700 | 52–60 | 65–75 |
| 190 | 2,470–2,850 | 55–63 | 69–79 |
| 200 | 2,600–3,000 | 58–66 | 72–83 |

## How Low Should You Go?

As discussed earlier, some fat is necessary for good health. Therefore, at least 15 percent of your calories should come from fat. Of course, if you eat a balanced diet rich in whole, natu-

ral foods, it would be difficult to eat less than this anyway. On the other hand, if you eat a diet rich in fat-free refined and processed foods, you could be at risk for a deficiency of essential fats, as well as deficiencies of other essential nutrients. This is why the recipes in this book so often use whole grains and other natural foods, and minimize the use of refined and processed foods. Realize, too, that a very low-fat diet is not for everyone. If you have a specific medical problem, be sure to check with your physician or nutritionist before making any dramatic dietary changes.

## The Role of Carbohydrates

Carbohydrates provide the body with the energy it needs to function. And some of the healthiest diets in the world—Asian diets, for instance—are built on a foundation of carbohydrate-rich foods. It is important to understand, though, that to be healthful, a high-carbohydrate diet must be properly planned—and the typical American version is not what the doctor ordered. In fact, the American diet, which contains an overabundance of nutrient-poor refined carbohydrates like white flour and sugar, actually *hastens* the onset of disorders like cancer, heart disease, and diabetes, and is a major contributing factor to the rising rate of obesity.

What types of carbohydrates should be included in a long-life diet? Carbohydrate-rich foods like vegetables, fruits, whole grains, and legumes are nature's best sources of the fiber, vitamins, minerals, antioxidants, and phytochemicals that are essential for promoting optimal health. In fact, these foods are some of the most powerful preventive medicines available. For instance, simply by choosing whole grains over refined grains, you may cut your risk of heart disease and diabetes by 30 percent. By eating generous amounts of vegetables and fruits, you can reduce your risk of developing many cancers by half. When you add the benefits of eating whole grains to those of eating vegetables, fruits, and legumes, it's easy to see how choosing a diet rich in unrefined carbohydrates can greatly extend both the quality and the quantity of your life.

## The Role of Protein

Protein is essential for building and repairing the body's tissues and for maintaining a strong immune system. Without protein, the body would not be able to manufacture hormones, antibodies, enzymes, and muscle tissues. Moreover, having a little protein in each meal will keep you feeling full and satisfied for a longer period of time.

Unfortunately, many people fall short of meeting their protein needs. Why? In an effort to reduce fat and cholesterol, they choose to eat less meat, or even give it up entirely. And while it is not necessary to obtain your protein from meat, you *must* substitute a protein-rich alternative. Many people do not do this.

How do you know if you are getting enough protein? Researchers have long recommended a daily intake of 0.36 gram of protein per pound of ideal body weight as a healthy amount for most adults. This amounts to 54 grams of protein per day for a 150-pound person. However, there is growing evidence that protein requirements may be higher for people over the age of fifty, with some researchers recommending 0.45 to 0.57 gram of protein per pound for people in this age group. This means that a 150-pound person could need as much as 68 to 85 grams of protein per day. As the following table shows, a well-planned, balanced diet can easily provide enough protein.

### Protein Content of Selected Foods

| Food | Amount | Protein |
|------|--------|---------|
| Chicken, fish, beef, pork | 3 ounces cooked | 21 g |
| Legumes | 1 cup cooked | 14 g |
| Tofu | 3 ounces | 13 g |
| Milk | 1 cup | 8 g |
| Cheese | 1 ounce | 8 g |
| Bread | 1 piece | 3 g |
| Rice, pasta, grains | ½ cup cooked | 3 g |
| Vegetables | ½ cup cooked | 2 g |
| Fruit | 1 piece | <1 g |

While it is essential that you get adequate protein for good health, you must also avoid going overboard and eating too *much* protein. Why? Diets too high in protein can cause calcium to be lost from the body, contributing to osteoporosis. (See Chapter 2 for more information on diet and osteoporosis.) High-protein diets also place an extra burden on the kidneys, which have the job of breaking down any protein that the body can not use. This is why people who have kidney disease are often encouraged to follow low-protein diets to slow the progression of their disease. Finally, high-protein diets are typically high in fat, cholesterol, and calories. And since meat displaces other foods like vegetables, fruits, and whole grains, heavy meat eaters also consume less of the fiber, vitamins, minerals, and phytochemicals that protect against disease and retard aging. Fortunately, by following the strategies outlined in the Guidelines for Good Eating presented on page 21, you will get all the protein your body needs for good health, but not more than your body can handle.

## The Role of Water

Although not often thought of as a nutrient, water is perhaps the most essential nutrient of all, for you could live only a few days without it. About 50 to 60 percent of your total body weight is water, and water has many varied functions throughout the body. For instance, water is the medium in which all of the body's chemical reactions occur, it transports nutrients to cells and removes waste products from the body, it lubricates the joints, and it helps regulate body temperature and blood pressure.

Even mild dehydration can lead to a myriad of health problems, including fatigue, a reduced ability to concentrate, poor skin tone, constipation, and kidney stones. Having a weight problem? Sufficient water intake is critical, since it helps suppress the appetite and promotes the metabolism of stored fat.

Despite the many critical functions of water, most people go through life dehydrated. How much water do you need? The average person needs eight 8-ounce glasses every day—more in hot weather and when exercising. If you are overweight, have an extra glass for every twenty-five pounds of excess weight. And don't wait until you feel thirsty to drink water, since the thirst mechanism is not finely tuned, and becomes even less so as we age.

What should you drink? Pure fresh water is your best choice. Caffeine-containing soft drinks, tea, and coffee can actually make matters worse, since caffeine is a diuretic and causes water to be lost from the body. As for caffeine-free soft drinks, tea, and coffee, they're fine in moderation. But keep in mind that pure water is still better because it contains no sugar, artificial sweeteners, or other additives. Always carry some water with you to drink throughout the day. After several weeks, you will probably find that your thirst mechanism has become more sensitive, and that you have actually begun to crave water.

## The Role of Calories

You now know about the four major nutrients. But before we go on to a discussion of vitamins, minerals, and other micronutrients, it is important to discuss another component of your diet—calories.

It is now increasingly recognized that calorie control is an essential strategy for promoting longevity. What do calories have to do with life span? To understand the connection, it helps to learn a little about calories and their effect on weight.

Three of the nutrients just discussed—fats, protein, and carbohydrates—each provide the body with the energy it needs to function, and this energy is measured in calories. Problems arise when you take in more calories than your body needs to burn for fuel. Any excess calories are then stored as fat. And, as you will learn in Chapter 2, as the amount of body fat rises, so does the risk of a variety of disorders, as well as that of premature death.

Clearly, there are good reasons to keep calories under control. What's the best way to do this? First, be aware of portion sizes. The simple consumption of *too much food* may well be the number-one dietary problem in America. In recent years, foods like bagels and muffins have more than doubled in size. Sixty-four-ounce sodas, super-size fries, triple-decker burgers, and all-you-can-eat buffets have become the norm. As a result, on the average, Americans eat about 300 calories more per day than they did a couple of decades ago—and the incidence of obesity has risen accordingly.

Watching your fat intake is another important strategy for controlling calories. With 9 calories per gram, fat has more than twice the calories of carbohydrates and protein. This is why you double the calories in a potato by turning it into French fries, triple the calories in pasta by tossing it in a creamy sauce, and increase the calories ten-fold by making cabbage into cole slaw. It's easy to see how a high-fat diet can blow your calorie budget in a hurry. While fat-free versions of mayonnaise, salad dressings, dairy products, and meats are substantially lower in calories than their full-fat counterparts, be aware that not all fat-free foods are also low in calories. Fat-free candies, cookies, and other junk foods often contain just as many calories as their full-fat counterparts. And unfortunately, because these foods are fat-free, people often eat twice as much as they normally would. Don't fall into this very common trap! Read labels and compare fat and calorie counts. Then fill your shopping cart accordingly.

No discussion of calories and longevity would be complete without a mention of the vast amount of research that has been done on caloric restriction and the aging process. Scientists have discovered that limiting animals to 70 percent of their usual caloric intake lengthens life span and prevents or delays the onset of many age-related diseases. Animals who are fed calorie-restricted diets exhibit more energy, maintain stronger immune systems, have greater mental acuity, and have healthier levels of blood pressure, blood sugar, and blood cholesterol than do animals that are allowed to eat all they want. And while most people are not willing to restrict their calories by 30 percent for the rest of their lives—nor do scientists even know if this would be healthful for humans— you can enjoy many of these same benefits if

you simply control your calories enough to maintain a healthy body weight. If better weight control is one of your goals, see the table on page 11 for help in setting up a realistic and healthy budget for both calories and fat. Chapter 2 provides more tips for reaching and maintaining a healthy body weight.

## Key Anti-Aging Nutrients

More than forty nutrients are known to be essential for life, and it seems certain that countless more will be discovered in the future. While all of these nutrients are important, some merit special attention in this chapter because they play central roles in promoting health and longevity—and because they are in short supply in many people's diets. Let's learn more about these important anti-aging nutrients.

### Antioxidants

Antioxidants include vitamin C, vitamin E, and the carotenoids, such as beta-carotene. Many phytochemicals are antioxidants, as well. (To learn about phytochemicals, see the inset "Feasting on Phytochemicals" on page 15.) In addition, the minerals selenium, copper, and zinc are necessary for some enzymes that function as antioxidants.

As already discussed, antioxidants are very important in preventing diseases and premature aging, as they detoxify destructive free radicals. But like the nutrients previously discussed, antioxidants are in short supply in many diets. Why? Vitamin E, like many other nutrients, is processed out of foods. In addition, people who consume large amounts of polyunsaturated fats—like those found in refined vegetable oils, margarine, and mayonnaise—have increased requirements for this nutrient. A diet that is rich in whole grains, wheat germ, and moderate amounts of nuts and seeds helps provide vitamin E, as well as minerals like selenium, copper, and zinc, which are essential for the production of antioxidant enzymes.

As for vitamin C, the carotenoids, and phytochemicals, fresh fruits and vegetables are the best sources of these nutrients. Unfortunately, most people fall short of the recommended five or more servings per day.

## Calcium

Calcium is one of the major minerals in the body, and 99 percent of the body's calcium is stored in the bones, where it helps form the bones' structure. Because of its role in bone health—and because of the increasing prevalence of osteoporosis—calcium has received much attention in recent years. As a result, many people have started taking calcium supplements. But it may be dangerous to view calcium as a magic bullet in the war against osteoporosis. Why? A number of diet and lifestyle factors besides calcium affect bone health, and these must also be considered if your bones are to utilize calcium most effectively. (See Chapter 2 for more information about osteoporosis.)

Besides its role in maintaining healthy bones, calcium has other important functions in the body. For instance, calcium is involved in muscle contraction, blood clotting, the conduction of nerve impulses, and the maintenance of normal blood pressure. Additionally, researchers believe that by reducing certain bile acids, high calcium intakes protect against colon cancer.

Unfortunately, most people, and especially women, fall short of the recommended daily intake of 1,000 milligrams of calcium, not to mention the 1,200 milligrams a day advocated for people over the age of fifty. Yet it's really not difficult to get the calcium you need from your diet. The inset "Boosting Your Dietary Calcium," found on page 17, shows that people who consume two to three servings of nonfat or low-fat dairy products daily, plus a variety of other healthy foods, can meet this requirement with ease.

## Chromium

The mineral chromium works with insulin to transport glucose from the blood into the cells. When a person is chromium-deficient, insulin

## *Feasting on Phytochemicals*

*Indoles, flavonoids, polyphenols, isothiocyanates, and lignans. If you saw them listed as ingredients on a food label, you might be alarmed. But these strange-sounding compounds aren't artificial ingredients, they're phytochemicals—beneficial substances that occur naturally in a wide variety of plant foods. Although scientists have not classified phytochemicals as essential nutrients—and are just beginning to understand how they work—it is clear that many of these compounds are potent antioxidants, and can fight cancer, heart disease, and many other disorders. The fact is that phytochemicals may be some of our most powerful weapons in the war against premature aging.*

*Researchers are not even close to identifying all of the beneficial phytochemicals that exist in foods, and they probably never will identify all of them. So the only way to be sure you are getting a good balance of these substances is to eat generous amounts of vegetables, fruits, whole grains, and legumes. Many phytochemicals are actually plant pigments, so if you choose a colorful array of fruits and veggies, you'll know you're getting a variety of these disease-fighting compounds. The following table presents just a sampling of the phytochemicals that have so far been identified, as well as the source and known functions of each compound.*

### Phytochemical Sources and Functions

| Phytochemical | Food Sources | Functions |
|---|---|---|
| Allium Compounds | Garlic, onions, leeks, and chives. | Protects against cancer, prevents blood clot formation, and lowers cholesterol. |
| Anthocyanins | Red grapes, red cabbage, radishes, eggplant, cranberries, raspberries, and red wine. | Acts as an antioxidant, protects LDL cholesterol from oxidation, and prevents blood clot formation. |
| Ellagic acid | Strawberries, raspberries, apples, grapes, walnuts, and whole grains. | Acts as an antioxidant, and protects against cancer. |
| Flavonoids | Wine, green tea, black tea, fruits, vegetables, nuts, and whole grains. | Acts as an antioxidant, fights tumor growth, prevents blood clot formation, and acts as an anti-inflammatory. |
| Indoles and Isothiocyanates | Cruciferous vegetables such as broccoli, cauliflower, cabbage, and rutabaga. | Stimulates enzymes that protect against cancer. |
| Isoflavones | Soy foods. | Acts as an antioxidant, fights cancer, reduces symptoms of menopause, and helps normalize high and low estrogen levels. |
| Lignans | Flaxseeds, berries, whole grains, and soybeans. | Acts as an antioxidant, reduces symptoms of menopause, and fights cancer. |
| Limonene | Citrus fruits, especially the rind. | Stimulates enzymes that protect against cancer. |
| Lutein | Greens, broccoli, and celery. | Acts as an antioxidant, and protects against cataracts and macular degeneration. |
| Lycopene | Tomatoes, pink grapefruit, and guava. | Acts as an antioxidant, and protects against prostate cancer. |
| Phytates | Whole grains and legumes. | Fights cancer. |
| Quercitin | Red and yellow onions, kale, broccoli, red grapes, cherries, and apples. | Fights cancer, and protects LDL cholesterol from oxidation. |
| Resveratrol | Red grapes and peanuts. | Acts as an antioxidant, and protects against heart disease. |

does not work as effectively, and the pancreas churns out extra insulin in an effort to compensate. Over time, these high insulin levels can raise blood triglycerides, lower HDL cholesterol, and raise blood pressure. Left unchecked, these unhealthy levels can lead to diabetes.

The recommended daily intake of chromium is 50 to 200 micrograms. Yet 90 percent of Americans are believed to consume less than even the lower recommended intake. Why is chromium so lacking in people's diets? Unprocessed carbohydrate-rich foods, like whole

# Boosting Your Dietary Calcium

*Although dairy products are the best known source of calcium, other foods add calcium to the diet, as well. Realize, though, that calcium is not absorbed equally well from all foods. For instance, some plant foods contain oxalates and phytates—compounds that bind calcium and make it unavailable for absorption. This makes the calcium in spinach only about 5-percent absorbable. On the other hand, the calcium in low-oxalate vegetables such as broccoli and kale is over 50-percent absorbable. About 32 percent of the calcium found in milk can be absorbed by the body, and about an equal percentage of the calcium from soy foods is absorbed. Finally, dried beans have an intermediate absorption rate of about 17 percent. The following table lists the calcium content of selected foods. Both these calcium contents and the absorbability factor should be taken into account as you choose calcium-rich foods for your diet.*

### Calcium Content of Foods

| Food | Amount | Calcium |
|------|--------|---------|
| Nonfat yogurt | 1 cup | 450 mg |
| Skim milk | 1 cup | 300 mg |
| Tofu (firm) | 4 ounces | 259 mg |
| Soymilk | 1 cup | 200–400 mg |
| Cheese | 1 ounce | 150–200 mg |
| Bok choy | 1 cup cooked | 158 mg |
| White beans | 1 cup cooked | 131 mg |
| Acorn squash | 1 cup baked | 108 mg |
| Mustard greens | 1 cup cooked | 104 mg |
| Kale | 1 cup raw | 90 mg |
| Pinto beans | 1 cup cooked | 89 mg |
| Broccoli | 1 cup cooked | 72 mg |
| Spinach | 1 cup raw | 55 mg |
| Black beans | 1 cup cooked | 47 mg |

grains and molasses, naturally supply the chromium needed for their own metabolism. When these foods are processed into refined grains and sugars, though, the chromium is removed.

How do you know if you are chromium-deficient? Unfortunately, there is no easy laboratory test to determine this. But if you take a look at your eating habits, you will get a good idea of your chromium intake. Do you eat refined grains like white rice, white bread, and other products made from refined flour, instead of whole grain products? Do you eat sugary foods on a regular basis? If the answers to these questions is "yes," you may be chromium-deficient. When you eat refined grains and sugars, you must borrow from your body's stores of chromium to break these foods down. And when the body's stores become depleted, the health problems mentioned above can develop.

The recipes in this book use ingredients like whole grain flours, oats, bran, and wheat germ as much as possible. By using these whole foods and limiting sugar, you can keep your chromium stores intact. To further insure a good supply of chromium, be sure to make other chromium-rich foods—seafood, mushrooms, molasses, prunes, nuts, and brewer's yeast, for instance—a regular part of your diet.

## Copper

The mineral copper is essential for a healthy heart and cardiovascular system. Copper is also a component of the enzyme superoxide dismutase, which detoxifies free radicals in the body. Unfortunately, most people consume markedly less than the recommended 1.5 to 3 milligrams per day. To make matters worse, diets high in fructose (a sweetener widely used in sodas, candies, and other sweet treats) and sucrose (white table sugar) interfere with the body's ability to use copper. The result? Many researchers believe that marginal copper deficiency is a prevalent and significant contributor to the high rate of cardiovascular disease in the United States.

How can you make sure that you get enough copper? Like other minerals, copper is lost in the processing of grains, so choose whole grains rather than their refined counterparts. Legumes, seafood, nuts and seeds, and vegetables are other good sources of copper. A limited intake of sugar and sweets made with high-fructose corn syrup and other fructose sweeteners is also essential for good copper status.

## Folate

One of the B-complex vitamins, folate, also known as folic acid, has become one of the most talked about nutrients of recent years. One reason is folate's role in keeping arteries free of the plaque that can lead to atherosclerosis. You see, folate, along with vitamins $B_6$ and $B_{12}$, is needed to break down an amino acid known as homocysteine. And researchers believe that high levels of homocysteine in the blood accelerate the rate at which plaque is deposited on artery walls. In fact, one study found that people who had low levels of blood folate and high levels of homocysteine were twice as likely to have plaque-clogged arteries as were people with normal levels. And based on numerous studies of folate, homocysteine, and cardiovascular disease, scientists have estimated that up to 50,000 deaths per year could be prevented if people simply consumed enough folate!

Besides keeping arteries clear, folate promotes health and fights aging in several other ways. Folate is necessary for the manufacture of DNA (the genetic material present in every cell of the body), and therefore is necessary to keep cells healthy. A deficiency of folate may cause DNA and chromosomal damage, contributing to the initiation and progression of cancer. Need another reason to increase your folate intake? B vitamins, including folate, are essential for maintaining normal brain function. Studies have shown that people who have low levels of folate and other B vitamins, along with high levels of homocysteine, have impaired memory and perform poorly on certain tests of thinking ability.

Where do you get folate? Think foliage. Fresh leafy greens like spinach and romaine lettuce are rich in folate, with each two-cup serving providing close to half the recommended daily intake. This makes fresh green salads one of the best ways to get your folate. Asparagus, broccoli, Brussels sprouts, oranges, strawberries, legumes, whole grains, and wheat germ are other good sources. Despite its wide occurrence in foods, folate deficiency is the most common vitamin deficiency in the world. Why? Most people eat too few vegetables. To make matters worse, folate is easily destroyed by heat, light, and exposure to air, so cooking can destroy up to half of a food's folate content. Reheating leftovers destroys even more.

So a diet that supplies at least five servings of fresh vegetables and fruits daily is your best strategy for getting the recommended daily amount of 400 micrograms of folate. Most multivitamins also supply this much folate, making a multivitamin a good insurance policy. A word of caution is in order when you take folate supplements, though. Don't go overboard. Taking large amounts of folate can mask a vitamin $B_{12}$ deficiency, letting it progress to the point of irreparable damage. This is why vitamin supplements that contain more than 1,000 micrograms of folate are available by prescription only.

## Iron

Unlike the other nutrients mentioned in this section, many people get too much iron in their diets—and this can actually *accelerate* the aging process. Why? Excess iron can react with oxygen in the body to produce free radicals. And this, as discussed earlier, can lead to the cell damage associated with aging. In addition, excess iron stores have been linked to an increased risk of cardiovascular disease, cancer, and other disorders.

As people become older, they need less iron than they did during times of growth and reproduction. In fact, people over the age of fifty need only about 10 milligrams of iron per day, compared with the 15 milligrams needed by younger adults. In addition, because the body has a limited ability to excrete iron, any iron consumed in excess of the body's needs builds up in the tissues.

Some people are especially vulnerable to the toxic effects of iron. One out of 250 people has an inherited genetic disorder called hemochromatosis, which causes the body to absorb and store large amounts of iron. Over the years, the extra iron accumulates in the heart, brain, liver, and pancreas, causing damage. Unfortunately, this condition is rarely diagnosed before age fifty, when symptoms begin to develop, so most people are not aware that they have it.

Where might unneeded iron come from? Ready-to-eat breakfast cereals are one of the biggest culprits because in many cases, each serving is fortified with up to 100 percent of the recommended daily intake of 18 milligrams. People who eat these foods regularly could be getting too much iron. In addition, many people take a multivitamin containing 100 percent of the RDI (Reference Daily Intake) for iron, adding to the problem. To keep your iron intake within reasonable limits, avoid fortified breakfast cereals that contain more than 25 percent of the RDI for iron (check the Nutrition Facts label), and avoid taking a multivitamin that contains more than 9 milligrams of iron.

Realize that some people actually suffer from iron deficiency, which can arise from health problems such as bleeding ulcers and other conditions that cause blood loss. If fact, due to the blood lost during menstruation, many women of child-bearing age are anemic from a deficiency of iron. Therefore, your physician might actually recommend iron supplements to bring your stores of this mineral up to a healthy level.

## Magnesium

An activator of over 300 enzymes, this mineral is involved in many aspects of metabolism. Included among these functions is the regulation of blood pressure, which requires not just magnesium, but also sodium, calcium, and potassium. For this reason, a magnesium deficiency can contribute to high blood pressure. Strong bones are also dependent on an adequate supply of magnesium. In fact, over half of the body's magnesium is stored in the bones.

Unfortunately, most people do not consume enough of this important nutrient. And if you are taking a multivitamin, you can't assume that you are getting enough magnesium, as most brands contain only 25 percent of the recommended 400 milligrams per day. Why might you be magnesium-deficient? Like other minerals, magnesium is processed out of refined foods. A healthful, balanced diet of whole foods, though, can help insure that you get enough magnesium. Good sources include whole grains, bran cereals, wheat germ, legumes, nuts and seeds, and bananas. And since magnesium is a component of chlorophyll—the substance that gives vegetables their green color—green vegetables are another good source.

## Selenium

As a component of the antioxidant glutathione peroxidase, selenium works closely with vitamin E to help the body fight free radicals. One recent study also found that selenium may offer powerful protection against cancer. In fact, people who took a 200-microgram selenium supplement daily were found to be only half as likely to develop or die from cancers of the colon, lung, and prostate, as people who took a placebo (fake) supplement.

Does your diet provide an adequate amount of selenium? Since the selenium content of foods depends on the selenium content of the soil in which the foods are grown, it's hard to be sure. However, whole grains are usually a good source, since they are grown in areas of the country that do have selenium-rich soil. Want even more selenium? Brazil nuts, grown in the selenium-rich soil of the Amazon, far surpass all other foods for selenium content. On average, one large nut provides 140 micrograms, or twice the recommended daily amount of 70 micrograms. Seafood is another good source of this essential nutrient.

Like many other nutrients, selenium is essential for life in *small amounts*. In large doses, though, it is toxic. So if you take selenium supplements, be moderate and do not take more than 200 micrograms per day. Taken in too high a dose for too long a time, this nutrient can cause loss of hair and fingernails, nausea, nerve damage, and other problems.

## Vitamin $B_{12}$

Also known as cobalamin, this nutrient performs a variety of functions in the body. Perhaps most significant in our discussion of longevity is that $B_{12}$ helps maintain the sheath that surrounds and protects the nerve fibers which transmit electrical impulses to the brain. Therefore, a lack of vitamin $B_{12}$ can lead to dementia, mental confusion, and, in extreme cases, a creeping paralysis of nerves and muscles. This vitamin also works with other B vitamins, such as folate and $B_6$, to dismantle

homocysteine, an amino acid that accelerates the development of cardiovascular disease.

Vitamin $B_{12}$ is present only in animal products, including lean meats, seafood, and poultry; low-fat and nonfat dairy products; and eggs. For this reason, vegans—vegetarians that eat no animal products—must take a supplement to meet their needs of 2.4 micrograms a day. As some people age, they become less able to absorb vitamin $B_{12}$, and so may require extra supplementation, or even $B_{12}$ shots. Older people who are having memory problems or mental confusion should be tested for vitamin $B_{12}$ deficiency.

## Zinc

Although zinc has many anti-aging roles, this mineral is probably best known for its role in maintaining a healthy immune system. Zinc is also required for the function of many enzymes throughout the body, including those involved in creating DNA—and, therefore, healthy cells. Zinc enzymes are also involved in maintaining healthy bones, muscle proteins, skin, and hair. And as a component of the antioxidant enzyme superoxide dismutase, zinc helps fight free radicals. Finally, because insulin is stored in zinc crystals in the pancreas, this mineral is involved in blood sugar control as well as in many aspects of carbohydrate metabolism.

Zinc tends to accompany the protein in foods, so the richest sources of zinc include shellfish (especially oysters), lean meats, and legumes. Nuts, seeds, wheat germ, and whole grains are also good sources of zinc. Like other minerals, zinc is lost in the refining of grains, so a balanced, whole foods diet is vital to keep zinc stores high.

Because many adults do not eat enough protein-rich food—especially as they grow older—and because many also eat refined grains, they often fall short of the recommended daily intake of 15 milligrams of zinc. Large doses of calcium supplements have been found to suppress zinc absorption, and may contribute to zinc deficiency in some people. A multivitamin containing 100 percent of the RDI for zinc provides a good insurance policy against this.

Be aware that large doses of zinc are toxic, and can interfere with the body's use of copper, reduce HDL cholesterol levels, and suppress the immune system. So do not take more than 15 milligrams of supplemental zinc daily unless the supplement is prescribed by a health professional. As little as 25 milligrams can cause nausea in some people, while larger doses can cause severe stomach upset and vomiting.

## *Do You Need Dietary Supplements?*

You have just learned about a few of the nutrients that are essential for promoting health and longevity. There are many more, but as you've read, there is one lifestyle component that insures your getting plenty of *all* of these essential nutrients, and this component is a diet that is rich in vegetables, fruits, whole grains, and legumes, and low in sugar, refined grains, and overly processed foods.

Should you take nutritional supplements? A growing body of evidence suggests that supplementation is, indeed, prudent. For instance, studies have shown that people who take vitamin E live longer and have less heart disease. Additionally, studies have shown that taking a daily multivitamin significantly improves immune function as people get older. Many researchers recommend the following as a basic and prudent daily supplementation regimen:

❏ A low-potency multivitamin—one that provides 100 percent of the RDI for a broad range of vitamins and minerals

❏ 100 to 200 micrograms of chromium, if it is not supplied by your multivitamin

❏ 100 to 400 international units of vitamin E

❏ 500 to 1,000 milligrams of vitamin C

❏ Enough calcium to bring your daily intake to 1,000 milligrams if you are under fifty years of age, and 1,200 milligrams if you are over fifty

❏ 200 to 400 milligrams of magnesium, if it is not supplied by your multivitamin

When taking supplements, always be sure to take them with a meal—not on an empty stomach—as this will enhance absorption.

Since certain medical conditions and medications interact adversely with nutrition supplements, you should always check with your physician before taking nutritional supplements. And do not be overzealous with nutritional supplements, as too much of a nutrient can be as bad—sometimes worse!—than an insufficient amount. Finally, remember that a healthy diet should be your primary source of nutrients, as there is no pill that can rival the balance of nutrients naturally found in foods.

## GUIDELINES FOR GOOD EATING

You have just learned about the roles played by fat, carbohydrates, and protein in promoting a long and healthy life. And you have learned the importance of a number of vitamins and minerals. But how do you put these principles into practice in your daily life? One of the easiest ways is to use the government-established Food Guide Pyramid as a meal-planning guide. (See the figure on page 22.) Beware, though—unless you make the right choices within each of the six food groups, your diet will fall short of the essential nutrients that fight aging and disease. Let's take a look at the guidelines that will allow you to use this tool to meet your nutritional needs.

## Eat Two to Three Servings of Protein-Rich Foods Every Day

As you know by now, an adequate intake of protein is critical for maintaining lean body mass and muscular strength, and for keeping your immune system going strong. Fortunately, whether you are a sworn meat eater or a vegetarian, there are plenty of ways to meet your protein requirements while keeping harmful fats and calories under control.

If you do eat meat, you will be happy to know that a wide selection of ultra-lean cuts of red meat, pork, poultry, and even lunch meats and sausages are now available to choose from. This means you can have your protein without a counterproductive dose of fat. Chapter 3 will guide you in selecting these low-fat products. Where do fish and seafood fit in? These foods range from practically fat-free to moderately fatty. However, the oil in fish provides essential omega-3 fatty acids. Therefore, all kinds of fish—even the more oily ones like salmon and

mackerel—are considered healthful, and are excellent alternatives to meat and poultry. In fact, fish should be substituted for meat at least twice a week.

Prefer not to eat meat? Plenty of protein-rich plant-based alternatives are available. And even if you are a meat eater, these vegetarian alternatives should constitute at least *half* of your protein choices. Why? Plant foods are naturally low in fat and contain no cholesterol. In addition, plant foods supply dietary fiber and phytochemicals that meats, poultry, and seafood do not.

Some of the best and most widely available alternatives to meat are legumes—dried beans, peas, and lentils. Beside being rich in protein and nutrients, legumes are loaded with soluble fibers that both lower cholesterol and help stabilize blood sugar levels. One type of legume that is gaining popularity in this country is the soybean. Once relegated only to health foods stores, tofu, tofu crumbles, texturized vegetable protein (TVP), and even burgers and crumbled ground meat alternatives made with soy protein are now widely available in grocery stores. Chapter 3 provides more information on selecting these healthful meat alternatives.

You will notice that the Food Guide Pyramid also includes nuts as a meat alternative. And while nuts do provide protein, you would have to eat a quarter cup of nuts or 2 tablespoons of nut butter to equal the protein in one ounce of meat. Unfortunately, this amount of nuts or nut butter also provides close to 200 calories and 20 grams of fat! So unless you can afford the calories and fat, it's best not to go overboard on nuts.

## Eat Two to Three Servings of Calcium-Rich Foods Every Day

As you learned earlier in the chapter, calcium is essential for maintaining strong bones and

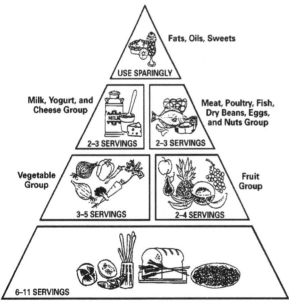

The Food Guide Pyramid

normal blood pressure, and for performing many other vital functions in the body. Yet most people's diets fall short of the recommended 1,000 to 1,200 milligrams per day. Why? Many people avoid calcium-rich dairy products, believing them to be high in fat and calories. While this used to be true, these days, a plethora of no- and low-fat reduced-calorie dairy products are widely available.

Prefer not to eat dairy products? No problem. But you must substitute other calcium-rich foods such as calcium-fortified soymilk, soy cheese, soy yogurt, and tofu. As a bonus, soy products also contain phytochemicals and nutrients that help protect against osteoporosis, cancer, and heart disease. Many green leafy vegetables—including kale and bok choy—are also loaded with calcium. Legumes, too, add significant amounts of calcium to the diet. The inset "Boosting Your Dietary Calcium," found on page 17, provides additional guidelines for adding calcium to your diet.

## Eat at Least Five Servings of Fruits and Vegetables Every Day

Fruits and vegetables offer a bounty of nutrients, fiber, and phytochemicals—all powerful preventive medicines against cancer, heart disease, and many other health problems. Since not all of the protective substances present in these foods have been identified, and some of them probably never will be, it is impossible to get all the benefits of fruits and vegetables from vitamin pills. So fruits and vegetables should be served in generous amounts at every meal.

Sadly, studies show that the average American eats only three to four servings of vegetables and fruits each day. Even worse, much of the time, these foods are laden with butter, margarine, cheese sauce, or other fats. But, as the remaining chapters in this book will show, getting your five-a-day is not as

hard as you may think. Also, you may not realize that a serving is really quite small. A medium-sized piece of fruit, a half cup of cooked or raw fruit or vegetables, a cup of leafy salad greens, a quarter cup of dried fruit, or three-fourths of a cup of fruit juice each constitute a serving. So if you include at least one cup of fruit or vegetables at each meal, you will be well on your way to five-a-day. Finally, remember that five servings are the minimum recommended amount. To maximize your health, aim for seven to nine servings.

## Choose Whole Grains Over Refined Grains

Grain products like bread, cereal, rice, and pasta form the base of the Food Guide Pyramid, with six to eleven servings recommended daily. But you should know that not all grains are created equal. To get the most from this food group, it is essential to choose *whole grain products*—products such as 100-percent whole grain breads and cereals, oats, barley, brown rice, and bulgur wheat. Why? In recent years, whole grains have emerged as one of the foremost protective foods. In fact, several major studies have shown that people who frequently eat whole grains are about 30 percent less likely to develop heart disease and diabetes than people who eat mostly refined grains. This should come as no surprise. Many of the nutrients that are present in whole grains—magnesium, chromium, copper, folate, vitamin E, and fiber, for instance—are known to be essential for the protection of the cardiovascular system and the metabolism of carbohydrates. In addition, whole grains contain lignans, flavonoids, and other health-promoting phytochemicals, the benefits of which are just being recognized.

Unfortunately, most people are not reaping the health benefits of whole grains. In fact, a whopping 83 percent of all grains eaten by Americans are refined. Refining strips grains of most of their fiber, vitamins, and minerals, and causes a 200- to 300-fold loss of phytochemicals. Therefore, a diet based on refined products can actually hasten the development of heart disease, diabetes, cancer, and premature aging.

The good news is that when made properly, breads, muffins, casseroles, breakfast foods, side dishes, soups, and even desserts can include wholesome whole grains. The inset "Great Grains," found in Chapter 4, will introduce you to a variety of versatile, fiber-rich grain products that can be found in your grocery store, and the recipes in this book will show you how to use these and other foods to create hearty and wholesome dishes in your own kitchen.

## Limit Your Use of Table and Cooking Fats

Fats used for cooking and baking—butter and margarine, for instance—and fats added at the table—such as oily salad dressings, mayonnaise, and butter—can really add up. In fact, in their full-fat versions, just one tablespoon of any of these products will add about 10 grams of fat to your meal. The good news is that for each of these foods, there is now a no- or low-fat alternative that can help you greatly reduce or eliminate the fats you use in cooking, in baking, and at the table. Chapter 3 will introduce you to many of these exciting new products, and the recipes in this book will show you how to use them to create great-tasting dishes that you will want to make time and time again.

## Eat Sugar Only in Moderation

When people start reducing their fat intake, often, without really thinking about it, they greatly increase their sugar intake. This is easy to understand. Stroll down the aisles of your local grocery store, and you will see a mind-boggling array of fat-free cookies, brownies, ice creams, and other goodies. While these products may contain little or no fat, they usually contain as much sugar as their high-fat counterparts, and sometimes more!

What health threats are posed by sugar? First and foremost, sugar contains no nutrients, and, when eaten in excess, can actually deplete your body's stores of chromium, the B vitamins, and other vitamins and minerals. Second, it has been found that high-sugar diets are often deficient in nutritious foods. Third, by overwhelming the taste buds and increasing the taste threshold for sweet flavors, diets rich in sugary foods can cause you to lose your taste for the more subtle flavors of wholesome, natural foods. Finally, sugary foods are usually loaded with calories, making them a real menace if you're watching your weight.

The good news is that, in moderation, sugar can be enjoyed without harm to your health. What's a moderate amount? No more than 10 percent of your daily intake of calories should come from sugar. For a person who needs 2,000 calories a day to maintain his or her weight, this amounts to an upper limit of 50 grams, or 12.5 teaspoons—about a quarter cup—of sugar a day. If you need only 1,600 calories a day, your upper limit would be 40 grams, or 10 teaspoons. Naturally, a diet that is lower in sugar is even better. To put your sugar budget into perspective, the table on the next page lists the sugar content of selected foods.

## Limit Your Sodium Intake to 2,400 Milligrams Per Day

A limited sodium intake has many benefits, ranging from better-controlled blood pressure to stronger bones. But of all the guidelines for

## Sugar Content of Selected Foods

| Food | Amount | Sugar (grams) | Sugar (tsp) |
|------|--------|---------------|-------------|
| Jellybeans | ½ cup | 79 | 20 |
| Soft Drink | 12-ounces | 38 | 9½ |
| Chocolate Cake With Icing | ⅟₁₆ cake | 34 | 8½ |
| Nonfat Ice Cream | 1 cup | 32 | 8 |
| Apple Pie | ⅛ pie | 24 | 6 |
| Chocolate Bar | 1½ ounces | 24 | 6 |
| Fat-Free Brownie | 1 brownie | 18 | 4½ |
| Fat-Free Cereal Bar | 1 bar | 17 | 4½ |
| Fruit Toaster Pastry | 1 pastry | 16 | 4 |
| Low-Fat Cream Filled Sandwich Cookie | 2 cookies | 12 | 3 |

good eating, this one can be the most difficult to follow, since many low-fat and fat-free foods contain extra salt. Fortunately, with a just a little effort, even this dietary goal can be met. The most effective sodium-control strategy is to avoid using salt for cooking and at the table. Believe it or not, just one teaspoon of salt contains 2,300 milligrams of sodium—almost your entire daily allowance—so it pays to put the salt shaker away. Another effective strategy is to limit your intake of high-sodium processed foods. Read labels, and choose the lower-sodium frozen meals, canned goods, broths, cheeses, and other products. Also, whenever you make a recipe that contains high-sodium cheeses, processed meats, or other salty ingredients, be sure not to add any extra salt. The recipes in this book will show you how to balance high-sodium products with low-sodium ingredients, herbs, and spices to make dishes that are low in sodium but high in flavor.

While the guidelines for good eating are few in number, they can make a big difference in your diet, providing you with most, if not all, of the nutrients you need to look and feel your best. And you'll find that the tips presented throughout this book make it surprisingly easy to follow these guidelines and build a healthful, enjoyable diet.

# 2.

## Fine-Tuning Your Diet to Fight Health Disorders

Chapter 1 presented the basic dietary strategies for promoting optimal health and longevity, and touched on the role of diet in the prevention of certain chronic diseases. In this chapter, you will learn more about the impact that diet has on specific health problems that may be of personal concern. As you will discover, the low-fat, high-nutrient diet discussed in Chapter 1 can do more than prevent disorders. Especially when the intake of key nutrients is optimized, a healthy diet can help control or even help reverse the progression of problems like cardiovascular disease and osteoporosis—disorders that can affect both the quality and the length of your life.

### ARTHRITIS

An estimated 40 million Americans suffer from arthritis, or inflammation of the joints. Most of them are over forty-five years of age. There are many kinds of arthritis. In this chapter, we will look at osteoarthritis and rheumatoid arthritis, the most common forms of this disorder.

### Osteoarthritis

By far, the most common type of arthritis is osteoarthritis, which is sometimes referred to as "wear and tear" arthritis. In osteoarthritis, the cartilage that cushions the ends of the bones wears thin, allowing bones to rub together, and causing pain and stiffness. Many people are affected by this disorder to some degree by the age of seventy.

Diet is an important consideration for both preventing and treating osteoarthritis, especially with regard to weight. Obesity is a well-documented risk factor for osteoarthritis, since extra weight means extra wear and tear on the joints. If you are overweight, it is well worth the effort to trim down. In one study, researchers found that middle-aged women who lost an average of eleven pounds reduced their risk of developing osteoarthritis by over 50 percent.

If you already have osteoarthritis, weight loss can provide some relief from pain and slow the progression of the disease. A diet high in antioxidant-rich foods may also slow the progression of osteoarthritis. In a recent study, researchers who tracked people with osteoarthritis discovered that those who consumed the most vitamin C were three times less likely to suffer a progression of the disorder than were people with low vitamin C intakes. Foods high in beta-carotene and vitamin E also appear to slow the progression of osteoarthritis. These same researchers discovered that getting plenty of vitamin D may also help keep osteoarthritis from worsening. In

27

fact, people with poor vitamin D status are three times more likely to become progressively worse than are people who get plenty of vitamin D.

## Rheumatoid Arthritis

Rheumatoid arthritis, the second most common form of arthritis, causes inflammation in the lining of the joints, resulting in swelling and pain. In most cases, the symptoms of this disorder first appear between the ages of twenty-five and fifty.

Besides maintaining a healthy body weight, people with this disorder should pay close attention to the kind of fat they eat. Why? As discussed in Chapter 1, certain fats called omega-6 fatty acids can alter body chemistry to favor inflammation, while others—omega-3 fatty acids—help fight inflammation. Therefore, diets high in omega-6 fats, including animal fats and certain vegetable oils, can worsen the symptoms of rheumatoid arthritis. Diets high in omega-3-rich fish oils can help ease symptoms.

How much omega-3 fat should you eat? Consuming as little as 2.6 grams of omega-3 fatty acids daily can reduce pain and stiffness—sometimes enough to eliminate the need for medication. In most cases, it takes three to four months to realize the benefits of omega-3 therapy. As the following table shows, making fish a regular part of your diet can help you easily incorporate this healthy nutrient into your diet.

While as little as 2.6 grams of omega-3 fat has been shown to relieve the pain and stiffness of rheumatoid arthritis, some studies have used three to four times this amount to get benefits—an amount most people find obtainable only by taking fish oil supplements. If you do decide to try fish oil supplements, you should do so only under the care of your physician, as large doses of omega-3 fatty acids can interfere with the actions of certain

### Omega-3 Content of Selected Fish

| Fish (4 ounces cooked) | Omega-3 Fat |
|---|---|
| Halibut | .8 g |
| Herring | 2.2 g |
| Mackerel | 3.0 g |
| Mullet | 1.1 g |
| Oysters | 1.6 g |
| Pompano | 2.3 g |
| Salmon (wild) | 2.5 g |
| Sardines (not oil packed) | 2.1 g |
| Sea trout | 1.5 g |
| Tuna | 1.7 g |
| Whitefish | 2.1 g |
| Yellowtail | 2.1 g |

drugs and with certain medical conditions. Furthermore, some fish oil supplements have been found to contain potentially toxic levels of vitamins A and D, as well as environmental contaminants. Clearly, these supplements must be chosen with care.

Flaxseeds are a rich source of omega-3 fat, as well, with 2 tablespoons providing about 3 grams. However the omega-3 fat in flax is not as potent as that in fish. The good news is that once eaten, the omega-3 fat in flax and other plant foods can be transformed by the body into fats that are identical to those found in fish. Zinc—and possibly other nutrients—are required for this transformation, so if you are not well-nourished, you may not get the full benefit of the omega-3 fats in plant foods.

Many people with rheumatoid arthritis also respond positively to an individually tailored vegetarian diet. However, at this point, no one is sure whether the benefits come from the avoidance of certain foods—such as meats, which are rich in omega-6 fats—or from the inclusion of more nutrient- and phytochemical-rich plant foods. One thing is certain, though: A healthful, well-balanced diet that includes daily servings of fish and flax may be one of your best defenses against rheumatoid arthritis.

Although people with arthritis are often

inclined to take it easy, exercise is critical in the treatment of both osteoarthritis and rheumatoid arthritis. Daily flexibility exercises can help prevent stiffness, and strengthening exercises are necessary to keep muscles strong enough to provide support for joints. A qualified exercise physiologist or physical therapist can prescribe the right exercises for you.

## CANCER

What you eat has a profound effect on your chances of developing cancer. In fact, up to 70 percent of all cancers are thought to be diet-related.

The first and foremost dietary recommendation for preventing cancer is to eat abundant amounts of unrefined plant foods, including at least five to nine servings of vegetables and fruits every day. Just doing this can cut the risk of many cancers in half. The reason? Vegetables and fruits are loaded with antioxidants and phytochemicals that fight cancer. And, along with whole grains and legumes, these foods also supply plenty of fiber, which helps sweep carcinogens out of the digestive tract before they have a chance to initiate cancer.

Do certain kinds of vegetables and fruits offer more protection than others? In general, fresh raw vegetables of *all* kinds seem to offer more protection than do cooked vegetables. Vegetables that appear to be especially beneficial include onions and garlic; carrots; spinach, kale, and other leafy greens; cruciferous vegetables like broccoli, cauliflower, cabbage, and Brussels sprouts; and tomatoes. Other protective produce includes citrus fruits, sweet potatoes, and winter squash.

Another essential cancer-prevention strategy is to limit your intake of high-fat foods. Why? Researchers believe that high-fat diets increase the risk of developing cancer in a number of ways. First, high-fat diets often lead to obesity, which causes the body to secrete more

of the hormones estrogen and insulin—substances that can promote the development of some forms of cancer. Second, people who eat high-fat diets tend to eat too few vegetables, fruits, and other cancer-fighting plant foods. Third, people who eat high-fat diets tend to eat more meat, high intakes of which are associated with colon and other cancers.

Are certain fats more cancer-promoting than others? Both saturated and polyunsaturated fats promote the development of various cancers. When consumed in large amounts, omega-6 polyunsaturated fats like safflower oil, sunflower oil, and corn oil are especially potent cancer promoters. On the other hand, the polyunsaturated omega-3 fat in fish actually offers protection against cancer. (Use the guidelines presented in Chapter 1 to help you to achieve a healthy dietary balance of omega-6 to omega-3 fat.) Monounsaturated fats like olive oil do not appear to promote cancer.

Environmental contaminants such as pesticides and agricultural chemicals, as well as food dyes, preservatives, and other additives, are another area of concern to anyone who wishes to reduce the risk of cancer. Fortunately, several strategies that complement the dietary guidelines already presented can be used to avoid unnecessary exposure to these substances. First, eat low on the food chain—in other words, eat more plant foods and fewer animal foods. Why? Agricultural chemicals that are applied to feed crops accumulate in the tissues of the farm animals that consume them. This means that animal foods generally contain higher concentrations of environmental contaminants than do plant foods. Since these chemicals are especially concentrated in the fatty portions of the meat, you can further minimize your exposure by choosing lean meats and by trimming away all visible fat. Second, thoroughly wash your produce before eating or cooking it. If your produce is waxed—and many apples, cucumbers, eggplants, and other fruits and vegetables are—peel

# Food Additives—A Cause for Concern?

Hundreds of additives—from dyes and preservatives to thickeners, fat substitutes, and more—are present in our foods. And while many additives are harmless or even beneficial, others are potential carcinogens. The following discussion will help you identify and avoid those additives that may pose a threat to your health.

**Artificial Sweeteners.** Although approved by the FDA, artificial sweeteners like saccharin, aspartame, and acesulfame-K continue to be surrounded by controversy. The best policy is to avoid them. Unfortunately, many people hear this advice and interpret it to mean they should resume drinking sugared sodas and using liberal amounts of sugar, instead. And while some sugar is fine in your diet, it's still a nutrient-poor food and should be limited.

**Fat Substitutes.** Most fat substitutes are composed of harmless plant-based thickeners, as well as plant fibers and fruit purées. These products safely and naturally add thickness and body to fat-free and low-fat products, and hold in moisture, too. The safety of one fat substitute, however, is controversial. Olestra—which is sometimes called by the brand name Olean—is a synthetic combination of sucrose (sugar) and fatty acids. Olestra cannot be absorbed by the body, and so provides no calories. And unlike other fat substitutes, olestra can be used for frying, and so is an ingredient in some fat-free potato chips and other snack foods. Finally, olestra confers the flavor and feel of fat to foods. But olestra is not without its problems. You see, this fat substitute binds with fat-soluble nutrients like vitamins A, D, E, K; the carotenoids; and perhaps other nutrients not yet identified, and carries them out of the body. Because olestra causes malabsorption of nutrients, it is fortified with vitamins A, D, E, and K—but not with carotenoids or any other nutrients. Many researchers fear that eating olestra-containing products will cause blood levels of carotenoids to become dangerously low, setting the stage for heart disease and other health problems. If that's not enough to worry about, olestra also causes diarrhea in some people.

**Food Dyes.** Purely cosmetic, dyes are not necessary in foods, yet most processed foods contain some sort of coloring agent. Fortunately, some food colors are perfectly safe. Examples of safe and natural colors are turmeric (a ground spice), anatto (the reddish seed of a tropical tree), beta-carotene, and beet juice extract. On the other hand, many artificial colors are suspected carcinogens and should be avoided. Artificial colors are easy to spot on food labels since they usually have names like yellow dye number 5, red dye number 3, blue dye number 2, and the like.

**Preservatives.** Preservatives are added to foods to prevent rancidity or to retard the growth of bacteria and mold. Although preservative-free foods are your best bet, it's definitely safer to consume a few preservatives than it is to eat rancid, bacteria-ridden, or moldy food! Fortunately, some preservatives are quite safe. Examples are citric acid, ascorbic acid (vitamin C), and alpha-tocopherol (vitamin E)—all of which are added to foods to prevent the oxidation or rancidity of fats and oils. Some preservatives to avoid include BHA and BHT, both of which are suspected carcinogens. Nitrites, added to many cured meats, are also a cause for concern. While not directly carcinogenic, nitrites react with proteins in the digestive tract to form carcinogenic substances known as nitrosamines. Keep in mind, though, that this reaction is blocked by vitamin C. So when you eat cured meats such as low-fat bacon, sausage, or ham, be sure to include a vitamin C-containing food like tomatoes or citrus in your meal. It should be noted that in recent years, manufacturers have greatly reduced the amount of nitrites added to foods, making them safer choices. However, because cured meats are still very high in sodium, they should be eaten only in moderation.

**Thickeners.** Many foods these days contain thickeners that add body. These additives are especially common in fat-free and low-fat products such as mayonnaise, salad dressings, margarine, and sour cream—products in which water has replaced some of the fat. Fortunately, most thickeners are very safe. Examples include carrageenean and agar, which are made from sea vegetables; guar gum, xanthan gum, and pectin, which are vegetable gums; and modified food starch, which is made from rice, wheat, corn, tapioca, or potatoes.

the produce, as waxes cannot be washed away. Of course, your best bet is to purchase organic foods—including both meat and produce—whenever possible. What about the chemicals added to foods during processing? It is a simple matter to avoid overly processed foods. If your diet is rich in vegetables, fruits, whole grains, and legumes, there will be little room left for processed foods, anyway. The inset "Food Additives—A Cause for Concern?" on page 30 provides more information on additives in foods.

There are many complex interactions between nutrients, substances in foods, hormones, obesity, and the development of cancer. But the basic strategy for preventing cancer is very simple—eat a low-fat, low-meat diet with lots of fruits, vegetables, whole grains, and legumes. Does this kind of diet sound familiar? It should. It's the same diet that protects against heart disease and most other chronic disorders.

## CARDIOVASCULAR DISEASE

Cardiovascular disease continues to be the number-one killer of Americans. Yet it has been well established that lifestyle changes—and especially dietary changes—can do a good deal not only to arrest the progression of cardiovascular disorders, but even to reverse them. This section will look at the two most common types of cardiovascular disease: atherosclerosis and high blood pressure.

### Atherosclerosis

The most common form of cardiovascular disease is atherosclerosis, a condition in which cholesterol deposits called *plaques* form on artery walls. As discussed in the Chapter 1, a diet high in saturated fats, trans fats, and cholesterol encourages the development of these plaques.

Although atherosclerosis can become a life-threatening disorder, problems can start long before the condition progresses to this point. As arteries become lined with plaque, they become hard and inelastic, raising blood pressure. When plaques begin to line the blood vessels of the brain, they restrict blood flow and oxygen to the brain, reducing mental alertness. And when plaques form in arteries that supply the sexual organs, impotence can result. To make matters worse, plaque-lined arteries increase the tendency of blood to form dangerous clots as it passes through, and when these clots get lodged in an artery that supplies the heart or brain, a heart attack or stroke can result.

Unfortunately, the well-intentioned person who switches over to a diet high in polyunsaturated fats may just add to the problem. How? As explained in Chapter 1, certain polyunsaturated fats are rich in omega-6 fatty acids, which alter body chemistry to favor the development of blood clots and high blood pressure. In addition, a diet too high in polyunsaturated fat encourages the development of free radicals, which can accelerate cardiovascular disease. As for monounsaturated fats, although they have no known harmful effects on the cardiovascular system, when too much is consumed, they can contribute to weight gain, and thus place a greater strain on the heart and blood vessels.

While avoiding excess fat is an essential strategy for fighting cardiovascular disease, eating more fiber is just as critical. In a recent study, researchers who looked at the eating habits of 43,000 men found that those whose diets contained an average of 29 grams of fiber per day had a 41-percent lower risk of heart attack than men who ate only 12 grams of fiber daily.

What is it about fiber that protects against heart disease? A number of things. First, soluble fiber—found in foods like fruits, vegetables, legumes, and barley—helps lower blood cholesterol levels. (To learn more about choles-

# *Understanding Your Blood Cholesterol Level*

*A high blood cholesterol level is a strong risk factor for heart disease. Fortunately, the guidelines presented in this book for a healthful, low-fat diet can dramatically reduce blood cholesterol levels for most people. Everyone over age twenty should have their cholesterol tested at least once every five years—more often, if necessary. This inset will explain what blood cholesterol is and what the results of a cholesterol test mean.*

*Cholesterol circulates in the bloodstream in particles called lipoproteins. Two kinds of lipoproteins should be measured when you get your blood cholesterol tested. Low-density lipoproteins (LDL) are also known as "lethal" or "bad" cholesterol. These cholesterol-rich particles transport cholesterol throughout the bloodstream to the cells of the body, where it is needed for various uses. If the LDL are loaded down with more cholesterol than the cells can use, the excess can collect on artery walls forming plaques, which can eventually block arteries and cause a heart attack or stroke. High-density lipoproteins (HDL), are also known as "healthy" or "good" cholesterol because these particles carry cholesterol away from the cells and back to the liver for recycling or disposal.*

*As you might guess, the worst case scenario would be to have a high LDL cholesterol and a low HDL cholesterol. In this situation, lots of cholesterol is being shipped into the bloodstream, and not enough is being shipped back to the liver for disposal—which makes plenty of cholesterol available for forming plaques in the blood vessels. The following table categorizes cholesterol, LDL, and HDL levels according to risk of heart disease.*

### *Cholesterol, Lipoproteins, and Heart Disease Risk in Adults*

| Fraction Measured | Low Risk | Intermediate Risk | High Risk |
|---|---|---|---|
| *Total cholesterol* | *Less than 200* | *200–239* | *240 & above* |
| *LDL cholesterol* | *Less than 130* | *130–159* | *160 & above* |
| *HDL cholesterol* | *60 and above* | *35–59* | *Less than 35* |

*Since the balance of LDL to HDL in your blood determines how much cholesterol is available to be deposited in blood vessels, your cholesterol test will probably also list the LDL/HDL ratio or the cholesterol/HDL ratio. For the lowest risk you should have:*

❑ *An LDL/HDL ratio of 3 or less—which means that you have no more than 3 times as much bad cholesterol as good cholesterol.*

❑ *A cholesterol HDL ratio of 4.5 or less—which means that you have no more than 4.5 times as much total cholesterol as good cholesterol.*

*High blood cholesterol is just one of a number of risk factors for heart disease. Other risk factors include smoking, high blood pressure, diabetes, family history, obesity, and a sedentary lifestyle. Dietary changes can dramatically reduce blood cholesterol and reduce your risk of heart disease, primarily by lowering LDL cholesterol. You can raise your HDL cholesterol mainly by exercising, by maintaining a healthy body weight, and by not smoking.*

terol levels, see the inset "Understanding Your Blood Cholesterol Level" above.) Second, fiber helps reduce insulin secretion, thus protecting against insulin resistance, which worsens cardiovascular disease. Third, fiber-rich foods are so filling that people are less likely to overeat or to fill up on empty-calorie foods, and thus become overweight. Last but not least, fiber-rich foods like vegetables, fruits, legumes, and whole grains are loaded with nutrients and phytochemicals that protect against cardiovascular disease. For instance, antioxidants like vitamin E, vitamin C, and the carotenoids deactivate the destructive free radicals that promote heart disease. Nutrients like folate, copper, chromium, and selenium are essential for maintaining a healthy heart and blood vessels. And potassium, calcium, and magnesium can help keep blood pressure in check. Sadly, because most people consume too few vegetables and fruits, their diets are deficient in the nutrients needed for heart health.

So far, we have looked at ways in which the proper diet can help prevent atherosclerosis. But can a heart-healthy diet *reverse* the process once it has begun? Yes. In a landmark study, cardiologist Dean Ornish proved that people who adopt a very low-fat meatless diet combined with moderate exercise and stress management can dramatically reduce their blood cholesterol levels and actually begin to dissolve the plaques that line their arteries. Dr. Ornish's diet limits fat to 10 percent of calories, and restricts cholesterol to 5 milligrams per day; is rich in unprocessed foods such as vegetables, fruits, whole grains, and legumes; and includes nonfat dairy products and egg whites. In contrast, Dr. Ornish's study found that the conventional recommended "heart-healthy" diet—which gets 30 percent of its calories from fat, and allows up to 300 milligrams of cholesterol daily—only *slows* the progression of heart disease.

## High Blood Pressure

One in four adult Americans has high blood pressure. Among people age sixty-five and over, the rate increases to more than one out of two. And since high blood pressure, also called *hypertension*, usually produces no outward symptoms, many people are not even aware that they have it. But don't let the absence of outward symptoms fool you. The heart must work harder to pump the blood through the cardiovascular system of a hypertensive person, so even a slightly elevated blood pressure can increase the chance of heart attack or stroke.

What exactly is high blood pressure? When you have your blood pressure measured, you are actually determining the measurement of the force exerted by the blood on the walls of your blood vessels. Two numbers are used to measure this force. The top number, or *systolic blood pressure*, is the pressure inside the arteries when the heart contracts. The bottom number, or *diastolic blood pressure*, is the pressure inside the arteries when the heart relaxes between beats. What is a normal blood pressure reading? In general, normal is considered to be around 120/80. When these numbers reach 140/90, a person is considered to have high blood pressure, meaning that there is abnormally high pressure in the arteries.

While anyone can develop high blood pressure, heredity makes some people more likely to experience it. But this does not mean that you are helpless, as many other contributing factors *are* within your control. Excess weight is one of the biggest risk factors, as it raises your risk by two- to six-fold. The typical American diet is another major contributor. This diet is high in fat and calories, which lead to obesity; provides too much omega-6 fat, favoring the development of high blood pressure; is too high in sodium, which causes fluid retention; is too low in the minerals needed to regulate blood pressure; and tends to lead to the development of atherosclerosis, which raises the pressure in blood vessels by making them hard and inelastic. Other lifestyle factors that can raise your risk of developing high blood pressure include smoking, excessive alcohol intake, a sedentary lifestyle, and poor stress management.

What can you do about high blood pressure? First, follow the Guidelines for Good Eating presented in Chapter 1. This will provide you with plenty of the calcium, potassium, and magnesium essential for keeping blood pressure under control, and at the same time will limit your sodium—a mineral that causes fluid retention and elevated blood pressure. Second, control calories to allow for gradual weight loss, if necessary. Losing just ten pounds can significantly reduce blood pressure in many people. Third, exercise regularly. This will not only keep your cardiovascular system strong and assist with weight loss, but will also help you better deal with stress, a potent contributor to high blood pressure. Finally, don't smoke or drink alcohol excessively. Taken together, these simple measures are so powerful that they can eliminate the need for medication in many people.

## DIABETES

An estimated 16 million Americans have diabetes, and only half of them are even aware of it. This is a shame, because diabetes is one of the most preventable of all diseases. Ninety percent of the people who get diabetes develop the disease during adulthood, usually past the age of forty. And for the vast majority of these people, poor nutrition, combined with a sedentary lifestyle, is a major contributing factor to the onset of the disease.

The most obvious dietary component that people think of when diabetes comes to mind is sugar, as diabetes causes blood sugar concentrations to become abnormally high. But, surprisingly, excess fat is often equally problematic. Why? High-fat diets are the primary cause of obesity, and obesity is the underlying cause of most cases of Type II (adult onset) diabetes. How does obesity lead to diabetes? As a person becomes overweight, his or her cells become less sensitive to insulin, the hormone that is responsible for keeping blood sugar levels under control. As body fat stores grow, the pancreas must secrete more and more insulin to keep blood sugar levels in check. Over time, blood insulin levels become chronically elevated and a condition known as *insulin resistance* develops. Left untreated, cells become so resistant to insulin that they can no longer adequate-

ly remove sugar from the blood. At this point, diabetes results. To make matters worse, once a person has developed diabetes, a high-fat diet poses a threat to much more than weight. You see, largely because of insulin resistance, diabetes affects the way the body metabolizes fat, causing fat and cholesterol to build up more in the blood than they would in a nondiabetic person. For this reason, diabetes is a risk factor for heart disease.

Choosing healthful foods that have a gentle effect on blood sugar is the cornerstone of diabetes treatment. This means eating balanced meals that include plenty of unrefined fiber-rich foods like whole grains, legumes, vegetables, and fruits. These foods contain chromium, magnesium, zinc, B-complex vitamins, and other nutrients that help the body metabolize carbohydrates. Fibrous foods also require more chewing and are more filling and satisfying than refined foods—a real boon to people who are trying to lose weight. As a bonus, soluble fibers—found in oats, barley, legumes, and some other foods—slow down the rate at which food is digested and absorbed, helping to stabilize blood sugar levels.

In addition to optimizing their consumption of whole foods, many people with diabetes use the glycemic index to help with meal planning. A way of ranking carbohydrate-rich foods based on how they affect blood sugar levels—and, therefore, on how much insulin the pancreas must secrete—the glycemic index can also be helpful in treating insulin resistance. Mounting evidence indicates that a diet emphasizing high-fiber, low-glycemic index foods cannot only help keep diabetes under control, but also prevent diabetes from developing in the first place. Researchers who tracked the eating habits of 65,000 women found that women who frequently consume refined carbohydrates like white bread, white rice, and sugar, are two and a half times more likely to develop diabetes than are women who eat fiber-rich diets with a low glycemic load. When investigators looked at the kinds of high-fiber foods the women were eating, whole grains emerged as being especially protective. The inset "Using the Glycemic Index to Enhance Health," found on page 36, presents more information on this topic.

Besides planning meals that do not raise blood sugar levels excessively, people with diabetes have to be especially careful to eat the right number of calories to maintain their desired body weight, as overeating in general will promote weight gain and elevate blood sugar levels. But the best foods for people with diabetes are the same as those for everyone else—foods that are low in harmful fat, high in fiber, and rich in nutrients. Where does sugar fit in? Research has shown that people with diabetes can include some sugar in their diets. However, because all carbohydrates are converted to sugar in the body, sugar must be substituted for other carbohydrate foods, not simply added to the diet. And since sugar is a nutrient-poor food, this practice should be kept to a minimum.

Most important, everyone with diabetes should meet with a registered dietitian or other qualified professional who can help devise an eating plan tailored to individual needs.

## MENOPAUSE-RELATED PROBLEMS

Although a stage of life, and not a disorder, menopause is discussed in this chapter because if not properly managed, it can lead to premature health problems. In addition, diet and lifestyle have a major bearing on how you feel during the years leading up to menopause, and on your quality of life thereafter.

Some time in their forties, most women begin experiencing fluctuating and declining estrogen production—a stage of life known as *perimenopause*. This drop in estrogen triggers a variety of symptoms, including hot flashes,

night sweats, fatigue, forgetfulness, and mood swings. By age fifty-one, most women produce so little estrogen that they stop menstruating, signaling the onset of menopause. For women who have had their ovaries surgically removed, menopause is abrupt and immediate, regardless of age. In either case, as estrogen levels drop, the risk for two major diseases—cardiovascular disease and osteoporosis—rises sharply.

To reduce the effects of menopause, many women turn to hormone-replacement therapy. Some women, however, prefer to avoid such therapy because of its association with an increased risk of breast cancer. Fortunately, diet may provide many of the benefits of hormone therapy—without the side effects.

How can diet ease menopause? Certain plant foods contain compounds known as *phytoestrogens*. These plant estrogens can mimic the effects of human estrogen in the body, partly offsetting the effects of reduced estrogen production by the ovaries. Researchers believe that regular consumption of soy foods—which are loaded with phytoestrogens known as *isoflavones*—is one reason why women following traditional Asian diets are only a third as likely to report menopausal symptoms as are women following an American diet. (See the inset "Isoflavones in Soy Foods" on page 37.)

How much soy do you have to eat to reduce menopausal symptoms? Aim for one to two servings per day. This is easy to accomplish if you use soymilk on cereal and in and baking, use soy cheese and yogurt as snacks and in recipes, sprinkle soy nuts over salads, toss tofu into casseroles and stir-fries, and substitute textured vegetable protein or Tofu Crumbles for part or all of the ground meat in recipes. One study found that women who adopted a soy-rich diet—one that provides a half cup of soy flour per day—experienced a 40-percent reduction in hot flashes in a matter of weeks.

Although soy foods are the best known

# Using the Glycemic Index to Enhance Health

The glycemic index is a ranking of carbohydrate-containing foods based on their potential to raise blood sugar levels. Why would this index be useful? People with diabetes are the most obvious beneficiaries. By being able to choose carbohydrate-containing foods that have a gentle effect on blood sugar, diabetics can exert more control over their condition. But this index can benefit others, as well. For the person with insulin resistance, foods that have a milder effect on blood sugar mean lower blood insulin levels, which in turn can help reduce levels of blood cholesterol and triglycerides, as well as blood pressure. For the person with hypoglycemia (low blood sugar), foods that result in less insulin secretion mean a reduced likelihood that blood sugar levels will drop too low. And since low-glycemic foods cause less fluctuation in blood sugar levels, they are also more satisfying.

To use the glycemic index in planning meals and snacks, start by choosing foods with low to moderate indexes—foods in the range of 25 to 50. Realize that individual responses to high-carbohydrate foods can vary, and that some people can be more liberal in their choices than others. You'll want to experiment to find what works for you.

When eating higher-glycemic foods, eat only moderate portions as part of a balanced meal. For instance, have a baked potato with a serving of lean meat and a fresh green salad. By combining a high-glycemic food with lower-glycemic choices, you will lower the index of the meal as a whole. If you were to eat only a baked potato, you would have higher blood sugar and insulin levels.

The following table lists the glycemic index of common foods when compared with pure glucose.

## The Glycemic Index of Common Foods

| Food | Glycemic Index | Food | Glycemic Index | Food | Glycemic Index | Food | Glycemic Index |
|---|---|---|---|---|---|---|---|
| **Cereal** | | **Dairy Products** | | **Grains and Breads** | | **Legumes** | |
| All Bran | 51 | Low-fat ice cream | 50 | Barley | 25 | Lima beans | 32 |
| Bran Buds | 58 | Skim milk | 32 | Brown rice | 66 | Navy beans | 38 |
| Bran Chex | 58 | Sweetened | 33 | Buckwheat | 54 | Pinto beans | 39 |
| Cheerios | 74 | low-fat yogurt | | Bulgur wheat | 48 | Split peas | 32 |
| Corn Flakes | 80 | Unsweetened | 14 | French bread | 95 | | |
| Crispix | 87 | low-fat yogurt | | Kaiser roll | 73 | **Sugars** | |
| Grape-Nuts | 67 | Whole milk | 27 | Millet | 71 | Fructose | 23 |
| Muesli | 66 | | | Rye bread | 65 | Glucose | 100 |
| Nutrigrain | 66 | **Fruits** | | Spaghetti (white) | 55 | Honey | 73 |
| Oat bran | 50 | | | Spaghetti | 37 | Lactose | 46 |
| Oatmeal (old-fashioned) | 49 | Apple juice | 41 | (whole wheat) | | (milk sugar) | |
| Oatmeal (quick-cooking) | 65 | Apples | 36 | White bagel | 72 | Sweet potatoes | 54 |
| Puffed Wheat | 74 | Bananas | 53 | White bread | 70 | Sucrose | 65 |
| Rice Chex | 89 | Cherries | 22 | White rice | 72 | | |
| Shredded Wheat | 67 | Grapefruit | 25 | Whole wheat bread | 69 | **Vegetables** | |
| Total | 76 | Grapefruit juice | 48 | | | Baked potatoes | 85 |
| | | Orange juice | 46 | **Legumes** | | Corn | 55 |
| **Crackers** | | Oranges | 43 | | | New potatoes | 62 |
| | | Peaches | 28 | Baked beans | 48 | Parsnips | 97 |
| Kavli crisbread | 65 | Pears | 36 | Black-eyed peas | 42 | Peas | 48 |
| Melba toast | 70 | Pineapples | 66 | Butter beans | 31 | Sweet potatoes | 54 |
| Rice cakes | 82 | Plums | 24 | Chickpeas | 33 | Sucrose | 65 |
| Ryevita | 69 | Raisins | 64 | Kidney beans | 27 | (white table sugar) | |
| Stoned Wheat Thins | 67 | Watermelons | 72 | Lentils | 29 | | |

# Isoflavones in Soy Foods

Soy foods are by far the richest known source of health-promoting isoflavones. Due to their soy-rich diet, the Japanese have the highest intake of isoflavones in the world, consuming up to 200 milligrams per day. Researchers believe that this is one reason for the exceptional health and longevity of the Japanese people. Indeed, not just in Japan, but throughout Asia, many people enjoy the health benefits of isoflavones, consuming about 45 milligrams per day. In contrast, most Americans consume less than 5 milligrams per day.

Most soy foods are good sources of isoflavones. Exceptions are soy sauce and soy oil, which are poor sources. Processed foods like soy hot dogs and soy ice cream tend to be lower in isoflavones because they are frequently diluted with nonsoy ingredients. To help you boost your intake of these healthful phyto-chemicals, the following table lists the approximate isoflavone content of various soy foods.

### Isoflavone Content of Selected Foods

| Food | Amount | Isoflavones |
|------|--------|-------------|
| Miso | 2 tablespoons | 10 mg |
| Soy flour | $^1/_4$ cup | 35 mg |
| Soy hot dog | 2 ounces | 9 mg |
| Soymilk | 1 cup | 40 mg |
| Soy nuts | $^1/_4$ cup | 40 mg |
| Soybeans, boiled | $^1/_2$ cup | 35 mg |
| Tofu | $^1/_2$ cup | 40 mg |
| Tofu yogurt | 1 cup | 38 mg |
| TVP | $^1/_4$ cup dry | 35 mg |

source of phytoestrogens, other foods contain these compounds, too. *Lignans*, a class of phytoestrogen found in legumes, whole grains, vegetables, fruits, flaxseeds, and sea vegetables, are also getting a lot of attention. Flaxseeds are by far the most concentrated source of lignans, providing up to eight hundred times more of this phytoestrogen than other plant foods. (For ideas on including these nutty-tasting seeds in your diet, see page 63.)

Although soy foods and flaxseeds get the most attention as sources of phytoestrogens, realize that it's also important to include a wide variety of vegetables, fruits, whole grains, and legumes in your diet. Many unprocessed plant foods contain lignans—although in smaller amounts than are found in flax. However, since these foods make up a larger part of your diet, their contribution is still very significant. In addition, many plant foods are rich in *bioflavonoids*, the compounds that give color to a wide variety of vegetables and fruits. These, too, possess some phytoestrogen activity.

One of the most common problems of menopausal women is weight gain. And even women who do not gain weight during this time usually experience negative changes in body composition. One study found that as women go through menopause, they gain an average of five and a half pounds of body fat, while losing almost seven pounds of lean body mass. Since muscle burns more calories than fat, this change in body composition is accompanied by a 100-calorie-per-day drop in metabolic rate—an amount that would cause a ten-pound weight gain per year if not compensated for by a reduction of caloric intake or an increase in exercise.

Can anything be done to prevent the muscle loss and fat gain that accompanies menopause? Plenty. Because hormone-replacement therapy helps combat these changes in body composition, many researchers believe that the phytoestrogen-rich diet discussed earlier could provide similar benefits. Researchers have also found that some muscle loss occurs simply because many women over fifty do not eat enough protein, which is needed to maintain and repair muscles. Finally, studies show that during the menopausal years, women become less physically active—to the tune of about 130 calories per day. And, by far, this is the biggest factor contributing to the problem of muscle loss and fat gain in menopausal and postmenopausal women.

Exercise physiologists strongly recommend a weight-training program as the first line of defense against muscle loss and fat gain. This— supplemented by a variety of other exercises, such as walking, biking, tennis, and golf—will help maintain healthy body composition and body weight, as well as reduce your risk for osteoporosis and cardiovascular disease. There is no doubt that exercise, combined with a balanced diet rich in phytoestrogens and other important nutrients, can make an enormous difference in the quality of your postmenopausal years.

## OSTEOPOROSIS

Osteoporosis, which literally means "porous bones," is actually a loss of normal bone density that can ultimately lead to bone breakage. As people live longer, this disorder is becoming increasingly prevalent.

Women typically begin losing bone mass in their fifties. This process accelerates with menopause, and then becomes more gradual afterwards. One out of every two women will eventually suffer a fracture related to osteoporosis. Men are at a lower risk for osteoporosis than women because they don't start losing bone mass until they reach their sixties or later. And since men usually start out with larger, denser bones than women, it takes longer for symptoms to develop. About 20 percent of the estimated 28 million Americans who are threatened by osteoporosis are men. (See "Risk Factors for Osteoporosis" on page 39.)

The good news is that there are many simple strategies you can use to prevent your bones

from deteriorating, and to even add back some bone mass if you already have experienced some bone loss. First, we'll look at some of the nutrients involved in bone health. Note that some of the following nutrients will enhance bone health, while others, if consumed in excessive amounts, can actually cause bones to become weaker.

*Boron.* Involved in the regulation of bone-strengthening hormones such as estrogen, testosterone, and vitamin D, this mineral has a protective effect on bones. Boron also helps the body conserve calcium and magnesium for bone building. Rich sources of boron include fruits, nuts, leafy green vegetables, and legumes. Perhaps this is why studies show that people who eat plenty of vegetables and fruits have a lower risk of osteoporosis. Because boron works so closely with calcium and magnesium in forming bones, many calcium-magnesium supplements also include 1 to 3 milligrams of this mineral for added benefit.

*Calcium.* Any discussion of osteoporosis must include a discussion of calcium, since 99 percent of the body's calcium is stored in the bones, where it helps form the bones' structure. The other 1 percent resides in the blood and other body fluids, where it is used for muscle contraction and other essential functions. Based on the body's needs, calcium is constantly moving back and forth between the bones and blood. If you do not get enough calcium in your daily diet to maintain normal blood levels of this nutrient, the bones will release some of their stored calcium, normalizing the blood levels. This means that over a number of years, people who consistently consume too little calcium can literally drain their bones of this essential mineral, causing them to become weak and porous.

Unfortunately, most women consume an average of only 640 milligrams of calcium per

---

# Risk Factors for Osteoporosis

*A variety of factors contribute to osteoporosis. Fortunately, many of these factors, such as lack of exercise and cigarette smoking, are within your control. If you do have some of the risk factors that are beyond your control—a family history of osteoporosis, for instance—you'll want to pay special attention to those factors that you can change. The following factors will help you determine your risk of experiencing osteoporosis.*

- ❑ *Family history of osteoporosis*
- ❑ *Postmenopausal estrogen levels*
- ❑ *Increasing age, and related reduced synthesis of vitamin D and absorption of calcium*
- ❑ *Female gender*
- ❑ *Caucasian or Asian race*
- ❑ *Being underweight*

- ❑ *Lack of exercise*
- ❑ *Nutritional deficiencies, such as insufficient calcium intake*
- ❑ *Nutritional excesses, such as excessive protein and sodium intake*
- ❑ *Cigarette smoking*
- ❑ *Excessive alcohol consumption*
- ❑ *Overuse of prescription drugs such as steroids and thyroid hormone*

---

day, while men consume 880 milligrams. This means that both groups are falling short of the recommended dietary intake of 1,000 to 1,200 milligrams. When you consider that some researchers are recommending up to 1,500 milligrams of calcium for postmenopausal women not taking estrogen, the picture looks even worse.

Before you start stocking up on calcium supplements, realize that, despite the common view that calcium is a magic bullet in the war against osteoporosis, it is not the only key to healthy bones. A variety of other nutrients—discussed in this section—work with calcium to build and strengthen bones. If these nutrients are lacking, you can take all the calcium in the world and still not achieve optimal bone health.

*Magnesium.* This mineral may be just as important as calcium in maintaining bone health, as magnesium strengthens the calcium-containing crystals that form the bone matrix. Magnesium also activates an enzyme that stimulates bone growth, and is involved in vitamin D metabolism, which is necessary for calcium absorption.

Without adequate magnesium, bones are more fragile, brittle, and susceptible to breaking. Studies have shown not only that most people's diets are deficient in magnesium, but that magnesium supplementation can increase bone mass and prevent fractures in women with osteoporosis.

Because calcium and magnesium work closely together, many researchers recommend a dietary calcium-magnesium ratio of 2 to 1. This means that if your daily diet provides 1,000 milligrams of calcium, it should also provide 500 milligrams of magnesium. Researchers are concerned that the widespread practice of taking calcium supplements without magnesium may be creating a nutrient imbalance that prevents bones from reaching their maximum potential.

Many brands of calcium supplements also contain magnesium, making these supplements a better choice than those containing calcium alone. If you are one of the many people who suffer from constipation when taking calcium supplements, you will be happy to know that magnesium helps prevent this unpleasant side effect.

*Protein.* As you learned in Chapter 1, it is important to eat two to three servings of protein-rich foods every day to repair body tissues, maintain muscle mass, and keep your immune system strong and healthy. However, also keep in mind that an *excessive* intake of protein can contribute to bone loss by causing calcium to be excreted in the urine.

On the other hand, mounting evidence indicates that the consumption of protein-rich soy foods can actually boost bone strength. How? Although the protein in soy foods—foods like tofu, texturized vegetable protein, and soybeans—does cause some calcium loss, this loss is much milder than that caused by the protein in meats. Soy foods also contain phytochemicals that act as estrogens in the body to inhibit bone loss. As a bonus, soybeans are a natural source of an easy-to-absorb form of calcium. Many brands of tofu also contain extra calcium, which is used as a thickening agent.

*Sodium.* Most people are aware that sodium can raise blood pressure, but few people know that sodium can also contribute to bone loss. How? High-sodium diets cause more calcium to be excreted in the urine. The typical American consumes 4,000 to 5,800 milligrams per day, an amount that causes 100 to 150 milligrams of calcium to be lost daily. Over time, this can really add up.

*Vitamin D.* Adequate amounts of this vitamin-hormone are fundamental to the prevention of osteoporosis. Why? Vitamin D must be present for the body to absorb calcium. This means that even if you load up on calcium-rich foods and supplements, if there is not enough vitamin D present, your bones will not benefit from your calcium intake. Where do you get vitamin D? Your primary source of this nutrient is sun exposure. The skin contains a substance that changes into vitamin D when exposed to sunlight. Therefore, people who spend most of their time indoors or who use strong sunscreens outdoors may not make enough of this nutrient. To make matters worse, as people age, their skin contains less of this vitamin D precursor, increasing the risk of deficiency. And, indeed, low levels of blood vitamin D are common in elderly women. A few foods—such as fortified skim and low-fat milk, fortified breakfast cereals, and fatty fish—contain some vitamin D. Your best bet, though, is to take a multivitamin, most of which provide 400 international units of this nutrient—100 percent of the recommended daily amount. In some cases, your physician may recommend up to 600 to 800 milligrams of supplemental vitamin D daily.

This section has touched on some of the nutrients that are involved in bone health. Besides the nutrients mentioned above, many others—such as folate, vitamin K, fluoride, zinc, manganese, silicon, copper, and vitamin C—are also needed to maintain strong bones. How can you put all of these recommendations into practice in your daily diet? Simply follow the Guidelines for Good Eating found in Chapter 1. A diet based on these guidelines will provide plenty of bone-building nutrients without an overabundance of calcium-wasting protein or sodium. In addition, avoid more than two servings a day of caffeine-containing beverages, including coffee, tea, and cola. Caffeine increases calcium excretion from the body.

If you want further insurance, a multivitamin can help guarantee your getting enough vitamin D and trace minerals. Your health-care provider may also recommend calcium supplements to bring your total calcium intake to 1,000 to 1,500 milligrams per day. But if you consistently follow the Guidelines for Good Eating, you should be getting close to 1,000 milligrams of calcium from your diet, anyway.

Finally, if you are to maximize your bone health, you must remain active. Weight-bear-

# Determining Your Ideal Body Weight

There are a number of ways to determine your healthiest weight, and to discover if, by current standards, you are overweight. One of the simplest means used by professionals is the body mass index (BMI), which describes body weight in relation to height. Simply put, as a person's weight increases, so does his or her BMI.

You can easily determine your own BMI using the following formula:

$$\frac{Weight\ (pounds)}{Height\ (inches)^2} \times 705 = BMI$$

To use this formula, just follow these steps. Let's assume, for the sake of this example, that you are 5 feet, 4 inches tall, and weigh 121 pounds.

**1.** First, calculate your height in inches, and square it—in other words, multiply the number by itself. In our example, your height is 64 inches. So:
$$64 \times 64 = 4,096$$

**2.** Now, write down your weight in pounds. In our example, your weight is 121 pounds.

**3.** Divide the smaller number (in this case, 121) by the larger number (4,096), rounding off your answer to the nearest hundredth:
$$121 \div 4,096 = .03$$

**4.** Multiply your final number—.03—by 705:
$$.03 \times 705 = 21$$

In this example, your BMI is 21. Don't have a calculator on hand? The table found in the second column will tell you your BMI at a glance.

Now that you know what your BMI is, you probably want to know what it means. BMIs between 19 and 25 are associated with the longest, healthiest life spans. Researchers have discovered that the weight that offers the greatest protection against cardiovascular disease, the biggest killer of Americans, corresponds to a BMI of 22.6 for men, and 21.1 for women. A BMI of 25 to 29.9 places you in the overweight category, and a BMI of 27 or greater is associated with an increased incidence of premature death. A BMI of 30 or more indicates a serious classification of obesity.

### Body Mass Index

| BMI | 20 | 21 | 22 | 23 | 24 | 25 | 26 | 27 | 28 | 29 | 30 |
|---|---|---|---|---|---|---|---|---|---|---|---|
| **Height** | | | | | **Weight in Pounds** | | | | | | |
| 5'0" | 102 | 107 | 112 | 117 | 122 | 127 | 132 | 138 | 143 | 148 | 153 |
| 5'1" | 106 | 111 | 117 | 122 | 127 | 132 | 138 | 143 | 148 | 154 | 159 |
| 5'2" | 109 | 114 | 120 | 125 | 130 | 135 | 141 | 146 | 152 | 158 | 163 |
| 5'3" | 113 | 119 | 124 | 130 | 135 | 141 | 146 | 152 | 158 | 164 | 169 |
| 5'4" | 117 | 123 | 129 | 135 | 141 | 146 | 152 | 158 | 164 | 170 | 176 |
| 5'5" | 120 | 126 | 132 | 138 | 144 | 150 | 156 | 162 | 168 | 174 | 180 |
| 5'6" | 124 | 131 | 137 | 143 | 149 | 156 | 162 | 168 | 174 | 180 | 187 |
| 5'7" | 127 | 134 | 140 | 147 | 153 | 159 | 166 | 172 | 178 | 185 | 191 |
| 5'8" | 132 | 139 | 145 | 152 | 158 | 165 | 172 | 178 | 185 | 191 | 198 |
| 5'9" | 135 | 142 | 149 | 155 | 162 | 169 | 176 | 182 | 189 | 196 | 203 |
| 5'10" | 140 | 147 | 154 | 161 | 168 | 175 | 182 | 189 | 196 | 203 | 210 |
| 5'11" | 143 | 150 | 157 | 164 | 171 | 179 | 186 | 193 | 200 | 207 | 214 |
| 6'0" | 148 | 155 | 162 | 170 | 177 | 185 | 192 | 199 | 207 | 214 | 221 |
| 6'1" | 151 | 158 | 166 | 174 | 181 | 189 | 196 | 204 | 211 | 219 | 226 |
| 6'2" | 156 | 164 | 171 | 179 | 187 | 195 | 203 | 210 | 218 | 226 | 234 |
| 6'3" | 159 | 167 | 175 | 183 | 191 | 199 | 207 | 215 | 223 | 231 | 239 |
| 6'4" | 164 | 172 | 181 | 189 | 197 | 205 | 214 | 222 | 230 | 238 | 246 |

*Source: Centers for Disease Control; Department of Agriculture.

Realize that if you are very muscular and/or have dense bones, your BMI is likely to be higher than the standards recommend. This does not mean that you are not healthy—quite the opposite, in fact. If you fall into this category, you can get a better idea of what your ideal body weight should be by having your percentage of body fat measured. A health professional such as an exercise physiologist can do this for you. The body fat percentages associated with the lowest health risks are between 12 and 20 percent for men, and 20 to 30 percent for women.

Before making any final decisions about your ideal body weight, consult your physician, nutritionist, or another appropriate health-care professional. If you have been overweight for many years, a realistic body weight may be somewhat higher than the BMI norms. But realize that if you can lose even a few pounds, you will reap significant health benefits.

ing exercises—including weight training, walking, racquet sports, and vigorous house and yard work—stimulate bones to absorb nutrients and use them to become denser and stronger.

## WEIGHT PROBLEMS

The problem of excess weight gain has reached epidemic proportions in the United States, with 55 percent of adult Americans now being considered overweight. The good news is that inappropriate weight gain is a problem that is well within your control.

You may have heard that weight gain is simply a part of growing older. Certainly, creeping weight gain during the adult years has become the norm for Americans, so many people have come to accept it as an inevitable result of a falling metabolism. Is this true? Only to a point. The truth is that most of the drop in metabolism that people experience during middle age and beyond comes from inactivity and the resulting loss of muscle mass. Therefore, it is largely preventable. Health experts recommend that you try to hold your weight steady and avoid gaining more than eleven pounds throughout your lifetime.

There is good reason for the experts to be so concerned about weight gain. It is now well known that the amount of body fat you store directly affects the length and quality of your life. The fact is that obesity-related medical conditions are the second leading cause of death in America, resulting in 300,000 lost lives each year. People who remain lean throughout life live longer because they are at a much lower risk for heart disease, high blood pressure, diabetes, and some types of cancer than are their overweight counterparts.

How does excess weight increase the risk of disease and premature death? Much of the increased risk centers on insulin, a hormone that the pancreas secretes as part of the diges-

tive process. Insulin allows the cells to utilize digestive carbohydrates for energy, and performs many other vital functions in the body. However, as people become overweight, their cells become resistant to insulin, forcing the pancreas to secrete more and more of this hormone to get the job done. As a result, blood insulin levels become chronically elevated and insulin resistance develops—a condition that was discussed earlier in this chapter, on page 34. Insulin resistance raises blood levels of a harmful kind of fat known as triglycerides, decreases levels of heart-protective HDL cholesterol, and raises blood pressure—all of which increase the risk of cardiovascular disease. Left untreated, insulin resistance can also turn into diabetes.

Of course, insulin resistance is not the only problem caused by obesity. Excess weight also increases the workload of the heart; strains the body's joints, increasing the risk or severity of arthritis; causes gallbladder disease; and increases the risk of some kinds of cancer.

Can anything be done about these weight-related problems? Yes. In most cases, a sensible weight-loss program is the best medicine. For instance, as the person with insulin resistance loses weight, insulin levels drop, greatly improving and sometimes even reversing this condition. Equally vital is exercise, which makes cells more responsive to insulin, thus reducing the amount that the pancreas must churn out. The inset "Using the Glycemic Index to Enhance Health," found on page 36, provides more strategies for controlling insulin resistance.

It is clear that if you are overweight, it is worth the effort needed to reduce your weight to a healthy level. Even losing a relatively small amount of weight can yield health benefits. For instance, a weight loss of just 20 percent can reduce the risk of cardiovascular disease by 40 percent in people who are obese. And losing as little as ten pounds can significantly reduce blood pressure—as well as the need for blood

# Secrets of Successful Weight Loss

On any given day, about 25 percent of American men and 45 percent of American women are trying to lose weight. Dieters spend more than $33 billion each year on weight-loss products and services, yet the weight problem among Americans is only getting worse. Why? It's simple—diets don't work. And if you consider the typical dieter's scenario, it's easy to see why. In their zeal to get off to a quick start, many dieters choose highly restrictive diets or eat ridiculously small amounts of food—so little food, in fact, that they feel weak, hungry, and deprived. Many dieters also spend long hours in the kitchen, chopping, measuring, and cooking special diet foods, only to find that after a few weeks, the diet is just too much work to continue. Whatever the reason for the failure, 95 percent of all dieters abandon their diets before reaching their goal weight, and quickly regain the lost weight—plus a few additional pounds.

What's a dieter to do? Relax. Forget about special weight-loss diets, stop being a slave to the scale, and, above all, be patient. Concentrate on developing healthier habits, and weight loss will follow. Weight that is lost gradually, as the result of modest lifestyle changes, is much more likely to stay off than weight lost on a quick-fix diet. Here are some simple tips that will help you get started on the road to successful weight loss.

❑ Choose low-fat, fiber-rich foods. As explained in Chapter 1, watching your fat grams will help keep calories under control. And eating plenty of fiber—in foods like vegetables, fruits, whole grains, and legumes—will help keep you feeling full and satisfied. In fact, serving large portions of vegetables and fruits at each meal is definitely one of the secrets of successful weight loss. Why? Besides being high in fiber and super-nutritious, vegetables are very low in calories. People who skip the vegetables and fruits at a mere 25 to 50 calories per cup, and pile on extra rice or pasta at 200 calories per cup, may find weight loss slower than they expected. (Realize that starchy vegetables like corn, peas, lima beans, and potatoes contain about the same amount of calories as pasta and rice, so be careful not to overdo portions of these veggies.)

❑ Eat balanced meals. One of the biggest mistakes that people make when they adopt a low-fat diet is that they entirely cut out protein-rich foods, such as fish, poultry, lean meats, legumes, soy products, egg whites, and low-fat dairy products. Instead, they go overboard on the pasta, bread, and starches. While it's important to avoid eating an excessive amount of protein, including some protein in each meal will help keep you feeling fuller longer, and will provide the essential amino acids needed to maintain and repair the body. An easy way to be sure you are getting a balanced meal is to mentally divide your plate into fourths. Then fill a quarter of your plate with a protein-rich food, another quarter with a starchy food, and the remaining half with vegetables and fruits.

❑ Limit sugar. Sugary foods—even fat-free versions—are loaded with calories. Sugary foods also contain few or no nutrients and, when eaten in excess, can deplete your body of essential nutrients like chromium and the B-complex vitamins. Read labels for sugar content, keeping in mind that every four grams of sugar is equal to one teaspoon.

❑ Eat at least three meals per day, spacing them out evenly. Eating just one or two meals a day slows your metabolism, and increases the likelihood that your meals will be stored as body fat. Eating several meals throughout the day helps keep your metabolism going strong.

❑ Do not overwhelm yourself with cooking, weighing, and measuring foods. Try one or two new low-fat recipes a week. When you find a recipe that works for you, make it a regular part of your diet. Continue experimenting with new recipes and new foods at your own pace, phasing in the new and phasing out the old. Before you know it, you will have designed your own personal low-fat diet.

❑ Eat when you are hungry, but learn the difference between hunger and other physical sensations. People often overeat because they get hunger confused with feelings of thirst, fatigue, or stress. If you keep properly hydrated with six to eight glasses of water each day, get enough rest, and work to keep stress under control, you will be less likely to overeat.

❏ *Eat slowly. As you eat, hormones and other chemicals are generated by your digestive system. These chemicals eventually make their way to the brain, which then lets you know you have had enough to eat. Since it takes about twenty minutes for this to happen, people who eat quickly consume more food and more calories than they need before they begin to feel full.*

❏ *Exercise regularly. The two main predictors for weight-loss success are low-fat eating and exercise—and one is just as critical as the other. Exercise not only directly burns calories, but also helps you gain muscle. This, in turn, raises your metabolism and improves your ability to burn fat and calories all day long. As a bonus, exercise helps reduce stress, a major cause of overeating. By both decreasing your dietary fat and calories and exercising regularly, you will maximize your chance for long-term success.*

*Small changes like the ones described above can make a big fat difference in your weight. For instance, by eliminating just 100 calories from your diet on a daily basis—the equivalent of one tablespoon of butter, mayonnaise, or other fat—you can lose ten pounds in a year. By eating a turkey sandwich for lunch instead of a deluxe cheeseburger, you can lose twenty pounds in a year. Substitute water for those two sugary sodas a day, and lose thirty pounds. Or walk five miles a week, and lose seven pounds. Changes like these, maintained for long periods of time, take weight off permanently. Need more help with your weight-loss program? A registered dietitian, nutritionist, or other qualified health professional can help you determine a healthy goal weight, and guide you in modifying your diet and lifestyle in a way that will allow you to reach your goal.*

pressure medications—in many people. How do you know what a healthy body weight is for you? The inset "Determining Your Ideal Body Weight," found on page 41, can help you decide. The inset "Secrets of Successful Weight Loss," beginning on page 43, will help you reach your ideal body weight through easy-to-accomplish lifestyle changes.

You have just seen how you can use the nutrients and phytochemicals in foods to help prevent and treat the diseases that target people in their later years. You may have noticed a common thread throughout these discussions—that a well-balanced low-fat diet rich in vegetables, fruits, legumes, and whole grains is the best medicine for the vast majority of health concerns facing people today. The rest of this book will introduce you to the ingredients and recipes that will make healthful eating a most enjoyable adventure.

# 3.

# Ingredients for a
# Longer Life

The previous chapters have shown how simple dietary changes can enhance both the length and the quality of your life. This chapter, along with the recipes presented in Part II, will allow you put these principles into practice by guiding your selection of the specific foods you need to maximize your health. In the pages that follow, we will take a look at the ingredients that will transform your pantry into a virtual pharmacy of healing foods. These foods will enable you to create dishes that will make healthful low-fat eating a most enjoyable adventure.

## LOW-FAT AND NONFAT CHEESES

Cheese is an excellent source of calcium and high-quality protein. Unfortunately, these nutrients often come packaged with a large dose of artery-clogging saturated fat. But take heart—an amazing array of fat-free and low-fat cheeses is now also available. These products will allow you to enjoy the foods you love while keeping your fat intake to a healthy minimum. Let's learn about some of the cheeses you will be using in your low-fat recipes.

**Cottage Cheese.** Although often thought of as a diet food, full-fat cream cheese has 5 grams of fat per 4-ounce serving, making it far from diet fare. Instead, choose nonfat or low-fat cottage cheese. Puréed until smooth, these healthful products make a great base for dips and spreads, and add richness and body to casseroles, quiches, cheesecakes, and many other recipes. Select brands with 1 percent or less milkfat, such as Breakstone's Free and Light n' Lively nonfat. Most brands of cottage cheese are quite high in sodium, with about 400 milligrams per half cup, so it is best to avoid adding salt whenever this cheese is a recipe ingredient. As an alternative, use unsalted cottage cheese, which is available in some stores.

Another option when buying cottage cheese is dry curd cottage cheese. This nonfat version is made without the "dressing" or creaming mixture. Minus the dressing, cottage cheese has a drier consistency; hence its name, dry curd. Unlike most cottage cheese, dry curd is very low in sodium. Dry curd cottage cheese can be substituted cup-for-cup for nonfat or low-fat cottage cheese in your favorite recipes—although you sometimes might want to add a tablespoon or two of milk to compensate for the drier consistency. Look for a brand like Breakstone's Dry Curd.

**Cream Cheese.** Cream cheese has long been touted as a lower-fat alternative to butter, but with 10 grams of fat per ounce, it is far from low-fat fare. Fortunately, light alternatives abound. Choose from Neufchâtel cheese, with 6

45

# *Cooking With Nonfat and Low-Fat Firm and Hard Cheeses*

*If you have been cooking with nonfat cheeses for a while, you may have noticed that some brands do not melt as well as their full-fat counterparts. So what do you do when you want to prepare a cheese sauce, a cheese soup, or another smooth and creamy dish? One option is to use a finely shredded brand of nonfat cheese. Often referred to on the package label as "fancy" shredded cheese, these finely shredded nonfat cheeses melt better than coarsely shredded brands— although they still may not melt completely. Or use a process nonfat cheese. Process cheeses are specially made to melt, so they will work in any sauce recipe. Most process cheeses tend to be quite high in sodium and artificial ingredients, but you can avoid a sodium overload when using these cheeses by leaving out the salt and avoiding the use of other high-sodium ingredients in your recipe. As for artificial ingredients, you can avoid these by choosing a brand like Lifetime, which contains none. What about reduced-fat cheeses? Most brands melt nicely, and can be substituted for full-fat brands in any sauce recipe, with very little difference in taste or texture.*

*What's your best choice for casseroles, lasagna, and pizza? Both nonfat and low-fat brands can be used, although low-fat brands like Sargento Light have more "stretch" as a pizza topping. As for topping salads, tacos, or a bowl of chili or black bean soup, any of the nonfat or low-fat shredded brands work nicely. Only your waistline will know the difference.*

grams of fat per ounce; light cream cheese, with 3 to 5 grams of fat per ounce; and nonfat cream cheese, with no fat at all. Like Neufchâtel and light cream cheese, nonfat cream cheese may be used in dips, spreads, and sauces. Look for brands like Philadelphia Free and Healthy Choice, and use the block-style cheese for best results when following recipes. The softer tub-style nonfat cream cheese should be reserved for spreading on bagels and other foods.

**Feta Cheese.** With 6 grams of fat per ounce, this semi-soft cheese has about a third less fat than most other kinds of cheese, and is considered moderately high in fat. However, a little bit goes a long way, so when used moderately in recipes that contain little or no other fats, you can enjoy this product without blowing your fat budget. An even better choice, though, is a reduced-fat brand like Athenos reduced-fat feta cheese. Now widely available in grocery stores, this product has only 4 grams of fat per ounce. Nonfat feta cheese is also available in some grocery stores.

**Firm and Hard Cheeses.** Both low-fat and nonfat cheeses of many types—including Cheddar, Monterey jack, mozzarella, Parmesan, provolone, and Swiss—are widely available in grocery stores. Reduced-fat cheeses generally have 3 to 6 grams of fat and 60 to 80 calories per ounce, while nonfat cheeses contain about 40 calories per ounce and no fat at all. Compare this with whole milk varieties, which contain 9 to 10 grams of fat and 100 to 110 calories per ounce, and you'll realize your savings. Look for brands like Alpine Lace, Cracker Barrel 2% Reduced Fat, Healthy Choice, Kraft 2% Milk Reduced Fat, Kraft Free, Lifetime, Sargento Light, Jarlsberg Lite Swiss, and Weight Watchers. The inset above provides tips for using these low- and no-fat cheeses in your favorite dishes.

**Parmesan Cheese.** Parmesan typically contains 8 grams of fat and 400 milligrams of sodium per ounce. As is true of most cheeses, reduced-fat and nonfat versions of Parmesan are available, including Kraft Free and Weight Watchers. But a little bit of this flavorful cheese goes a long way, so when used moderately in recipes that call for few or no other high-fat ingredients, even the "real thing" will not blow your fat budget. Some of the recipes in this book specifically call for nonfat Parmesan, some call for regular Parmesan, and still others give you a choice. Why? Nonfat Parmesan works beautifully in sauces and creamy soups, where it adds thickness and body. It also works well in casseroles and recipes like lasagna. However, it is too dry to be used as a topping for casseroles and other dishes. In these instances, a few tablespoons of regular Parmesan will produce the best results.

**Ricotta Cheese.** Ricotta is a mild, slightly sweet, creamy cheese that may be used in dips, spreads, and traditional Italian dishes like lasagna. As the name implies, nonfat ricotta contains no fat at all. Low-fat and light ricottas, on the other hand, have 1 to 3 grams of fat per ounce, while whole milk ricotta has 4 grams of fat per ounce. Look for brands like Frigo Fat-Free, Polly-O Free, Maggio Nonfat, Sorrento Fat-Free, and Sargento Light. Many stores and regional dairies offer their own fat-free brands, as well.

**Soft Curd Farmer Cheese.** This soft, spreadable white cheese makes a good low-fat substitute for cream cheese. Brands made with skim milk have about 3 grams of fat per ounce compared with cream cheese's 10 grams. Soft curd farmer cheese may be used in dips, spreads, and cheesecakes, and as a filling for blintzes. Some brands are made with whole milk, so read the label before you buy. Look for a brand like Friendship Farmer Cheese.

**Yogurt Cheese.** A good substitute for cream cheese in dips, spreads, and cheesecakes, yogurt cheese can be made at home with any brand of yogurt that does not contain gelatin, modified food starch, or vegetable gums like carrageenan and guar gum. These ingredients will prevent the yogurt from draining properly. Yogurts that contain pectin will drain nicely and can be used for making cheese. Simply place the yogurt in a funnel lined with cheesecloth and let it drain into a jar in the refrigerator for eight hours or overnight. When the yogurt is reduced by half, it is ready to use. The whey that collects in the jar may be used in place of the liquid in bread and muffin recipes.

**Nondairy Cheese Alternatives.** If you choose to avoid dairy products because of a lactose intolerance, or if you would like to enjoy more of the health benefits of soy foods, you'll be glad to know that low-fat and reduced-fat cheeses made from soymilk are now available in a variety of flavors. Look for brands like TofuRella, Soya Kaas, and Nu Tofu. Low-fat cheeses made from nut milks and other nondairy products are also available, although they do not contain the health-promoting isoflavones that soy cheeses do. Look for brands like AlmondRella, VeganRella, and Smart Beat Fat Free Nondairy Slices. Be aware that some nondairy cheeses do contain casein, a milk protein that you may want to avoid.

## OTHER LOW-FAT AND NONFAT DAIRY PRODUCTS

Of course, cheese isn't the only dairy product you use in your everyday cooking. How about the sour cream in dips, casseroles, and sauces, and the buttermilk in your favorite biscuits? Fortunately, there are low-fat and nonfat versions of these and other dairy products, as well.

**Buttermilk.** An essential ingredient in the low-fat kitchen, buttermilk adds a rich flavor and texture to all kinds of breads and baked goods, and lends a "cheesy" taste to sauces, dressings, frozen desserts, and many other recipes. Originally a by-product of butter making, this product should perhaps be called "butterless" milk. Most brands of buttermilk are from 0.5 to 2 percent fat by weight, but some brands are as much as 3.5 percent fat. Choose brands that are no more than 1 percent milkfat.

If you do not have any buttermilk on hand, a good substitute can be made by mixing equal parts of nonfat yogurt and skim milk. Alternatively, place a tablespoon of vinegar or lemon juice in a one-cup measure, and fill to the one-cup mark with skim milk. Let the mixture sit for five minutes before using.

**Evaporated Skim Milk.** This ingredient can be substituted for cream in sauces, gravies, quiches, puddings, and many other dishes. Not only do you save 620 calories and 88 grams of fat for each cup of evaporated skim milk you substitute for cream, but you add extra calcium, protein, potassium, and other nutrients to your recipe. If you don't have this product on hand, you can easily make a substitute by mixing $1/3$ cup of instant nonfat dry milk powder with $7/8$ cup of skim or low-fat milk. This will yield one cup of evaporated milk substitute.

**Milk.** One gallon of whole milk contains 128 grams of fat, the equivalent of almost two sticks of butter! And while you may not drink a gallon at a time, the fat you consume from milk can really add up. What are the best milk choices? Choose skim (nonfat) milk for the very least fat. Next in line is 1-percent low-fat milk, with about 2.5 grams ($1/2$ teaspoon) of fat per cup. What about 2-percent milk? Formerly called 2-percent low-fat milk, this product must now be called *reduced-fat milk*. Why? By legal definition, a low-fat product can have no more than 3 grams of fat per serving. With 5 grams of fat per cup, 2-percent milk is not low-fat. People who cannot tolerate milk sugar (lactose) will be glad to know that most supermarkets stock Lactaid milk in a nonfat version. Nonfat Lactaid milk may be used in place of milk in any recipe.

**Nonfat Dry Milk.** Like evaporated skim milk, this product adds creamy richness, as well as important nutrients, to quiches, cream soups, sauces, custards, and puddings. For a richer taste and texture in a variety of dishes, add a tablespoon or two of dry milk powder to each cup of skim or low-fat milk used. You can also mix $1/3$ cup of nonfat dry milk powder with $7/8$ cup of skim or low-fat milk, and use the resulting product as a substitute for cream. Just be sure to always use *instant* dry milk powder, as this product will not clump.

**Nondairy Milk Alternatives.** If you would like to reap more of the health benefits of soy foods, try one of the many brands of low-fat, calcium-fortified soymilk that are now available. These products have a light, nutty flavor and can be substituted for dairy milk in any recipe, adding health-promoting isoflavones to your diet. If you do not like the flavor of soymilk, try low-fat vanilla soymilk, which has a slightly sweet, nutty flavor. Vanilla soymilk can be used as a beverage, on cereal, or in cooking.

Health foods stores and some grocery stores also carry several brands of milk alternatives made from rice, almonds, and oats. These products have a creamy, mild flavor similar to that of milk. The plain, unflavored versions are good for topping cereal and for cooking. Flavors such as vanilla, chocolate, and mocha are also available. Whatever flavor you choose, be sure to get a low-fat, calcium-fortified version.

**Sour Cream.** As calorie- and fat-conscious people know, full-fat sour cream contains 48 grams of fat and almost 500 calories per cup! Use nonfat sour cream, though, and you'll eliminate at least half of the calories and all of the fat. Made from cultured nonfat milk thickened with vegetable gums, nonfat sour cream beautifully replaces its fatty counterpart in dips, spreads, sauces, and many other dishes.

All brands of nonfat sour cream can be substituted for the full-fat versions in dips, dressings, and other cold dishes. However, some brands will separate when added to hot dishes like sauces and gravies. For these recipes, use brands like Land O Lakes and Breakstone's, both of which hold up well during cooking.

**Yogurt.** Yogurt adds creamy richness and flavor to sauces, baked goods, and casseroles. And, of course, it is a perfect base for many dips and dressings. Like some brands of nonfat sour cream, however, yogurt will curdle if added to hot sauces or gravies. To prevent this, first let the yogurt warm to room temperature. Then stir 1 tablespoon of cornstarch or 2 tablespoons of unbleached flour into the yogurt for every cup of yogurt being used. You will then be able to add this tasty ingredient to your dish without fear of separation.

In your low-fat cooking, select brands of yogurt with 1 percent or less milkfat. As an alternative to dairy yogurt, try soy yogurt, which is available in health foods stores and many grocery stores.

## FAT-FREE AND LOW-FAT SPREADS AND DRESSINGS

Like dairy products, spreads and dressings have long been a major source of fat and calories in many people's diets. Happily, many low-fat and nonfat alternatives to your high-fat favorites are now available. Let's learn a little more about these fat-saving products.

**Butter and Margarine.** Which is better, butter or margarine? Neither should have a prominent place in your diet. Butter is a concentrated source of artery-clogging saturated fat, while margarine contains harmful trans fats. In addition, both are pure fat and loaded with calories. If you are used to spreading foods with butter or margarine, though, you can easily reduce your dietary fat by switching to a

nonfat or reduced-fat spread, and using it sparingly. Every tablespoon of nonfat margarine that you substitute for regular margarine or butter will save you 11 grams of fat and 85 to 95 calories. Replacing regular butter or margarine with a reduced-fat version will save 4 to 7 grams of fat and 40 to 70 calories per tablespoon.

Although you cannot sauté with nonfat and low-fat spreads, you can use these products for many of your other cooking needs. For instance, most brands melt well enough to be tossed with steamed vegetables, pasta, or rice dishes. In many cases, you can also bake with light butter and reduced-fat margarine. Simply replace the desired amount of full-fat butter or margarine with three-fourths as much of a light brand. For baking, select a light spread that contains 5 to 6 grams of fat per tablespoon, as brands with less fat generally do not perform well for this use.

Another fat-free alternative to butter and margarine is butter-flavored sprinkles. Made mostly of cornstarch with natural butter flavor, products like Butter Buds and Molly McButter come in handy shaker containers for sprinkling onto moist foods like baked potatoes and steamed vegetables. Butter Buds also comes in packets that can be mixed with water to make a pourable butter substitute.

**Mayonnaise.** Nonfat and reduced-fat mayonnaise are highly recommended over regular mayonnaise, which provides 10 grams of fat per tablespoon. How can mayonnaise be made without all that oil? Manufacturers use more water and vegetable thickeners to create creamy spreads that can replace the full-fat versions in all of your favorite recipes. Look for brands like Hellman's Low-Fat, Kraft Free, Miracle Whip Free, Smart Beat, and Weight Watchers.

**Salad Dressings.** Available in a wide variety of flavors, from balsamic and raspberry vinaigrettes to ranch and Italian, fat-free dressings contain either no oil or so little oil that they have less than 0.5 gram of fat per 2-tablespoon serving. Compare the no- and low-fat products with their full-fat counterparts, which provide 12 to 18 grams of fat per serving, and your savings are clear. Use these dressings instead of oil-based brands to dress your favorite salads or as a delicious basting sauce for grilled foods. Beware, though—many fat-free dressings are quite high in sodium, so compare brands and flavors, and choose those that are on the lower end of the sodium range. Another option is to dress your salads only with flavored vinegars. Try raspberry, rice, balsamic, herb, and red wine vinegars. And keep in mind that most vinegars are salt-free as well as fat-free.

## OILS

Like butter and margarine, the oils used in cooking, baking, and salad dressings can blow your fat budget in a hurry. Many people are confused about oils because liquid vegetable oils have long been promoted as being "heart-healthy." The reason? These oils are low in artery-clogging saturated fat, and contain no cholesterol. Unfortunately, many people also assume that these products are low in total fat and calories, and therefore may be used liberally. Not so. The fact is that *all* oils are pure fat. Just one tablespoon of any oil has 13.6 grams of fat and 120 calories. Vegetable oils do provide the essential fats that are needed for good health, but a couple of teaspoons of polyunsaturated vegetable oil—such as safflower, sunflower, corn, or soy—or a couple of tablespoons of nuts or seeds can supply enough essential fat for an entire day.

Believe it or not, you can use oil to slash the fat in many baked goods in half. Simply replace the butter or margarine in the original recipe with half as much oil. Then bake as usual, checking the product a few minutes before the end of the usual baking time.

Which vegetable oils are best? Those that are low in saturated fats and rich in monounsaturated fats—olive and canola oils, for instance—are the oils of choice these days. However, if you keep your use of all fats and oils to a minimum, any liquid vegetable oil, depending on your taste and cooking preferences, is fine. Some vegetable oils, though, are more useful to the low-fat cook than others. Here are a few oils you might consider buying on your next trip to the grocery store.

**Canola Oil.** Low in saturated fats and rich in monounsaturated fats, canola oil also contains a fair amount of linolenic acid, an essential omega-3 fat that most people do not eat in sufficient quantities. Canola oil has a very mild, bland taste, so it is a good all-purpose oil for cooking and baking when you want no interfering flavors.

**Extra Virgin Olive Oil.** Unlike most vegetable oils, which are very bland, olive oil adds its own delicious flavor to foods. Extra virgin olive oil is the least processed and most flavorful type of olive oil. And a little bit goes a long way, making this product a good choice for use in low-fat recipes. What about "light" olive oil? In this case, light refers to flavor, which is mild and bland compared with that of extra virgin oils. This means that you have to use more oil for the same amount of flavor—not a good bargain.

**Macadamia Nut Oil.** Like olive and canola oils, macadamia nut oil is low in saturated fats and rich in monounsaturated fats. And like canola oil, macadamia nut oil contains a fair amount of linolenic acid. An excellent all-purpose oil for cooking and baking, this product adds a delicate nutty flavor to foods.

**Sesame Oil.** Like olive oil, sesame oil can enhance the flavors of many foods. And when used in small amounts, this ingredient will add a distinctive taste to your dishes without blowing your fat budget.

**Unrefined Corn Oil.** Most of the vegetable oils sold in grocery stores today have been highly processed and refined, greatly extending their shelf life. Unfortunately, processing depletes oils of much of their natural nutty flavor and aroma—and of close to half of their vitamin E content. Most people grew up on these comparatively bland, tasteless refined oils, and have never even seen an unprocessed vegetable oil. They don't know what they're missing. Many stores stock at least one brand of unrefined oil, such as the widely available Spectrum unrefined corn oil. This amber-colored, buttery tasting oil is excellent for baking. And because it is so flavorful, a small amount is all you'll need in your low-fat recipes. Once opened, unrefined oils can turn rancid quickly. For this reason, you should purchase small bottles—a pint or less—and store the oil in the refrigerator.

**Walnut Oil.** With a delicate nutty flavor, walnut oil is another excellent choice for baking and cooking. This oil also contains a fair amount of the omega-3 fat linolenic acid. Most brands of walnut oil have been only minimally processed, so like unrefined corn oil, this oil should be kept in the refrigerator.

**Nonstick Vegetable Oil Cooking Spray.** Available unflavored and in butter and olive oil flavors, these products are pure fat. The advantage to using them is that the amount that comes out during a one-second spray is so small that it adds an insignificant amount of fat to a recipe. Nonstick cooking sprays are very useful to the low-fat cook to promote the browning of foods and to prevent foods from sticking to pots and pans.

## EGGS AND EGG SUBSTITUTES

From breakfast omelettes and French toast to quiches, casseroles, and puddings, eggs are star ingredients in many foods. But, as most people know, eggs are also loaded with cholesterol and fat. In fact, just one large egg uses up two-thirds of your daily cholesterol budget and provides 5 grams of fat. This may not seem like all that much until you consider that a three-egg omelette contains two days worth of cholesterol and 15 grams of fat—and that's without counting the cheese filling or the butter used in the skillet! The good news is that with the development of fat-free egg substitutes, you can now enjoy your favorite egg dishes with absolutely no fat or cholesterol at all.

Just what are egg substitutes? Contrary to what the term "substitute" implies, these products are made from 99 percent pure egg whites. The remaining 1 percent consists of vegetable thickeners and yellow coloring—usually beta-carotene or the plant-based coloring agents anatto or turmeric. You will find egg substitutes in both the refrigerated foods section and the freezer case. When selecting an egg substitute, look for fat-free brands like Egg Beaters, Better'n Eggs, Nu Laid, Scramblers, Second Nature, and The Right Egg. Many stores also have their own brand of fat-free egg substitute. Beware, though: Some brands contain vegetable oil, and so have almost as much fat as the eggs you are replacing.

You may wonder why some of the recipes in this book call for egg whites, while others call for egg substitute. In some cases, one ingredient does, in fact, work better than the other. For instance, egg substitute is the best choice when making quiches and custards. In addition, because they have been pasteurized (heat treated), egg substitutes are safe to use uncooked in eggnogs and salad dressings. On the other hand, when recipes require whipped egg whites, egg substitutes do not work.

In most recipes, egg whites and egg substitutes can be used interchangeably. Yet even in these recipes, one ingredient may be listed instead of the other due to ease of measuring. For example, while a cake made with three tablespoons of egg substitute would turn out just as well if made with three tablespoons of egg whites, this would require you to use one and a half large egg whites, making measuring something of a nuisance. When replacing egg whites with egg substitute, or whole eggs with egg whites or egg substitute, use the following guidelines:

---

1 large egg = 1 $\frac{1}{2}$ large egg whites

---

1 large egg = 3 tablespoons egg substitute

---

1 large egg white = 2 tablespoons egg substitute

---

## ULTRA-LEAN POULTRY, MEAT, AND VEGETARIAN ALTERNATIVES

Because of the high fat and cholesterol contents of meats, many people have sharply reduced their consumption of meat, have limited themselves to white meat chicken or turkey, or have totally eliminated meat and poultry from their diets. Happily, whether you are a sworn meat eater, someone who only occasionally eats meat dishes, or a confirmed vegetarian, plenty of lean meats, lean poultry, and excellent meat substitutes are now available. Here are some suggestions for choosing the leanest possible poultry and meat.

### Turkey

Although both chicken and turkey have less total fat and saturated fat than beef and pork, your leanest choice when buying poultry is turkey. What's the difference between the fat and calorie contents of chicken and turkey? While a 3-ounce portion of chicken breast without skin contains 139 calories and 3 grams of fat, the same amount of turkey breast without skin contains only 119 calories and 1 gram of fat.

All of the leanest cuts of turkey come from the breast, so that all have the same amount of fat and calories per serving. Below, you will learn about the cuts that you're likely to find at your local supermarket.

**Turkey Cutlets.** Turkey cutlets, which are slices of fresh turkey breast, are usually about $\frac{1}{4}$-inch thick and weigh about 2 to 3 ounces each. These cutlets may be used as a delicious ultra-lean alternative to boneless chicken breast, pork tenderloin slices, or veal.

**Turkey Medallions**. Sliced from turkey tenderloins, medallions are about 1 inch thick and weigh about 2 to 3 ounces each. Turkey medallions can be used as a substitute for pork or veal medallions.

**Turkey Steaks.** Cut from the turkey breast, these steaks are about $\frac{1}{2}$ to 1 inch in thickness. Turkey steaks may be baked, broiled, grilled, cut into stir-fry pieces or kabobs, or ground for burgers.

**Turkey Tenderloins.** Large sections of fresh turkey breast, tenderloins usually weigh about 8 ounces each. Tenderloins may be sliced into cutlets, cut into stir-fry or kabob pieces, ground for burgers, or grilled or roasted as is.

**Whole Turkey Breasts.** Perfect for people who love roast turkey but want only the breast meat, turkey breasts weigh 4 to 8 pounds each. These breasts may be roasted with or without stuffing.

**Ground Turkey.** Ground turkey is an excellent ingredient for use in meatballs, chili, burgers—in any dish that uses ground meat. When shopping for ground turkey, you'll find that different products have different percentages of fat. Ground turkey breast, which is only 1 percent fat by weight, is the leanest ground meat you can buy. Ground dark meat turkey made without the skin is 8 to 10 percent fat by weight.

Brands with added skin and fat usually contain 15 percent fat—which is higher than many kinds of ground beef. The moral is clear. Always check labels before making a purchase.

## Chicken

Although not as low in fat as turkey, chicken is still lower in fat than most cuts of beef and pork, and therefore is a valuable ingredient in low-fat cooking. Beware, though: Many cuts of chicken, if eaten with the skin on, contain more fat than some cuts of beef and pork. For the least fat, choose the chicken breast, and always remove the skin—preferably, before cooking.

Where does ground chicken fit in? Like ground turkey, ground chicken often contains skin and fat. In fact, most brands contain at least 15 percent fat, so read the labels before you buy.

## Beef and Pork

Although not as lean as turkey, beef and pork are both considerably leaner today than in decades past. Spurred by competition from the poultry industry, beef and pork producers have changed breeding and feeding practices to reduce the fat content of these products. In addition, butchers are now trimming away more of the fat from retail cuts of meat. The result? On average, grocery store cuts of beef are 27 percent leaner today than they were in the early 1980s, and retail cuts of pork are 43 percent leaner.

### *Choosing the Best Cuts and Grades*

Of course, some cuts of beef and pork are leaner than others. Which are the smartest choices? The table on this page will guide you in selecting those cuts that are lowest in fat.

While identifying the lowest-fat cuts of meat is an important first step in healthy cooking, be aware that even lean cuts have varying amounts of fat because of differences in grades.

In general, the higher and more expensive grades of meat, like USDA Prime and Choice, have more fat due to a higher degree of marbling—internal fat that cannot be trimmed away. USDA Select meats have the least amount of marbling, and therefore the lowest amount of fat. How important are these differences? A USDA Choice piece of meat may have 15 to 20 percent more fat than a USDA Select cut, and USDA Prime may have even more fat. Clearly, the difference is significant. So when choosing beef and pork for your table, by all means check the package for grade. Then look for the least amount of marbling in the cut you have chosen, and let appearance be your final guide.

### The Leanest Beef and Pork Cuts

| Cut (3-ounce cooked portion) | Calories | Fat |
|---|---|---|
| *Beef* | | |
| Eye of Round | 143 | 4.2 g |
| Top Round | 153 | 4.2 g |
| Round Tip | 157 | 5.9 g |
| Top Sirloin | 165 | 6.1 g |
| *Pork* | | |
| Tenderloin | 139 | 4.1 g |
| Ham (95% lean) | 112 | 4.3 g |
| Boneless Sirloin Chops | 164 | 5.7 g |
| Boneless Loin Roast | 165 | 6.1 g |
| Boneless Loin Chops | 173 | 6.6 g |

**Ground Beef.** No food adds more fat—and, most especially, saturated fat—to people's diets than ground beef. Just how fatty is ground beef? At its worst, it is almost one-third pure fat. And ground sirloin and round are not necessarily leaner. Terms like sirloin and round merely indicate the part of the animal from which the meat came, and not the amount of fat it contains.

The only way to be sure of fat content is to buy meat whose label provides some nutrition information. However, if your only choices are unlabelled packages of ground beef, choose the product that is darkest in color. As the fat content goes up, the color of ground beef becomes paler.

To obtain the leanest ground beef possible, you can select a piece of top round and have the butcher trim and grind it for you. Ground beef made this way will be about 95-percent lean. Most stores also carry prepackaged ground beef that is 93-percent lean. This is also an acceptable choice. In fact, you may be surprised to learn that 93-percent lean ground beef contains about half the fat of most ground turkey—which is about 85-percent lean—making the beef a better choice in this case.

## Lean Processed Meats

Because of our new fat-consciousness, low-fat bacon, ham, and sausage are now available, with just a fraction of the fat of regular processed meats. Some of these low-fat products are used in the recipes in this book. Here are some examples.

**Bacon.** Turkey bacon, made with strips of light and dark turkey meat, looks and tastes much like pork bacon. But with 30 calories and 2 grams of fat per strip, turkey bacon has 50 percent less fat than crisp-cooked pork bacon, and shrinks much less during cooking. Besides being a leaner alternative to regular breakfast bacon, turkey bacon may be substituted for pork bacon in Southern-style vegetables, casseroles, and other dishes.

Canadian bacon, which has always been about 95-percent lean, is another useful ingredient in the low-fat kitchen. Use this flavorful product in breakfast casseroles and soups, and as a topping for pizzas.

**Ham.** Low-fat hams are made from either pork or turkey. These products contain as little as 0.5 gram of fat per ounce. Of course, all cured hams, including the leaner brands, are very high in sodium. However, used in moderation—to flavor bean soups or breakfast casseroles, for instance—these products can be incorporated into a healthy diet. Just avoid adding further salt to your recipes.

**Lunchmeats.** Many varieties of ultra-lean lunchmeats are now available, including pastrami, corned beef, ham, and roast beef. These meats are ideal substitutes for fatty cold cuts in sandwiches and party platters. Keep in mind, though, that just like their full-fat counterparts, these meats are high in sodium, and so should be used in moderation. Be sure to choose brands that are at least 96-percent lean, and therefore contain no more than 1 gram of fat per ounce.

**Sausage.** A variety of low-fat smoked sausages and kielbasa—made from turkey or from a combination of turkey, beef, and pork—is now available. Per ounce, these products contain a mere 30 to 40 calories, and from less than 0.5 gram to 3 grams of fat. Compare this with an ounce of full-fat pork sausage, which contains over 100 calories and almost 9 grams of fat, and you'll see what a boon these new healthier mixtures are. Beware, though: While labeled "light," some brands of sausage contain as much as 10 grams of fat per 2.5-ounce serving. This is half the amount of fat found in the same-size serving of regular pork sausage, but is still a hefty dose of fat for such a small portion of food.

Whenever a recipe calls for smoked sausage or kielbasa, try a brand like Butterball Fat-Free, Healthy Choice, or Hillshire Farm 97-percent Fat-Free, all of which have less than 1 gram of fat per ounce. Louis Rich, Mr. Turkey, and Butterball are other good reduced-fat brands. When buying bulk ground turkey breakfast sausage, try brands like Louis Rich, which contains 75 percent less fat than ground pork sausage. Many stores also make their own fresh turkey sausage, including turkey Italian sausage. When buying fresh sausage, always check the package labels and choose the leanest mixture available.

## Vegetarian Alternatives

Most people know about using beans as a meat alternative, but not as many are familiar with the wide variety of soy-based meat alternatives that are widely available. Many of the recipes in Chapter 11 feature these versatile products, which will enhance your diet with protein as well as health-protective isoflavones. Let's take a look at some of the products that you will be using.

**Meatless Recipe Crumbles.** Made from soy and other vegetable proteins, these products can replace part or all of the ground meat in a variety of recipes. No longer limited to health foods stores, fat-free products like Harvest Burger for Recipes and Morningstar Farms Burger Style Recipe Crumbles can be found in the freezer case of most grocery stores. These products are precooked, so you simply thaw them and add them to recipes like sloppy Joes, chili, tacos, and casseroles. Use 2 cups of crumbles to replace 1 pound of ground meat. To use as a meat extender, mix 1 cup of crumbles with 8 ounces of cooked, crumbled ground meat.

**Texturized Vegetable Protein (TVP).** Made from defatted soy flour, this product, which can replace ground meat in many recipes, comes packaged as small nuggets that you rehydrate with water. TVP is sold in health foods stores and some grocery stores. To replace 1 pound of ground meat, pour $7/8$ cup of boiling broth or water over 1 cup of TVP. Let the mixture sit for about 5 minutes, or until the

liquid is absorbed. To use as a meat extender, rehydrate $1/2$ cup of the nuggets with 7 tablespoons of broth or water. Then mix with 8 ounces of cooked, crumbled ground meat.

**Tofu.** Made from soybeans in a process similar to cheese-making, tofu has long been a staple in Asian diets. Tofu's naturally bland flavor and unique texture enable it to absorb a wide variety of flavors—a characteristic that makes it a versatile product, indeed. From spicy stir-fries, savory burgers, tacos, and chili, to smooth and creamy dips, cheesecakes, and puddings, tofu can star in just about any dish, and can be substituted for many common cooking ingredients, from cheese to ground beef. Tofu does contain some fat—up to 5 grams per 3-ounce serving, depending on the type. However, many low-fat brands are also available. Look for tofu in the produce section of your supermarket, and in your local health foods store, too. (To learn more about choosing and using tofu, see the inset "Tofu Tips" on page 182.)

**Tofu Crumbles.** These precooked mildly seasoned bits of tofu come ready to use. Like meatless recipe crumbles, Tofu Crumbles can replace ground meat in a wide variety of recipes. Substitute one 10-ounce package—about 2 cups of crumbles—for a pound of cooked, crumbled ground meat. To use as a meat extender, mix a cup of crumbles with 8 ounces of cooked ground meat. Look for Tofu Crumbles in the tofu section of your grocery store.

## FISH AND OTHER SEAFOOD

Of the many kinds of fish and other seafood now available, some is almost fat-free, while some is moderately fatty. However, the oil in fish provides omega-3 fatty acids, a substance that most people do not eat in amounts sufficient for optimum health. The omega-3 fats in fish can help reduce blood triglycerides, lower

# *The Joy of Soy*

Although soy foods have been a staple of Asian diets for thousands of years, the rest of the world is just beginning to discover the tremendous health benefits and versatility of these ingredients. Nutritionists have long known that tofu, texturized vegetable protein, soy flour, soymilk, and soy cheese are rich in protein, vitamins, and minerals. But soy's most recent claim to fame centers on the fact that it is rich in a class of phytochemicals known as isoflavones. What do isoflavones have to offer? Researchers believe that they work in several ways to promote health and fight a wide range of diseases. Here are some examples of the power of isoflavones and soy foods.

**Cancer.** *Isoflavones may protect against both breast and prostate cancer. An isoflavone known as genestin is thought to be partly responsible for this protection, since it inhibits the growth of cancer cells. But these phytochemicals protect against cancer in another way, too. Chemically similar to the hormone estrogen, isoflavones compete with and block the activity of the body's natural estrogen. By acting as anti-estrogens, isoflavones—in a manner similar to that of the anti-cancer drug tamoxifen—may help fight the development of estrogen-dependent cancers like breast cancer. Researchers believe that frequent consumption of soy foods is one reason why Asian women have a quarter of the risk of dying from breast cancer that American women do.*

**Heart Disease.** *Studies have shown that the protein and isoflavones in soy foods directly reduces blood cholesterol. And, of course, when you substitute soy foods for high-fat, high-cholesterol meats, you get even more cholesterol-lowering benefits. Isoflavones also make arteries more elastic, and thus help the cardiovascular system work more efficiently. Finally, the antioxidants in soy foods may help protect LDL cholesterol from free radical damage. This is good news, because when free radicals oxidize LDL particles, they more readily form plaques in blood vessels.*

**Menopause.** *Asian women are only a third as likely as American women to complain of hot flashes and other symptoms of menopause. And researchers believe that the isoflavones in soy foods are partly responsible. During menopause, isoflavones, which are chemically similar to the body's natural estrogen, help offset the effects of declining estrogen levels.*

**Osteoporosis.** *Eating more vegetarian sources of protein can help reduce the risk for osteoporosis. How? First, while all protein causes calcium to be excreted in the urine, the protein in plant foods has a milder effect than the protein in animal foods. In addition, researchers believe that by acting in a manner similar to that of estrogen, the isoflavones in soy foods help bones retain their calcium, keeping them strong.*

Clearly, adding soy foods to your diet is a smart move. How much soy should you eat? As little as one serving of soy food per day—a half cup of tofu, texturized vegetable protein, or cooked soybeans, or a cup of soymilk—is associated with a reduced risk of cancer and heart disease. Two servings per day has been found to significantly reduce the symptoms of menopause. There are plenty of ways to include soy foods in your daily diet. Here are some ideas:

❑ *Substitute low-fat soymilk for dairy milk in baking and cooking.*

❑ *Use low-fat soymilk on cereal.*

❑ *Substitute Tofu Crumbles, texturized vegetable protein (TVP), or meatless recipe crumbles for part or all of the ground meat in chili, tacos, sloppy Joes, and casseroles. In most dishes, you can replace half of the ground meat without any detectable difference.*

❑ *Substitute low-fat soy cheese for dairy cheese in recipes.*

❑ *Substitute soy flour for 10 to 15 percent of the flour in baked goods. (Place 2 tablespoons of soy flour in a measuring cup; then fill the cup with your usual flour.) At this level, soy flour actually adds moistness and tenderness to baked goods. At higher levels, though, baked goods can brown excessively and develop an "off" flavor.*

❑ *Include tofu in recipes. (See Chapter 11 for ways to use tofu.)*

❑ *Add soy nuts—roasted soybeans—to casseroles, stir-fries, veggie burgers, and salads.*

blood pressure, and prevent the formation of deadly blood clots. This means that all kinds of fish, including the more oily ones like salmon, mackerel, mullet, and sardines, are considered healthful. In fact, eating just two meals of fish a week can help prevent heart disease.

Many commercial fish are now raised on "farms." How do these fish differ from the fish caught in their natural habitats? Farm-raised fish are higher in fat and calories than their wild counterparts. Most of the extra fat is unsaturated, though, so it won't contribute to heart disease. As for beneficial omega-3 fats, farm-raised and wild fish tend to contain about the same amounts.

What about the cholesterol content of shellfish? It may not be as high as you think it is. With the exception of shrimp and oysters, a 3-ounce serving of most shellfish contains about 60 milligrams of cholesterol—well under the daily upper limit of 300 milligrams. The same-size serving of shrimp has about 166 milligrams of cholesterol, which is just over half the recommended daily limit. Oysters have about 90 milligrams of cholesterol. However, all seafood, including shellfish, is very low in saturated fat, which has a greater cholesterol-raising effect than does cholesterol.

Fish is highly perishable, so it is important to know how to select a high-quality product. First, make sure that the fish is firm and springy to the touch. Second, buy fish only if it has a clean seaweed odor, rather than a "fishy" smell. Third, when purchasing whole fish, choose those fish whose gills are bright red in color, and whose eyes are clear and bulging, not sunken or cloudy. Finally refrigerate fish as soon as you get it home, and be sure to cook it within forty-eight hours of purchase.

## GRAINS AND FLOURS

Just because a food is fat-free or low-fat does not mean it is good for you. Fat-free products made from refined white flour and refined grains are practically devoid of fiber and other nutrients. Whole grains and whole grain flours, on the other hand, contain a multitude of vitamins, minerals, and phytochemicals. As a bonus, because they are fiber-rich foods, whole grains are much more filling and satisfying than refined products, so they can help you control your weight. Eating whole grains is truly one of the secrets of living longer and better, as more and more studies are finding that these foods are protective against cardiovascular disease, diabetes, and cancer. Fortunately, once accustomed to the heartier taste and texture of whole grains, most people prefer them over refined grains, which are bland and tasteless in comparison.

If you have never used whole grain flours before, a word should be said about storing these products. Since whole grain flours contain a very small amount of oil, they can more quickly become rancid than can their refined counterparts. For this reason, be sure to store them in the refrigerator or freezer. Not sure how to substitute whole grain flours for refined flours in your favorite recipes? The inset "Using Whole Grain Flours in Baking," found on page 59, will make it easy for you to successfully replace part or all of the refined flour with one of the healthy whole grain products discussed below.

**Barley.** This grain has a light, nutty flavor, making it a great substitute for rice in pilafs, soups, casseroles, and other dishes. Hulled or pearled barley, like brown rice, cooks in about 50 minutes. Quick-cooking barley is also widely available. With all the fiber of hulled barley, this product, available from both Mother's and Quaker, cooks in about 12 minutes. **Barley flour** is also available in health foods stores and some grocery stores. This mildly sweet flour is perfect for cakes, muffins, and other baked goods, and can replace up to a half of the wheat flour in these products.

**Brown Rice.** Brown rice is whole kernel rice, meaning that all nutrients are intact. With a slightly chewy texture and a nutty flavor, this grain makes excellent pilafs and stuffings. Brown rice does take twice as long as white rice to cook. But if you place the rice in the cooking water and refrigerate it overnight, or for at least 8 hours, the grain will cook in just 20 to 25 minutes. Several brands of quick-cooking brown rice—including Arrowhead Mills, Minute Brand, and Uncle Ben's—are also available. These brands can be made in 10 to 12 minutes. **Brown rice flour** is also available in many grocery stores and makes a nutritious addition to waffles, and baked goods, lending them a crunchy texture.

**Buckwheat.** Buckwheat is technically not a grain, but the edible fruit seed of a plant that is closely related to rhubarb. Roasted buckwheat kernels, commonly known as **kasha**, are delicious in pilafs and hot breakfast cereals. **Buckwheat flour**, made from finely ground whole buckwheat kernels, is delicious in pancakes, waffles, breads, and muffins.

**Cornmeal.** This grain adds a sweet flavor, a lovely golden color, and a crunchy texture to baked goods. Select whole grain (unbolted) cornmeal for the most nutrition. Your next best choice is bolted cornmeal, which is nearly whole grain. By contrast, degermed cornmeal is refined. If you find all of this confusing, just look at the Nutrition Facts label and choose a brand that contains at least 2 grams of fiber in each 3-tablespoon serving. Cornmeal may be fine, medium, or coarsely ground, and is available in white, yellow, and even blue colors. Keep in mind that the color of the cornmeal neither reflects its nutritional value nor indicates the degree to which it was refined.

**Kamut.** This ancient variety of wheat has made a comeback in recent years. **Kamut kernels**, which are also called berries, are about three times the size of wheat berries and have a delicate, buttery flavor and chewy texture. Kamut berries may be cooked whole and incorporated into pilafs, casseroles, and other dishes. Also available are **kamut flakes**, which can be cooked like oatmeal. In addition, many health food stores sell **kamut flour**, which can be substituted for regular whole wheat flour in yeast breads, quick breads, and other baked goods. Kamut is closely related to durum wheat, which is used for making pasta. For this reason, kamut makes a superior whole wheat pasta with a mild flavor and smooth texture.

**Millet.** A long-time staple in African and Asian diets, this tiny grain has a mild flavor and can be substituted for rice in almost any dish. It is also good as a hot breakfast cereal. Millet cooks in about 20 minutes. **Millet flour**, available in health food stores, can replace part of the wheat flour in baked goods.

**Oats.** Loaded with cholesterol-lowering soluble fiber, oats are for more than just a breakfast cereal ingredient. Use this healthful product to add a chewy texture and sweet flavor to your muffins, quick breads, pancakes, cookies, and crumb toppings.

Another fiber-rich product to look for is **oat bran**. Made of the outer part of the oat kernel, oat bran has a sweet, mild flavor and is a concentrated source of cholesterol-lowering soluble fiber. Great as a hot and hearty breakfast cereal, oat bran can also replace part of the flour in your low-fat baked goods, where it helps to retain moisture. Look for oat bran in the hot cereal section of your grocery store alongside the rolled oats. The softer, more finely ground products, including Quaker and Mother's, can be substituted for up to a third of the flour in baked goods. Coarsely ground oat brans, like Hodgson Mill, add a pleasantly chewy texture to muffins and cookies. When

# *Using Whole Grain Flours in Baking*

*Have a favorite bread, muffin, cake, or cookie recipe that you would like to make more healthful? Try adding the goodness of whole grain flour. A wide variety of fiber- and nutrient-rich whole grain flours are available for use in baking. Experiment with different kinds to see which you like best. Here are some guidelines that will allow you to substitute various whole grain flours for refined wheat (white) flour in your own favorite recipes.*

*1 cup refined wheat flour equals:*

❏ *1 cup unbleached flour*

❏ *1 cup whole wheat pastry flour*

❏ *1 cup minus 1 tablespoon white whole wheat flour*

❏ *1 cup minus 2 tablespoons regular whole wheat flour*

❏ *1 cup minus 3 tablespoons kamut flour*

❏ *1 cup barley flour*

❏ *1 cup brown rice flour*

❏ *1 cup millet flour*

❏ *1 cup oat flour*

❏ *1 cup spelt flour*

---

using a coarsely ground product, soak it in some of the recipe's liquid for about 15 minutes before adding it to the recipe.

Still another oat product to stock up on is **oat flour**. This mildly sweet flour is perfect for cakes, muffins, and other baked goods. Like oat bran, oat flour retains moisture in baked goods, reducing the need for fat. To add extra fiber and nutrients, substitute oat flour for up to half of the refined wheat flour in your own recipes. Look for Arrowhead Mills oat flour in grocery and health foods stores, or make your own oat flour by finely grinding quick-cooking rolled oats in a blender.

**Quinoa (keen'wa).** Rich in iron, magnesium, copper, vitamin B$_6$, and protein, quinoa has a unique light taste and a fluffy texture. It cooks in just 15 minutes, and is delicious in puddings and pilafs, and as a hot cereal. Be sure to rinse quinoa well with cool water before cooking to remove the bitter saponins—a natural repellent to birds and insects that coats the outside of the grain.

**Spelt.** Like kamut, spelt is a ancient variety of wheat that's gaining renewed interest. Spelt looks similar to whole grain wheat, but has a milder flavor. **Spelt berries**—whole spelt kernels—may be cooked whole and incorporated into pilafs, casseroles, and other dishes. Also available are **spelt flakes**, which can be cooked like oatmeal. In addition, many health food stores sell **spelt flour**, which can be substituted for regular whole wheat flour in yeast breads, quick breads, muffins, and other baked goods.

**Toasted Garbanzo Flour.** Made from ground garbanzo beans (chickpeas), this flour is rich in protein, fiber, and minerals. Replace up to 15 percent of the wheat flour in recipes with toasted garbanzo flour, and you'll enjoy a rich, nutty flavor. This product is also an excellent thickener for cream soups and gravies and can be used as a binder in veggie burgers, where it adds not only a distinctive taste, but also a protein boost. Look for toasted garbanzo flour in health foods stores.

**Unbleached Flour.** This is refined white flour that has not been bleached. Unbleached white flour lacks significant amounts of nutrients compared with whole wheat flour, but does contain more vitamin E than bleached flour. Arrowhead Mills, Gold Medal, Hodgson Mill, and Pillsbury's Best all make unbleached flour.

**White Whole Wheat Flour.** This is a good whole grain flour for all your baking needs, including yeast breads. Made from hard white wheat instead of the hard red wheat used to make regular whole wheat flour, white whole wheat flour contains all the fiber and nutrients of regular whole wheat flour, but is sweeter and lighter tasting than its red wheat counterpart. King Arthur white whole wheat flour is available in many grocery stores and by mail order.

**Whole Grain Wheat.** Available in many forms, this grain is perhaps easiest to use in the form of bulgur wheat. Cracked wheat that is pre-cooked and dried, bulgur wheat can be prepared in a matter of minutes and can replace rice in any recipe. Look for it in grocery and health foods stores.

**Whole Wheat Flour.** Made of ground whole grain wheat kernels, whole wheat flour includes the grain's nutrient-rich bran and germ. Nutritionally speaking, whole wheat flour is far superior to refined flour. Sadly, many people grew up eating refined baked goods, and find whole grain products too heavy for their taste. A good way to learn to enjoy whole grain flours is to use part whole wheat and part unbleached flour in recipes, and gradually increase the amount of whole wheat used over time. Most grocery stores stock Gold Medal, Pillsbury's Best, Hodgson Mill, Arrowhead Mills, or Heckers whole wheat flour. If you find these brands too heavy for your taste, try either whole wheat pastry flour or white whole wheat flour.

**Whole Wheat Pastry Flour.** When muffin, quick bread, cake, pastry, pancake, pie crust, and cookie recipes call for whole wheat flour, whole wheat pastry flour is the best choice. The reason? Made from a finely ground, soft (low-protein) wheat, whole wheat pastry flour has a milder, sweeter flavor and produces lighter,

softer-textured baked goods than regular whole wheat flour does. Look for Arrowhead Mills whole wheat pastry flour in health foods stores and many grocery stores. Keep in mind, though, that whole wheat pastry flour is not suitable for most yeast breads. Regular whole wheat and white whole wheat flours, which are higher in gluten, will allow your yeast breads to rise better.

## SWEETENERS

As discussed in Chapter 1, many people who adopt a low-fat diet end up eating unhealthy amounts of sugar—a practice that contributes to a myriad of health problems. But with just a little forethought, you *can* have your cake and eat it, too. Most of the recipes in this book contain 25 to 50 percent less sugar than traditional recipes do. Ingredients like fruit juices, fruit purées, and dried fruits; flavorings and spices like vanilla extract, nutmeg, cinnamon, and orange rind; and mildly sweet grains such as whole wheat pastry flour, oats, and oat bran are used to reduce the need for sugar while boosting nutritional value.

The recipes in this book call for moderate amounts of white sugar, brown sugar, and different liquid sweeteners. However, a large number of sweeteners are now available, and you should feel free to substitute one sweetener for another, using your own tastes, your desire for high-nutrient ingredients, and your pocketbook as a guide. (Some of the newer, less-refined sweeteners are far more expensive than traditional sweeteners.)

For best results, replace granular sweeteners with other granular sweeteners, and substitute liquid sweeteners for other liquid sweeteners. You can, of course, replace a liquid with granules, or vice versa, but adjustments in other recipe ingredients will have to be made. (For each cup of liquid sweetener substituted for a granulated sweetener, reduce the liquid by a quarter to a third of a cup.) Also be aware that each sweetener has its own unique flavor and its own degree of sweetness, making some sweeteners better suited to particular recipes.

Following is a description of some of the sweeteners commonly available in grocery stores, health foods stores, and gourmet shops. Those sweeteners that can't be found in local stores can usually be ordered by mail. (See the Resource List on page 229.)

**Apple Butter.** Sweet and thick, apple butter is made by cooking down apples with apple juice and spices. Many brands also contain added sugar, but some are sweetened only with juice. Use apple butter as you would honey to sweeten products in which a little spice will enhance flavor. Spice cakes, bran muffins, and oatmeal cookies are all delicious when made with apple butter.

**Brown Rice Syrup.** Commonly available in health foods stores, brown rice syrup is made by converting the starch in brown rice into sugar. This syrup is mildly sweet—about 30 to 60 percent as sweet as sugar, depending on the brand—and has a delicate malt flavor. Perhaps most important, brown rice syrup retains most of the nutrients found in the rice from which it was made. This sweetener is a good substitute for honey or other liquid sweeteners whenever you want to tone down the sweetness of a recipe.

**Brown Sugar.** This granulated sweetener is simply refined white sugar that has been coated with a thin film of molasses. Light brown sugar is lighter in color than regular brown sugar, but not lower in calories, as the name might imply. Because this sweetener contains some molasses, brown sugar has more calcium, iron, and potassium than white sugar. But like most sugars, brown sugar is no nutritional powerhouse. The advantage of using this sweetener instead of white sugar is that it is more flavorful and so often can be used in smaller quantities.

**Date Sugar.** Made from ground dried dates, date sugar provides copper, magnesium, iron, and B vitamins. With a distinct date flavor, date sugar is delicious in breads, cakes, and muffins. Because it does not dissolve as readily as white sugar does, it is best to mix date sugar with the recipe's liquid ingredients and let it sit for a few minutes before proceeding with the recipe. Date sugar is less dense than white sugar, and so is only about two-thirds as sweet. However, date sugar is more flavorful, and so can often be substituted for white sugar on a cup-for-cup basis.

**Fruit Juice Concentrates**. Frozen juice concentrates add sweetness and flavor to baked goods while enhancing nutritional value. Use the concentrates as you would honey or other liquid sweeteners, but beware—too much will be overpowering. Always keep cans of frozen orange and apple juice concentrate in the freezer just for cooking and baking. Pineapple and tropical fruit blends also make good sweeteners, and white grape juice is ideal when you want a more neutral flavor.

**Fruit Source.** Made from white grape juice and brown rice, this sweetener has a rather neutral flavor and is about as sweet as white sugar. Fruit Source is available in both granular and liquid forms. Use the liquid as you would honey, and the granules as you would sugar. The granules do not dissolve as readily as sugar does, so mix Fruit Source with the recipe's liquid ingredients and let it sit for a few minutes before proceeding with the recipe.

**Fruit Spreads, Jams, and Preserves.** Available in a variety of flavors, these products make delicious sweeteners. For best flavor and nutrition, choose a brand made from fruits and fruit juice concentrate, with little or no added sugar, and select a flavor that is compatible with the baked goods you're making. Use as you would any liquid sweetener.

**Honey.** Contrary to popular belief, honey is not significantly more nutritious than sugar, but it does add a nice flavor to baked goods. It also adds moistness, reducing the need for fat. The sweetest of the liquid sweeteners, honey is generally 20 to 30 percent sweeter than sugar. Be sure to consider this when making substitutions.

**Maple Sugar.** Made from dehydrated maple syrup, granulated maple sugar adds a distinct maple flavor to baked goods. Powdered maple sugar is also available, and can be used to replace powdered white sugar in glazes.

**Maple Syrup.** The boiled-down sap of sugar maple trees, maple syrup adds delicious flavor to all baked goods, and also provides some potassium and other nutrients. Use it as you would honey or molasses.

**Molasses.** Light, or Barbados, molasses is pure sugar cane juice boiled down into a thick syrup. Light molasses provides some calcium, potassium, and iron, and is delicious in spice cakes, muffins, breads, and cookies. Blackstrap molasses is a by-product of the sugar-refining process. Very rich in calcium, potassium, and iron, it has a slightly bitter, strong flavor, and is half as sweet as refined sugar. Because of its distinctive taste, more than a few tablespoons in a recipe is usually overwhelming.

**Sucanat.** Granules of evaporated sugar cane juice, Sucanat tastes similar to brown sugar. This sweetener provides small amounts of potassium, chromium, calcium, iron, and vitamins A and C. Use it as you would any other granulated sugar.

**Sugar Cane Syrup.** The process used to make sugar cane syrup is similar to that of making light molasses. Consequently, the syrup has a molasses-like flavor and is nutritionally comparable to the other sweetener.

## OTHER INGREDIENTS

Aside from the ingredients already discussed, a few more items may prove useful as you venture into healthful low-fat cooking. Some ingredients may already be familiar to you, while others may become new additions to your pantry.

**Barley Nugget Cereal.** Crunchy, nutty cereals, like Grape-Nuts nuggets, make a wholesome addition to crumb toppings, cookies, muffins, and other sweet treats whenever you want to reduce or eliminate the use of high-fat nuts. Fat-free and low-fat granola cereals can be used in the same way.

**Curry Paste.** A flavorful blend of curry spices mixed with canola oil, tamarind (the fruit of an Asian tree), and ground lentils, curry paste has a deeper, richer flavor than curry powder. Available in the imported foods section of many grocery stores and in specialty shops, this spicy seasoning is available in hot, medium, or mild varieties. Although curry paste contains oil, a teaspoon or two is generally enough to flavor an entire recipe, so it adds very little fat to your dish. Most brands of curry paste contain salt, but by avoiding the addition of other salty ingredients, you can keep sodium under control. If you do not have curry paste on hand, substitute an equal amount of curry powder and add a little extra salt to the recipe.

**Dried Fruits.** A wide variety of dried fruits are available for your cooking pleasure. Dried pineapple, apricots, peaches, cranberries, prunes, dates, and currants can be found in most grocery stores, while health foods stores and gourmet shops often carry dried mangoes, papaya, cherries, and blueberries. These foods add bursts of natural sweetness as well as flavor and texture to breads, desserts, salads, and many other dishes—without adding fat. If you cannot find the type of dried fruit called for in a recipe, feel free to substitute another type.

**Flaxseeds.** These small nutty-tasting seeds have long been a popular ingredient with bakers in Europe and Canada. But besides adding flavor and crunch to foods, flaxseeds contain a plethora of health-promoting nutrients. One of the richest known sources of omega-3 fatty acids, flaxseeds are also loaded with lignans, a type of phytoestrogen that may help prevent cancer and ease the symptoms of menopause. Widely available in health foods stores, flaxseeds are very economical and can be stored at room temperature for several months. Best of all, they can be easily incorporated into your diet.

Probably the easiest way to enjoy the goodness of flax is to sprinkle the seeds on hot or cold cereal. Or try adding them to bread and muffin batters, or to other baked goods.

Flaxseeds can also be ground into meal with a blender or food processor. The resulting product, which looks similar to wheat bran, can be sprinkled over cereal, just like the whole seeds. Flaxseed meal can also be substituted for up to a quarter of the flour in baked goods. The slightly sweet, nutty taste of flax enhances the flavors of muffins, breads, and other baked goods. And because the meal contains fibers and gums, it will actually improve the texture of your reduced-fat products. Just keep in mind that once ground into meal, the seeds can turn rancid quickly, so try to prepare the meal just before use. When you do have leftovers, store the meal in an opaque container in the refrigerator, and use it within a week.

Finally, if you're looking for a healthy egg substitute for use in your baked goods, flaxseeds may be the answer. The inset "Alternatives to Eggs in Baked Goods," found on page 128, provides directions for quickly and easily turning flaxseeds into a great replacement for eggs.

**Miso.** Miso is a rich-tasting salty paste made from fermented soybeans and grains. A seasoning staple in Japan for thousands of years, miso is used to flavor soups, sauces, dressings, and many other dishes. Miso comes in a variety of flavors and colors, ranging from mild, nutty-tasting, sweet white and yellow misos, to hearty red and full-bodied dark brown misos.

Like tofu, TVP, and many other soy foods, miso contains healthful isoflavones as well as a variety of vitamins and minerals. However, since this salty flavoring is typically used only in small amounts, it is not as significant a source of nutrients as tofu and other soy foods.

Use miso as you would other salty condiments like bouillon, anchovy paste, and soy sauce to flavor stocks, soups, sauces, dressings, marinades, and many other dishes. Dark miso complements the flavor of hearty soups, bean dishes, and savory gravies, while light miso is perfect in milder tasting sauces, soups, and dressings. Remember that miso is high in sodium, so use it sparingly. One tablespoon contains 600 to 1,000 milligrams of sodium—the equivalent of a quarter to a half teaspoon of salt.

The unpasteurized misos sold in health foods stores contain enzymes and bacteria that are thought to aid digestion and promote health. To preserve these enzymes and bacteria, add miso at the end of the cooking time whenever possible. For instance, if you are using miso to flavor a soup, remove a small amount of the soup, add the miso, and stir until smooth. Stir the mixture back into the pot, and serve immediately.

**Nuts.** It may surprise you to learn that the recipes in this book sometimes include nuts as an ingredient, or suggest them as an optional addition. True, nuts are high in fat. But when used in small amounts, these tasty morsels will not blow your fat budget, and will provide some of the essential fats, vitamins, and minerals needed for good health. Read more about the benefits of nuts on page 214.

**Soy Nuts.** Made from soaked soybeans that are roasted until browned and crisp, these crunchy treats look like roasted peanuts, and have a similar texture and a nutty flavor. Sprinkle them over salads or add to casseroles, stir-fries, and veggie burgers as you would any other nut. With about 100 calories and 5 grams of fat per quarter-cup serving, soy nuts have half the calories and 75 percent less fat than most other nuts. Soy nuts are also loaded with isoflavones.

**Wheat Germ.** The embryo of the wheat kernel, wheat germ is loaded with B vitamins, vitamin E, zinc, magnesium, and many other nutrients. Use this ingredient to add crunch and nutty flavor to a wide range of dishes.

Two kinds of wheat germ are commonly available in the cereal section of grocery stores—plain toasted and honey crunch. Try substituting toasted wheat germ for part of the flour in quick breads, muffins, and coffee cakes. It also makes a nutritious filler for meat loaves or burgers, and a crunchy coating for oven-fried foods. Honey crunch wheat germ, which has a more nugget-like texture than toasted wheat germ, makes an excellent substitute for chopped nuts—but with 90 percent less fat. It is also delicious sprinkled over cereal, fruit, or yogurt.

## ABOUT THE NUTRITIONAL ANALYSIS

The Food Processor II (ESHA Research) computer nutrition analysis system, along with product information from manufacturers, was used to calculate the nutritional information for the recipes in this book. Nutrients are always listed per one piece, one muffin, one cookie, one serving, etc.

Sometimes recipes give you options regarding ingredients. For instance, you might be able to choose between wheat germ and nuts, 95-percent lean ground beef and meatless recipe crumbles, or nonfat and low-fat mayonnaise. This will help you create dishes that suit your tastes. Just keep in mind that the nutritional analysis is based on the first ingredient listed.

This book is filled with creative dishes that naturally promote health and longevity. But more important, they are so simple, satisfying, and delicious that you will truly enjoy serving them to your family and friends. So get ready to create some new family favorites and to experience the pleasures and rewards of healthful, low-fat cooking.

# Part II

# Recipes for Long Life

# 4.

# Breakfasts for Champions

It is often said that breakfast is the most important meal of the day, and there are a number of reasons why this is true. First, eating breakfast helps rev up your metabolism, making it easier to maintain a healthy weight. Second, spreading your food intake among three or more meals throughout the day results in lower insulin, blood sugar, and blood cholesterol levels—all of which contribute to greater general health. Finally, breakfast offers a wonderful opportunity to add certain nutrient-rich foods to your diet.

One of the most important foods that should be featured in a long-life breakfast menu is whole grains. Why? Besides being rich in fiber, whole grains, unlike their refined counterparts, provide vitamin E, folate, copper, chromium, and magnesium, as well as a host of health-promoting phytochemicals. As a result, these foods have emerged as one of the foremost protective foods. Researchers believe that a diet abundant in whole grains greatly reduces the risk of both heart disease and diabetes, and significantly enhances overall health and well-being.

Within this chapter, you will find plenty of ways to enjoy wholesome whole grains. If cereal is your pleasure, choose from among a variety of hot and hearty cereals, or try a crunchy homemade granola or a nutrient-packed muesli. Either way, you will get a bowlful of old-fashioned goodness. Can pancakes and French toast be part of a wholesome breakfast menu? Most definitely. These recipes trim away unnecessary oil, butter, egg yolks, and salt, leaving your favorite treats just as delicious as always, but a great deal more healthful. In fact, you'll find that you need not discard even your best-loved egg dishes—as long as you know how to make them. Fat-free egg substitutes can replace the whole eggs in all of your omelettes and breakfast casseroles, providing protein without the fat or cholesterol. And low-fat cheeses, ultra-lean sausage, and other breakfast favorites can take their place at the breakfast table, too.

So heat up the griddle, and get ready for high-nutrient, taste-tempting breakfast foods that will not only get you out of bed, but will keep you going all morning long!

# Cinnamon-Vanilla French Toast

*For variety, substitute 12 oat bran or whole wheat English muffin halves or 12 pieces of presliced multigrain, oatmeal, or whole wheat bread for the bread called for in this recipe.*

### Yield: 12 slices

1¼ cups fat-free egg substitute

1 cup low-fat vanilla soymilk or evaporated skim milk

2 tablespoons maple syrup

½ teaspoon ground cinnamon

½ teaspoon vanilla extract

1 oblong loaf unsliced multigrain bread (about 6-x-12 inches, or 1 pound)

**1.** Place the egg substitute, milk, maple syrup, cinnamon, and vanilla extract in a blender, and process until well mixed. Pour into a shallow bowl, and set aside.

**2.** Slice twelve ¾-inch-thick pieces of bread from the loaf. (You will need only about three-fourths of the loaf.) Dip each bread slice in the egg mixture, turning to coat both sides and to thoroughly soak the bread.

**3.** Coat a griddle or large nonstick skillet with nonstick cooking spray, and preheat over medium heat until a drop of water sizzles when it hits the surface. (If using an electric griddle, preheat the griddle to 375°F.)

**4.** Arrange the bread slices on the griddle, and cook for about 2 minutes on each side, or until golden brown. As the slices are done, transfer them to a serving plate and keep warm in a preheated oven. Serve hot, topped with a warm fruit topping (page 71), maple syrup, or honey.

## NUTRITIONAL FACTS
(Per Slice)

| Cal: 99 | Carbs: 17 g | Chol: 0 mg | Fat: 0.7 g |
|---|---|---|---|
| Fiber: 2 g | Protein: 5.7 g | Sodium: 193 mg | |

# Banana French Toast

*Like Cinnamon-Vanilla French Toast (at left), this dish is just as delicious when made with English muffin halves or presliced bread.*

### Yield: 12 slices

1¼ cups fat-free egg substitute

1 cup sliced banana (about 1 large)

½ cup evaporated skim milk or low-fat soymilk

1½ teaspoons vanilla extract

¼ teaspoon ground nutmeg

1 oblong loaf unsliced multigrain bread (about 6-x-12 inches, or 1 pound)

**1.** Place the egg substitute, banana, milk, vanilla extract, and nutmeg in a blender, and process until smooth. Pour into a shallow bowl, and set aside.

**2.** Slice twelve ¾-inch-thick pieces of bread from the loaf. (You will need only about three-fourths of the loaf.) Dip each bread slice in the egg mixture, turning to coat both sides and to thoroughly soak the bread.

**3.** Coat a griddle or large nonstick skillet with nonstick cooking spray, and preheat over medium heat until a drop of water sizzles when it hits the surface. (If using an electric griddle, preheat the griddle to 375°F.)

**4.** Arrange the bread slices on the griddle, and cook for about 2 minutes on each side, or until golden brown. As the slices are done, transfer them to a serving plate and keep warm in a preheated oven. Serve hot, topped with maple syrup or honey. Garnish with a few banana slices and a sprinkling of pecans, if desired.

## NUTRITIONAL FACTS
### (Per Slice)

| | | | |
|---|---|---|---|
| Cal: 97 | Carbs: 16 g | Chol: 0 mg | Fat: 0.7 g |
| Fiber: 2 g | Protein: 6 g | Sodium: 180 mg | |

# Multigrain Pancakes

### Yield: 12 pancakes

1 cup plus 2 tablespoons whole wheat pastry flour

2 tablespoons yellow cornmeal

2 tablespoons oat bran

2 tablespoons toasted wheat germ

1 tablespoon sugar

1 teaspoon baking soda

1¾ cups nonfat or low-fat buttermilk

2 egg whites, lightly beaten, or ¼ cup fat-free egg substitute

**1.** Place the flour, cornmeal, oat bran, wheat germ, sugar, and baking soda in a large bowl, and stir to mix well. Add the buttermilk and the egg whites or egg substitute, and mix with a wire whisk to blend well.

**2.** Coat a griddle or large nonstick skillet with nonstick cooking spray, and preheat over medium heat until a drop of water sizzles when it hits the surface. (If using an electric griddle, preheat the griddle according to the manufacturer's directions.)

**3.** For each pancake, pour ¼ cup of batter onto the griddle, and spread into a 4-inch circle. Cook for about 1½ minutes, or until the top is bubbly and the edges are dry. Turn and cook for an additional minute, or until the second side is golden brown.

**4.** As the pancakes are done, transfer them to a serving plate and keep warm in a preheated oven. Serve hot, topped with honey, maple syrup, or a warm fruit topping (page 71).

## NUTRITIONAL FACTS
### (Per Pancake)

| | | | |
|---|---|---|---|
| Cal: 70 | Carbs: 13.2 g | Chol: 1 mg | Fat: 0.7 g |
| Fiber: 1.8 g | Protein: 3.8 g | Sodium: 151 mg | |

### Variation

To make Multigrain Banana Pancakes, add 1½ cups of sliced bananas to the batter, and proceed with recipe as directed to make 15 pancakes. Top with maple syrup or honey and a sprinkling of pecans, if desired.

## NUTRITIONAL FACTS
### (Per Pancake)

| | | | |
|---|---|---|---|
| Cal: 70 | Carbs: 14 g | Chol: 1 mg | Fat: 0.7 g |
| Fiber: 1.8 g | Protein: 3.2 g | Sodium: 121 mg | |

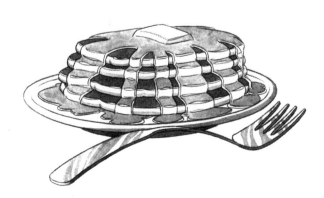

# Cottage-Apple Pancakes

## Yield: 20 pancakes

1⅓ cups whole wheat pastry flour
1 tablespoon sugar
1 tablespoon baking powder
1 cup skim milk or low-fat vanilla soymilk
1 cup nonfat or low-fat cottage cheese
¼ cup plus 2 tablespoons fat-free egg substitute
1¼ cups finely chopped peeled apple (about 2 medium)

1. Place the flour, sugar, and baking powder in a large bowl, and stir to mix well. Add the milk, cottage cheese, and egg substitute, and stir to mix well. Stir in the apples.

2. Coat a griddle or large nonstick skillet with nonstick cooking spray, and preheat over medium heat until a drop of water sizzles when it hits the surface. (If using an electric griddle, preheat the griddle according to the manufacturer's directions.)

3. For each pancake, pour 3 tablespoons of batter onto the griddle, and spread into a 3-inch circle. Cook for about 1½ minutes, or until the top is bubbly and the edges are dry. Turn and cook for an additional minute, or until the second side is golden brown.

4. As the pancakes are done, transfer them to a serving plate and keep warm in a preheated oven. Serve hot, topped with honey or maple syrup.

## NUTRITIONAL FACTS
### (Per Pancake)

| Cal: 48 | Carbs: 9 g | Chol: 1 mg | Fat: 0.2 g |
|---|---|---|---|
| Fiber: 1.3 g | Protein: 3.5 g | Sodium: 105 mg | |

# Blueberry-Yogurt Pancakes

## Yield: 14 pancakes

1½ cups whole wheat pastry flour
1 tablespoon baking powder
¾ cup skim milk or low-fat soymilk
1 cup nonfat or low-fat vanilla yogurt
2 egg whites, lightly beaten, or ¼ cup fat-free egg substitute
1¼ cups fresh or frozen blueberries

1. Place the flour and baking powder in a large bowl, and stir to mix well. Add the milk, yogurt, and egg whites or egg substitute, and mix with a wire whisk to blend well. Fold in the blueberries.

2. Coat a griddle or large nonstick skillet with nonstick cooking spray, and preheat over medium heat until a drop of water sizzles when it hits the surface. (If using an electric griddle, preheat the griddle according to the manufacturer's directions.)

3. For each pancake, pour ¼ cup of batter onto the griddle, and spread into a 4-inch circle. Cook for about 1½ minutes, or until the top is bubbly and the edges are dry. Turn and cook for an additional minute, or until the second side is golden brown.

4. As the pancakes are done, transfer them to a serving plate and keep warm in a preheated oven. Serve hot, topped with honey, maple syrup, or Warm Blueberry Topping (page 71).

## NUTRITIONAL FACTS
### (Per Pancake)

| Cal: 65 | Carbs: 13 g | Chol: 1 mg | Fat: 0.4 g |
|---|---|---|---|
| Fiber: 1.9 g | Protein: 3 g | Sodium: 122 mg | |

# Heartwarming Fruit Toppings

*Deliciously sweet syrups add that crowning touch to pancakes, waffles, and French toast. While all syrups are fat-free, they are generally almost pure sugar, and add up to 60 calories for each tablespoon used. Instead of the usual refined, sugary syrups, try one of the following fruit toppings over your breakfast treats. With less calories than even reduced-calorie syrups, these syrups are more natural, wholesome, and economical, too.*

## Warm Blueberry Topping

*For variety, substitute blackberries, raspberries, sliced strawberries, or halved pitted cherries for the blueberries.*

Yield: 1½ cups

¾ cup white grape juice, divided
1 tablespoon cornstarch
2 cups fresh or frozen blueberries
¼ cup sugar

1. Place 2 tablespoons of the juice and all of the cornstarch in a small bowl. Stir to dissolve the cornstarch, and set aside.
2. Place the blueberries, the remaining juice, and the sugar in a 1½-quart saucepan. Stir to mix well, and bring to a boil over medium-high heat. Reduce the heat to low, cover, and simmer, stirring occasionally, for about 5 minutes, or until the fruit is very soft.
3. Stir the cornstarch mixture, and add it to the pot. Cook, stirring constantly, for another minute or 2, or until the mixture is thickened and bubbly. Serve warm over pancakes, French toast, or waffles. Store any leftover sauce in the refrigerator for up to 3 days.

### NUTRITIONAL FACTS
(Per ¼-Cup Serving)

| Cal: 83 | Carbs: 21 g | Chol: 0 mg | Fat: 0.2 g |
|---|---|---|---|
| Fiber: 1.4 g | Protein: 0.5 g | Sodium: 5 mg | |

## Sweet Orange Syrup

Yield: 1½ cups

1 tablespoon cornstarch
1 cup orange juice
½ cup honey or molasses

1. Place the cornstarch and 2 tablespoons of the orange juice in a 1-quart saucepan, and stir to dissolve the cornstarch. Stir in first the remaining orange juice, and then the honey or molasses.

2. Place the pan over medium heat, and cook, stirring constantly, for about 3 minutes, or until the mixture is bubbly and slightly thickened.
3. Serve warm over pancakes, French toast, waffles, or polenta. Store any leftover sauce in the refrigerator for up to 3 days.

### NUTRITIONAL FACTS
(Per 2-Tablespoon Serving)

| Cal: 55 | Carbs: 13.5 g | Chol: 0 mg | Fat: 0 g |
|---|---|---|---|
| Fiber: 0 g | Protein: 0.2 g | Sodium: 1 mg | |

## Warm Apple Topping

Yield: 2 cups

1 cup apple juice, divided
1 tablespoon cornstarch
3 cups sliced peeled apples (about 4 medium)
¼ cup light brown sugar
¼ teaspoon ground cinnamon
Pinch ground nutmeg

1. Place 1 tablespoon of the apple juice and all of the cornstarch in a small bowl. Stir to dissolve the cornstarch, and set aside.
2. Place the apples, the remaining juice, and the brown sugar, cinnamon, and nutmeg in a 1-quart saucepan. Stir to mix well, and bring to a boil over high heat. Reduce the heat to low, cover, and simmer, stirring occasionally, for about 5 minutes, or until the apples are tender.
3. Stir the cornstarch mixture, and add it to the pot. Cook, stirring constantly, for another minute or 2, or until the mixture is thickened and bubbly. Serve warm over pancakes, French toast, or waffles. Store any leftover sauce in the refrigerator for up to 3 days.

### NUTRITIONAL FACTS
(Per ¼-Cup Serving)

| Cal: 59 | Carbs: 15 g | Chol: 0 mg | Fat: 0.1 g |
|---|---|---|---|
| Fiber: 0.8 g | Protein: 0.1 g | Sodium: 3 mg | |

# Baked Breakfast Polenta

Yield: 16 slices

3 cups water

3 cups skim milk

2 cups polenta, coarsely ground yellow cornmeal, or yellow corn grits

$\frac{1}{2}$ teaspoon salt

Nonstick butter-flavored cooking spray

$\frac{1}{2}$ cup fat-free egg substitute

$\frac{3}{4}$ cup plus 2 tablespoons toasted wheat germ

1. Place the water, milk, polenta, and salt in a 4-quart pot, and bring to a boil over high heat, stirring frequently. Reduce the heat to low, cover, and simmer, stirring every few minutes, for about 15 minutes, or until the polenta is very thick and begins to pull away from the sides of the pan when stirred.

2. Coat a 9-x-4-inch loaf pan with nonstick butter-flavored cooking spray, and spread the hot polenta evenly in the pan. Cover and refrigerate for several hours or overnight, or until the polenta is firm enough to slice.

3. When ready to prepare the recipe, unmold the polenta onto a cutting board, and slice into eighteen $\frac{1}{2}$-inch-thick slices. Place the egg substitute in a shallow bowl, and place the wheat germ in another shallow bowl.

4. Dip each polenta slice first in the egg substitute, and then in the wheat germ, turning to coat each side. Coat a large baking sheet with the cooking spray, and arrange the slices on the sheet. Spray the tops lightly with the cooking spray.

5. Bake at 400°F for 15 to 20 minutes, or until the polenta is hot on the inside and golden brown on the outside. Serve hot, topped with Sweet Orange Syrup (page 71), maple syrup, or honey.

## NUTRITIONAL FACTS
(Per Slice)

Cal: 116    Carbs: 21 g    Chol: 0 mg    Fat: 0.9 g
Fiber: 3.1 g    Protein: 5.8 g    Sodium: 103 mg

# Polenta Porridge

Yield: 4 servings

2 $\frac{1}{2}$ cups water

2 $\frac{1}{2}$ cups skim milk or low-fat vanilla soymilk

1 cup polenta, coarsely ground cornmeal, or yellow corn grits

$\frac{1}{2}$ cup golden raisins

1. Place the water and milk in a 3-quart pot. Stir in the polenta, cornmeal, or grits, and bring to a boil over medium heat, stirring frequently.

2. Reduce the heat to low, cover, and simmer, stirring every few minutes, for about 15 minutes, or until the mixture is thick and creamy. Add the raisins during the last few minutes of cooking.

3. Serve hot, topped with honey or maple syrup, if desired.

## NUTRITIONAL FACTS
(Per 1 $\frac{1}{8}$-Cup Serving)

Cal: 252    Carbs: 52.4 g    Chol: 2 mg    Fat: 0.8 g
Fiber: 5.1 g    Protein: 9.3 g    Sodium: 81 mg

# Cinnamon Apple-Raisin Granola

## Yield: 7 servings

1 ½ cups old-fashioned oats*
¼ cup plus 2 tablespoons wheat bran
¼ cup plus 2 tablespoons oat bran
1 teaspoon ground cinnamon
½ cup chopped pecans or walnuts (optional)
¼ cup frozen apple juice concentrate, thawed
3 tablespoons maple syrup or honey
2 tablespoons light brown sugar
¾ cup dark raisins

* Look for oats that cook in 5 minutes.

1. Place the oats, wheat bran, oat bran, cinnamon, and, if desired, the nuts in a medium-sized bowl, and stir to mix well. In a small bowl, stir together the juice concentrate, maple syrup or honey, and brown sugar. Add the apple juice mixture to the oat mixture, and stir until moist and crumbly.

2. Coat a nonstick 9-x-13-inch pan with nonstick cooking spray, and spread the mixture evenly in the pan. Bake at 325°F for about 30 minutes, or until the mixture is golden brown. Stir after the first 15 minutes of baking, and then after every 5 minutes until done.

3. Remove the pan from the oven, stir in the raisins, and allow the granola to cool to room temperature. (As the granola cools, it will become crisp.) Transfer the mixture to an airtight container, and store for up to 1 month.

## NUTRITIONAL FACTS
### (Per ½-Cup Serving)

Cal: 184    Carbs: 40 g    Chol: 0 mg    Fat: 1.6 g
Fiber: 4.4 g    Protein: 4.6 g    Sodium: 6 mg

# Marvelous Muesli

*This super-nutritious cereal is a snap to make.*

## Yield: 6 cups

2 ½ cups old-fashioned oats*
¾ cup Grape-Nuts nuggets
¾ cup honey crunch wheat germ
½ cup dried cherries, blueberries, or cranberries
½ cup chopped dried apricots
½ cup golden raisins
½ cup toasted chopped pecans, hazelnuts, Brazil nuts, or almonds (optional)

* Look for oats that cook in 5 minutes.

1. Place all of the ingredients in a large bowl, and stir to mix well. Transfer to an airtight container, and store for up to 1 month.

2. To serve, place ½ cup of the muesli in an individual serving bowl. Add ¾ cup of skim milk, nonfat vanilla or plain yogurt, or applesauce. Stir and let sit for 5 minutes before serving.

## NUTRITIONAL FACTS
### (Per ½-Cup Serving, Cereal Only)

Cal: 159    Carbs: 30 g    Chol: 0 mg    Fat: 1.7 g
Fiber: 4.4 g    Protein: 6 g    Sodium: 49 mg

# California Crunch Granola

## Yield: 8 servings

2 cups old-fashioned oats*

½ cup oat bran

¾ teaspoon ground cinnamon

½ cup chopped almonds, hazelnuts, or pecans (optional)

¼ cup honey

3 tablespoons frozen white grape juice concentrate, thawed

2 tablespoons light brown sugar

¼ cup plus 2 tablespoons golden raisins or chopped dates

¼ cup plus 2 tablespoons chopped dried apricots or dried cherries

* Look for oats that cook in 5 minutes.

1. Place the oats, oat bran, cinnamon, and, if desired, the nuts in a medium-sized bowl, and stir to mix well. In a small bowl, stir together the honey, juice concentrate, and brown sugar. Add the honey mixture to the oat mixture, and stir until moist and crumbly.

2. Coat a nonstick 9-x-13-inch pan with non-stick cooking spray, and spread the mixture evenly in the pan. Bake at 325°F for about 30 minutes, or until the mixture is golden brown. Stir after the first 15 minutes of baking, and then every 5 minutes until done.

3. Remove the pan from the oven, stir in the dried fruits, and allow the granola to cool to room temperature. (As the granola cools, it will become crisp.) Transfer the mixture to an airtight container, and store for up to 1 month.

## NUTRITIONAL FACTS
### (Per ½-Cup Serving)

Cal: 176    Carbs: 39 g    Chol: 0 mg    Fat: 1.7 g
Fiber: 3.8 g    Protein: 4.8 g    Sodium: 3 mg

# Creamy Rice Cereal

*This hearty breakfast cereal is a nutritious alternative to refined cereals like farina or cream of wheat. For variety, substitute millet for the rice.*

## Yield: 4 servings

1 cup brown rice

2 cups skim milk or low-fat vanilla soymilk

2 cups water

1. Place the rice in a blender or food processor, and process at medium speed for 1 minute, or until it has the texture of cornmeal.

2. Place the processed rice, milk, and water in a 2-quart pot, and cook over medium heat, stirring frequently, until the mixture begins to boil. Reduce the heat to low, cover, and simmer, stirring every couple of minutes, for about 10 minutes, or until the mixture is thick and creamy. Add a little more water or milk during the last few minutes of cooking if necessary.

3. Serve hot, topped with a little honey, brown sugar, or maple syrup and a sprinkling of raisins or chopped dried fruit, if desired.

## NUTRITIONAL FACTS
### (Per 1-Cup Serving)

Cal: 213    Carbs: 42 g    Chol: 2 mg    Fat: 1.5 g
Fiber: 1.7 g    Protein: 7.9 g    Sodium: 66 mg

# Breakfast Brown Rice Pudding

Yield: 4 servings

3 cups cooked brown rice
½ cup dark raisins, chopped dried apricots, or other chopped dried fruit
1 cup skim milk or low-fat vanilla soymilk
3–4 tablespoons maple syrup
Ground cinnamon or nutmeg

1. Place the rice, raisins or other fruit, milk, and maple syrup in a 2-quart pot, and stir to mix well. Bring to a boil over medium-high heat.
2. Reduce the heat to low, cover, and simmer, stirring occasionally, for 5 to 8 minutes, or until the raisins are plumped and most of the liquid has been absorbed. Serve hot, topping each serving with a sprinkling of the cinnamon or nutmeg.

### NUTRITIONAL FACTS
(Per 1-Cup Serving)

Cal: 235    Carbs: 52.4 g    Chol: 1 mg    Fat: 1.2 g
Fiber: 2.6 g    Protein: 5.5 g    Sodium: 40 mg

# Cinnamon-Apple Oatmeal

Yield: 4 servings

2 cups old-fashioned oats*
3 cups water
1 cup unsweetened apple juice
1 cup chopped peeled apple (about 1 large)
¼ cup dark raisins
¾ teaspoon ground cinnamon

* Look for oats that cook in 5 minutes.

1. Place all of the ingredients in a 2-quart pot, and stir to mix well. Bring to a boil over high heat. Then reduce the heat to low, cover, and simmer, stirring occasionally, until the oats are tender and the liquid has been absorbed. (Depending on the thickness of the oats, this will take from 5 to 15 minutes.)
2. Serve hot, topped with a little maple syrup or brown sugar and some skim milk or vanilla soymilk, if desired.

### NUTRITIONAL FACTS
(Per 1-Cup Serving)

Cal: 234    Carbs: 50 g    Chol: 0 mg    Fat: 2.6 g
Fiber: 5.2 g    Protein: 6.8 g    Sodium: 5 mg

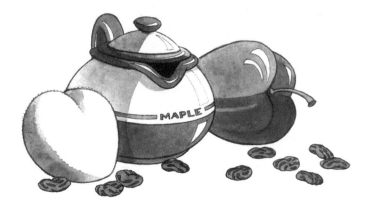

# *Great Grains*

*Grains play a prominent role in the world's most healthful cuisines. Naturally cholesterol-free and low in fat, grains—in their whole (unrefined) form—are also rich in health-promoting fiber, and contain a wealth of vitamins, minerals, and phytochemicals. That's why it is well worth the effort to learn how to add the goodness of whole grains to your diet. And once accustomed to the nutty flavors and satisfying texture of wholesome whole grains, most people prefer them over bland refined grains.*

*A wide variety of whole grains are available for use in breakfast cereals, salads, pilafs, stuffings, breads, and many other dishes. You'll find that most grocery stores stock several kinds, including barley, brown rice, buckwheat, and bulgur wheat. Natural foods stores carry a more extensive selection of whole grains, often in self-serve bulk bins.*

*The rest of this inset provides basic cooking directions for whole grains. In the table below, you will find the amount of water needed to cook one cup of the grain, the cooking time, and the yield once cooked. The cooking directions found below the table apply to most of the grains listed in the table. For those grains that must be cooked differently, the cooking directions have been provided within the table.*

## Grain Cooking Chart

| Grain (one cup) | Water | Cooking Time and Directions | Yield | Grain (one cup) | Water | Cooking Time and Directions | Yield |
|---|---|---|---|---|---|---|---|
| Barley (hulled or pearled) | $2^1/_2$ cups | 50–60 minutes. Follow cooking directions below. | 3 cups | Rye, cracked | $2^1/_2$ cups | 15–20 minutes. Follow cooking directions below, but stir occasionally. | 3 cups |
| Brown rice | $2^1/_2$ cups | 45–50 minutes. Follow cooking directions below. | 3 cups | Rye, rolled | 2 cups | 20 minutes. Follow cooking directions below, but stir occasionally. | $2^1/_2$ cups |
| Buckwheat groats or kasha | $2^1/_2$ cups | 15–20 minutes. Follow cooking directions below. | 3 cups | Rye, whole berries | $2^1/_2$ cups | 1–$1^1/_4$ hours. Follow cooking directions below. | 3 cups |
| Couscous | $1^1/_2$ cups | Bring the couscous and water to a boil, cover, and remove from the heat. Let sit for 5 minutes. | 3 cups | Spelt, whole berries | $2^1/_2$ cups | 1–$1^1/_4$ hours. Follow cooking directions below. | 3 cups |
| Kamut, whole kernels | 3 cups | $1^1/_2$–2 hours. Follow cooking directions below. | $2^3/_4$ cups | Wheat, bulgur | $1^1/_2$–2 cups, depending on brand | Place the bulgur in a large heatproof bowl, and pour the boiling water over it. Stir, cover, and let sit for 30–45 minutes, or until most of water is absorbed. Drain off any excess water. | $2^1/_2$ cups |
| Millet | 3 cups | 20 minutes. Follow cooking directions below. | $3^1/_2$ cups | | | | |
| Oats, old-fashioned | 2 cups | 5–20 minutes, depending on the oats' thickness. Follow cooking directions below, but stir occasionally. | 2 cups | | | | |
| Oats, quick-cooking | $1^3/_4$ cups | 1 minute. Follow cooking directions below. | 2 cups | Wheat, cracked | $2^1/_2$ cups | 15–20 minutes. Follow cooking directions below, but stir occasionally. | 3 cups |
| Oats, steel cut | $2^1/_2$ cups | 15–20 minutes. Follow cooking directions below, but stir occasionally. | 3 cups | Wheat, rolled | 2 cups | 20 minutes. Follow cooking directions below, but stir occasionally. | $2^1/_2$ cups |
| Quinoa | 2 cups | 10–15 minutes. Follow cooking directions below. | 3 cups | Wheat, whole berries | $2^1/_2$ cups | 1–$1^1/_4$ hours. Follow cooking directions below. | 3 cups |
| | | | | Wild rice | $2^1/_2$ cups | 50–60 minutes. Follow cooking directions below. | 3 cups |

## Cooking Directions

*Unless stated otherwise in the above table, the basic procedure for cooking grains is the same. Place the grain and water in a saucepan, and bring to a boil over high heat. Stir, reduce the heat to low, cover, and simmer for the specified amount of time. Do not stir during cooking, as this can make the grains gummy and sticky. When the grain has finished cooking, let it sit for 5 to 10 minutes covered; then fluff with a fork. You can halve the cooking time for long-cooking grains like barley, brown rice, and kamut by soaking the grain in its cooking water for 8 hours or overnight in the refrigerator.*

# Ham and Pepper Omelette

## Yield: 1 serving

2 tablespoons chopped ham or Canadian bacon, at least 97% lean

2 tablespoons chopped green bell pepper

2 tablespoons chopped red bell pepper

2 tablespoons chopped onion

1/2–3/4 cup fat-free egg substitute

3–4 tablespoons shredded nonfat or reduced-fat Cheddar cheese

Paprika (garnish)

1. Coat an 8-inch nonstick skillet with non-stick cooking spray. Preheat the skillet over medium heat, and add the ham, peppers, and onion. Cover and cook, stirring occasionally, for 2 to 3 minutes, or just until the vegetables are crisp-tender. Transfer the ham and vegetables to a small bowl, and cover to keep warm.

2. Respray the skillet, and place over medium-low heat. Add the egg substitute, and cook without stirring for about 2 minutes, or until the eggs are set around the edges. Use a spatula to lift the edges of the omelette, and allow the uncooked egg to flow below the cooked portion. Cook for another minute or 2, or until the eggs are almost set.

3. Arrange first the ham and vegetables, and then the cheese, over half of the omelette. Fold the other half over the filling, and cook for another minute or 2, or until the cheese is melted and the eggs are completely set.

4. Slide the omelette onto a plate, sprinkle some paprika over the top, and serve immediately.

## NUTRITIONAL FACTS
### (Per Serving)

| Cal: 139 | Carbs: 8.6 g | Chol: 12 mg | Fat: 0.6 g |
|---|---|---|---|
| Fiber: 1 g | Protein: 24 g | Sodium: 563 mg | |

# Apple Crunch Parfaits

*For variety, substitute diced peaches or apricots for the apples, and California Crunch Granola (page 74) for the Cinnamon Apple-Raisin Granola.*

## Yield: 4 servings

1 1/2 cups chopped peeled apple (about 2 medium)

2 cups nonfat or low-fat vanilla yogurt

3/4 cup Cinnamon Apple-Raisin Granola (page 73)

1. Place 3 tablespoons of chopped apples in the bottoms each of four 10-ounce balloon wine glasses or parfait glasses. Top with 1/4 cup of yogurt and 1 1/2 tablespoons of granola.

2. Repeat the layers, and serve immediately.

## NUTRITIONAL FACTS
### (Per Serving)

| Cal: 194 | Carbs: 40 g | Chol: 0 mg | Fat: 1 g |
|---|---|---|---|
| Fiber: 2.7 g | Protein: 7.7 g | Sodium: 82 mg | |

# Spring Vegetable Frittata

Yield: 4 servings

1 cup 1-inch pieces fresh asparagus spears

1/3 cup chopped red bell pepper

1/3 cup chopped onion

1 teaspoon dried fines herbes* or dried thyme

1/4 teaspoon ground black pepper

1 cup diced cooked new potatoes (about 5 medium)

2 cups fat-free egg substitute

2 tablespoons grated nonfat or regular Parmesan cheese

1 cup shredded nonfat or reduced-fat mozzarella or provolone cheese

* A blend of thyme, oregano, sage, rosemary, marjoram, and basil, fines herbes can be found in the dried spice section of most grocery stores.

**1.** Coat a 10-inch oven-proof skillet with non-stick cooking spray, and preheat over medium heat. Add the asparagus, red bell pepper, onion, fines herbs or thyme, and pepper. Cover and cook, stirring occasionally, for about 3 minutes, or until the vegetables are crisp-tender. Add a few teaspoons of water if the skillet becomes too dry.

**2.** Add the potatoes to the skillet, and stir to mix. Cover and cook over medium heat for 1 minute, or until the mixture is heated through. Add a little water if the skillet becomes too dry.

**3.** Reduce the heat to low, and pour the egg substitute over the potato mixture. Cook without stirring for about 12 minutes, or until the eggs are almost set.

**4.** Place the skillet under a preheated broiler, and broil for about 3 minutes, or until the eggs are set, but not dry. Sprinkle first the Parmesan and then the mozzarella or provolone over the top, and broil for another minute, or until the cheese is melted and lightly browned.

**5.** Cut the frittata into wedges, and serve hot.

## NUTRITIONAL FACTS
(Per Serving)

Cal: 162   Carbs: 16 g   Chol: 5 mg   Fat: 0.3 g
Fiber: 1.9 g   Protein: 24 g   Sodium: 425 mg

# Sausage and Potato Strata

Yield: 6 servings

3 cups sliced cooked potatoes (about 3 medium)

1 1/4 cups shredded nonfat or reduced-fat Cheddar cheese

1 cup diced low-fat smoked sausage or kielbasa (about 6 ounces), or 1 cup cooked, crumbled ground turkey sausage (about 8 ounces uncooked)

1 1/4 cups evaporated skim milk

1 1/4 cups fat-free egg substitute

**1.** Coat an 8-inch (2-quart) square baking pan with nonstick cooking spray, and arrange half of the potatoes over the bottom of the pan, slightly overlapping the slices. Sprinkle half of the cheese and then half of the sausage over the potatoes.

**2.** Place the evaporated milk and egg substitute in a medium-sized bowl, and whisk to mix well. Pour half of the egg mixture over the potato, cheese, and sausage layers. Repeat all of the layers.

3. Bake uncovered at 350°F for about 1 hour, or until the top is nicely browned and a sharp knife inserted in the center of the dish comes out clean. Remove the dish from the oven, and let sit for 15 minutes before cutting into squares and serving.

### NUTRITIONAL FACTS
(Per Serving)

| Cal: 196 | Carbs: 24 g | Chol: 17 mg | Fat: 0.9 g |
|---|---|---|---|
| Fiber: 1 g | Protein: 22.3 g | Sodium: 557 mg | |

# Turkey Breakfast Sausage Patties

*This versatile sausage mixture can also be used in recipes like Sausage and Potato Strata (page 78). To precook before adding to other dishes, just coat a large skillet with cooking spray, and preheat over medium heat. Add the sausage and cook, stirring to crumble, until the meat is no longer pink. Then drain on paper towels and use as desired.*

### Yield: 6 patties

1 pound ground turkey, 96% to 93% lean

1½ teaspoons ham-flavored bouillon granules

2 teaspoons dried sage

½ teaspoon dried thyme

¼ teaspoon ground black pepper

⅛ teaspoon cayenne pepper or crushed red pepper (optional)

1. Place all of the ingredients in a medium-sized bowl, and mix thoroughly. Cover and refrigerate for several hours or overnight to allow the flavors to blend.

2. Shape the mixture into six 3-inch patties. Coat a large skillet with nonstick cooking spray, and preheat over medium-low heat. Arrange the patties in the skillet and cook for 4 minutes on each side, or until nicely browned and no longer pink inside. Drain on paper towels, and serve hot.

### NUTRITIONAL FACTS
(Per Patty)

| Cal: 101 | Carbs: 0 g | Chol: 46 mg | Fat: 2.8 g |
|---|---|---|---|
| Fiber: 0 g | Protein: 17.6 g | Sodium: 226 mg | |

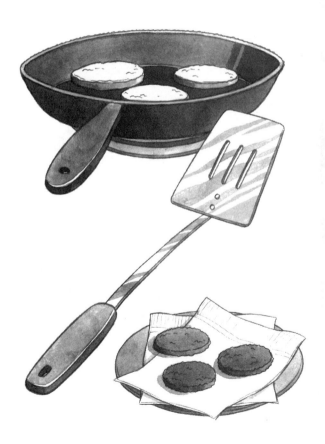

# 5.

# Hors D'Oeuvres With a Difference

You have decided to optimize your health through a nutrient-rich low-fat diet. Does that mean that you have to give up fun, festivity, and the fabulous foods that go along with it? Of course not! It's true that most traditional party favorites are loaded with fat and calories, but as you will see, the wide variety of low- and no-fat products that are now available enables smart partiers to whip up a healthful version of just about any festive food.

How are the recipes in this chapter different from their traditional versions? Reduced-fat and nonfat cheeses, ultra-lean meats, and nonfat sour cream and mayonnaise replace their full-fat counterparts in a variety of dips, spreads, and other party-perfect creations. You will be amazed by the big fat difference a few simple ingredient substitutions can make in traditional party favorites. For instance, a bowl of dip made with a cup of full-fat mayonnaise gets 1,582 calories and 186 grams of fat from the mayonnaise alone. When you prepare the same dip with a light mayonnaise,

you will cut the fat and calories by 50 to 80 percent. Use a nonfat mayonnaise, and you will eliminate *all* of the fat and 90 percent of the calories! Then scoop up your dip with a selection of low-fat whole grain crackers, breads, and nonfat chips, and you will have a wholesome snack that is every bit as tempting as its full-fat counterpart.

This chapter uses a variety of healthful ingredients to create a wide range of hot and cold hors d'oeuvres, both plain and fancy. From savory Mediterranean Meatballs and Oven-Fried Mushrooms to Party Pinwheels and Bueno Bean Dip, you will find a wealth of tempting tidbits and fabulous finger foods. Add some trays of fresh vegetables, a selection of in-season fruit, and plenty of low-cal beverages, and your menu will be the life of the party.

So send out the invitations, and get ready to treat friends and family to festive foods that are high on satisfaction, yet remarkably low in fat. Your guests will appreciate this more than you know.

# Oven-Fried Mushrooms

### Yield: 20 appetizers

20 medium whole fresh mushrooms
  (about 8 ounces)
Nonstick olive oil cooking spray

BATTER COATING
1/4 cup unbleached flour
1/4 cup fat-free egg substitute
3 tablespoons skim milk

CRUMB COATING
1/2 cup dried bread crumbs
3/4 teaspoon dried thyme
3/4 teaspoon ground paprika

DIPPING SAUCE
1/2 cup nonfat sour cream
2 tablespoons nonfat or reduced-fat
  mayonnaise
1 1/2 tablespoons finely chopped onion
1–2 teaspoons prepared horseradish

1. To make the batter coating, place the flour, egg substitute, and skim milk in a shallow bowl, and stir with a wire whisk until smooth. Set aside.

2. To make the crumb coating, place the bread crumbs, thyme, and paprika in a shallow bowl, and stir to mix well. Set aside.

3. Coat a large baking sheet with nonstick cooking spray. Dip each mushroom first in the batter coating and then in the crumb coating. Arrange the mushrooms in a single layer on the prepared pan.

4. Spray the mushrooms lightly with the olive oil cooking spray, and bake at 400°F for 8 minutes. Turn the mushrooms over, and bake for 7 to 9 additional minutes, or until nicely browned.

5. While the mushrooms are cooking, place the sauce ingredients in a small bowl, and stir to mix well.

6. Arrange the mushrooms on a serving platter, and serve hot, accompanied by the dish of sauce. Be aware that the centers of the mushrooms can be very hot when they first come out of the oven, so bite carefully.

### NUTRITIONAL FACTS
(Per Appetizer)

| | | | |
|---|---|---|---|
| Cal: 23 | Carbs: 4 g | Chol: 0 mg | Fat: 0.1 g |
| Fiber: 0.3 g | Protein: 1.2 g | Sodium: 36 mg | |

# Chutney Chicken Kabobs

### Yield: 18 appetizers

1 pound boneless skinless chicken breasts
1 can (15 ounces) unsweetened pineapple
  chunks in juice, undrained
1/4 cup mango chutney
2 tablespoons reduced-sodium soy sauce
1 1/2 teaspoons crushed fresh garlic
36 one-inch scallion pieces (white and light
  green parts only), or 36 green bell pepper
  strips (each 1-x-1/2 inch)

1. Rinse the chicken, and pat it dry with paper towels. Cut the chicken breasts lengthwise

into ⅓-inch-thick strips. (This will be easiest to do if the meat is partially frozen.) Place the strips in a shallow nonmetal container, and set aside.

**2.** Drain the pineapple, and place ¼ cup plus 2 tablespoons of the juice in a blender. Refrigerate the pineapple chunks until ready to assemble the kabobs.

**3.** To make the marinade, add the chutney, soy sauce, and garlic to the pineapple juice, and process for about 1 minute, or until smooth. Remove ¼ cup of the marinade, and refrigerate until ready to cook the kabobs. Pour the remaining marinade over the chicken strips, and toss to mix well. Cover the chicken and refrigerate for at least 3 hours, and up to 24 hours.

**4.** Just before making the kabobs, place 18 six-inch bamboo skewers in a shallow dish,

and cover with water. Allow the skewers to soak for 20 minutes. (This will prevent them from burning.)

**5.** Loosely weave 1 long and 1 short chicken strip, 2 pineapple chunks, and 2 pieces of scallion or green pepper onto each skewer. Grill the skewers over medium coals or broil 6 inches under a preheated broiler for about 3 minutes on each side, or until almost done. Baste the kabobs with the reserved marinade and cook for another minute or 2 on each side, or until the meat is nicely browned and no longer pink inside. Serve hot.

### NUTRITIONAL FACTS
#### (Per Appetizer)

| | | | |
|---|---|---|---|
| Cal: 42 | Carbs: 3.4 g | Chol: 15 mg | Fat: 0.3 g |
| Fiber: 0.3 g | Protein: 6 g | Sodium: 48 mg | |

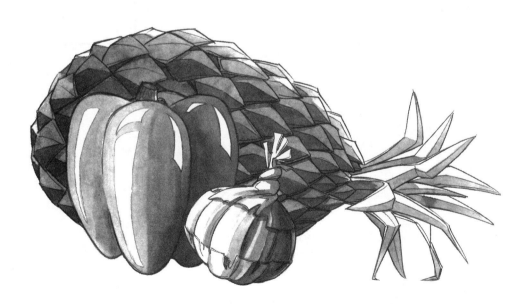

# Spinach and Cheese Strudels

### Yield: 24 appetizers

12 sheets (12 x 18 inches) phyllo pastry (about 10 ounces)
Nonstick butter-flavored cooking spray

FILLING
1 cup chopped fresh mushrooms
1 teaspoon crushed fresh garlic
$\frac{1}{2}$ teaspoon dried thyme
$\frac{1}{4}$ teaspoon coarsely ground black pepper
1 package (10 ounces) frozen chopped spinach, thawed and squeezed dry
$\frac{1}{2}$ cup nonfat or low-fat cottage cheese
$\frac{1}{4}$ cup fat-free egg substitute, or 2 egg whites, lightly beaten

$\frac{1}{4}$ cup grated nonfat or regular Parmesan cheese
1 cup shredded nonfat or reduced-fat mozzarella cheese

1. To make the filling, coat a large nonstick skillet with nonstick cooking spray, and preheat over medium heat. Add the mushrooms, garlic, thyme, and pepper, and stir to mix. Cover and cook, stirring occasionally, for about 3 minutes, or until the mushrooms are tender. Remove the skillet from the heat and stir in first the spinach, then the cottage cheese and egg substitute, and finally the Parmesan and mozzarella.

2. Spread the phyllo dough out on a clean, dry surface, with the short end facing you. Cut the phyllo dough lengthwise down the center to make 2 stacks, each measuring about 18 x 6 inches. Lay one stack on top of the other to make one 18-x-6-inch stack of 24 phyllo sheets. Cover the dough with plastic wrap to prevent it from drying out as you

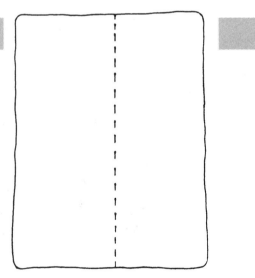

**a.** Cut the phyllo sheets into 2 long strips.

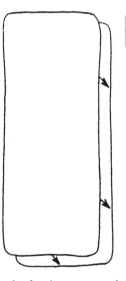

**b.** Lay 1 stack of strips on top of the other.

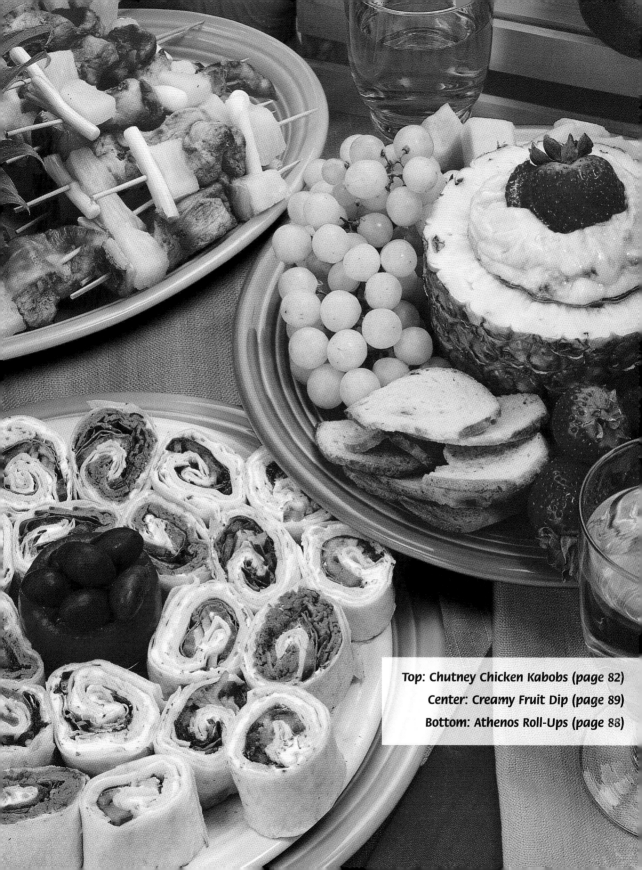

**Top: Chutney Chicken Kabobs (page 82)**
**Center: Creamy Fruit Dip (page 89)**
**Bottom: Athenos Roll-Ups (page 88)**

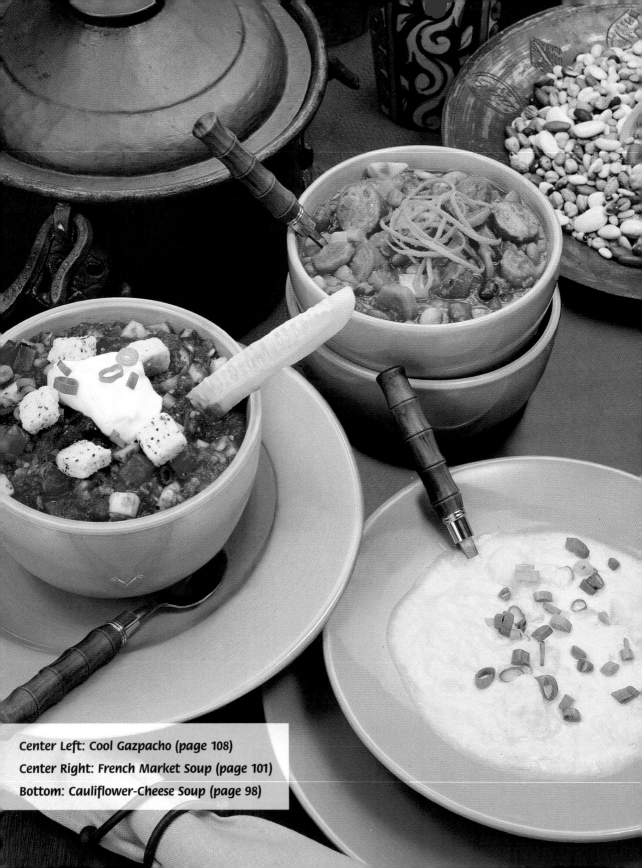

Center Left: Cool Gazpacho (page 108)
Center Right: French Market Soup (page 101)
Bottom: Cauliflower-Cheese Soup (page 98)

work. (Remove strips as you need them, being sure to re-cover the remaining dough.)

3. Remove 1 strip of the phyllo dough, and lay it flat on a clean dry surface. Spray the strip lightly with the cooking spray. Fold the bottom up to form a double layer of phyllo measuring approximately 9 x 6 inches.

4. Spread 1 slightly rounded tablespoon of filling over the bottom of the phyllo sheet, leaving a 1½-inch margin on each side. Fold the left and right edges inward to enclose the filling. Then roll the pastry up from the bottom, jelly-roll style. Repeat steps 3 and 4 with the remaining filling and phyllo sheets to make 24 strudels.

5. Coat a large baking sheet with nonstick cooking spray, and arrange the strudels on the sheets. Spray the top of each strudel lightly with the cooking spray.

6. Bake at 375°F for about 15 minutes, or until golden brown. Allow to cool for 10 minutes before serving warm.

## NUTRITIONAL FACTS
### (Per Appetizer)

| Cal: 51 | Carbs: 7.4 g | Chol: 0 mg | Fat: 0.7 g |
|---------|--------------|------------|------------|
| Fiber: 0.5 g | Protein: 3.7 g | Sodium: 129 mg | |

### Time-Saving Tip

To save time on the day you bake Spinach and Cheese Strudels (page 84) or Curried Vegetable Turnovers (page 86), prepare the pastries ahead of time to the point of baking, and arrange them in single layers in airtight containers, separating the layers with sheets of waxed paper. Then place the pastries in the freezer until needed. When ready to bake, arrange the frozen pastries on a coated sheet and allow them to sit at room temperature for 45 minutes before baking.

# Making Spinach and Cheese Strudels

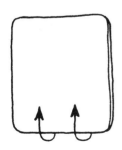

**c.** Fold the bottom of each strip up to double the strip.

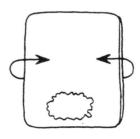

**d.** Spread the filling over the bottom of each strip. Fold the left and right edges inward.

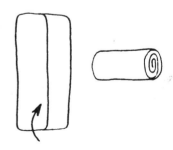

**e.** Roll the pastry up jelly-roll style.

# Curried Vegetable Turnovers

### Yield: 24 appetizers

12 sheets (12 x 18 inches) phyllo pastry (about 10 ounces)
Nonstick butter-flavored cooking spray

FILLING

¾ cup finely chopped carrots

¾ cup finely chopped celery (include the leaves)

¾ cup finely chopped onion

¾ cup finely chopped fresh mushrooms

¾ cup finely chopped peeled Yukon Gold or russet potatoes

⅓ cup vegetable or chicken broth

2–3 teaspoons curry paste

1. To make the filling, coat a large nonstick skillet with nonstick cooking spray, and preheat over medium heat. Add all of the filling ingredients, and stir to mix well. Cover and cook, stirring occasionally, for 8 to 10 minutes, or until the vegetables are tender. Add a little more broth during cooking if needed to prevent sticking. If there is excess liquid in the skillet at the end of cooking, cook uncovered for a minute or 2 to remove most of the moisture. Remove the skillet from the heat, and set aside to cool slightly.

2. Spread the phyllo dough out on a clean, dry surface, with the short end facing you. Cut the phyllo dough lengthwise into 4 long strips, each measuring about 18 x 3 inches. Cover the dough with plastic wrap to prevent it from drying out as you work. (Remove strips as you need them, being sure to re-cover the remaining dough.)

3. Remove 2 strips of phyllo dough and stack 1 on top of the other. Spray the strip lightly

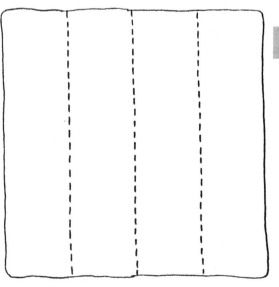

**a.** Cut the phyllo sheets into 4 strips.

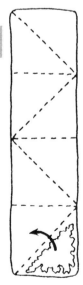

**b.** Fold the filled corner up and over.

## Making Curried Vegetable Turnovers

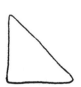

**c.** Continue folding to form a triangle.

with the cooking spray. Spread 1 rounded tablespoon of the filling over the bottom right-hand corner of the double phyllo strip. Fold the filled corner up and over to the left, so that the corner meets the left side of the strip. Continue folding in this manner until you form a triangle of dough. Repeat with the remaining filling and dough.

4. Coat a large baking sheet with nonstick cooking spray, and arrange the turnovers seam-side down on the sheet. Spray the top of each turnover lightly with cooking spray.

5. Bake at 375°F for about 15 minutes, or until golden brown. Allow to cool for 10 minutes before serving warm.

### NUTRITIONAL FACTS
(Per Appetizer)

| | | | |
|---|---|---|---|
| Cal: 44 | Carbs: 7.8 g | Chol: 0 mg | Fat: 0.9 g |
| Fiber: 0.6 g | Protein: 1 g | Sodium: 110 mg | |

# Corn and Pepper Quesadillas

Yield: 16 appetizers

4 flour tortillas (8-inch rounds), warmed to room temperature

1 cup shredded nonfat or reduced-fat Monterey jack cheese

½ cup well-drained diced roasted red bell peppers (half of a 7-ounce jar)

½ cup frozen whole kernel corn, thawed

Nonstick butter-flavored cooking spray

TOPPINGS

⅓ cup nonfat sour cream

3 tablespoons sliced scallions

1. Place the sour cream and scallions in separate serving dishes, and set aside.

2. Lay a tortilla out on a flat surface, and spread 2 tablespoons of the cheese over the *bottom half only* of the tortilla. Top the cheese with 2 tablespoons of the roasted red peppers, 2 tablespoons of the corn, and 2 more tablespoons of the cheese. Fold the top half of the tortilla over to enclose the filling. Repeat with the remaining ingredients.

3. Coat a large baking sheet with nonstick cooking spray, and arrange the folded tortillas on the sheets in a single layer. Spray the tops lightly with the nonstick cooking spray.

4. Bake at 425°F for 5 minutes. Turn the quesadillas over, and bake for 4 additional minutes, or until the tortillas are lightly browned and the cheese is melted.

5. To serve, place each quesadilla on a cutting board, and cut into 4 wedges. Arrange the wedges on a serving platter accompanied by the dishes of sour cream and scallions.

### NUTRITIONAL FACTS
(Per Appetizer)

| | | | |
|---|---|---|---|
| Cal: 52 | Carbs: 8 g | Chol: 0 mg | Fat: 0.8 g |
| Fiber: 0.2 g | Protein: 3.4 g | Sodium: 178 mg | |

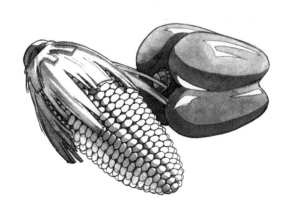

# Party Pinwheels

## Yield: 40 appetizers

2 blocks (8 ounces each) nonfat cream cheese, softened to room temperature

$^3\!/_4$ cup grated carrots (about 1$^1\!/_2$ medium)

$^1\!/_2$ cup finely chopped green bell pepper

$^1\!/_2$ cup chopped black olives

$^1\!/_2$ cup finely chopped scallions

2 tablespoons finely chopped fresh parsley

4 flour tortillas (10-inch rounds), warmed to room temperature

**1.** Place the cream cheese in a medium-sized bowl. Add the carrots, peppers, olives, scallions, and parsley, and stir to mix well.

**2.** Lay a tortilla out on a flat surface, and spread $^1\!/_2$ cup of the cheese mixture over the tortilla, extending the filling all the way to the top and bottom, but to within only 1 inch of the side edges. Starting from the bottom, roll the tortilla up tightly jelly-roll style. Repeat with the remaining tortillas and filling. Then wrap each roll separately in plastic wrap. Chill for at least 2 hours, and for up to 8 hours.

**3.** When ready to serve, unwrap the tortilla rolls, slice 1$^1\!/_4$ inches off each end, and discard the ends. Slice the rolls into $^3\!/_4$-inch slices and arrange on a serving platter. Allow the pinwheels to come to room temperature before serving.

## NUTRITIONAL FACTS
### (Per Appetizer)

| | | | |
|---|---|---|---|
| Cal: 30 | Carbs: 4 g | Chol: 0 mg | Fat: 0.5 g |
| Fiber: 0.4 g | Protein: 2.1 g | Sodium: 104 mg | |

# Athenos Roll-Ups

## Yield: 24 appetizers

1 block (8 ounces) nonfat cream cheese, softened to room temperature

1 teaspoon crushed fresh garlic

$^1\!/_2$ teaspoon dried oregano

4 flour tortillas (10-inch rounds), warmed to room temperature

8 ounces turkey breast or lean roast beef, thinly sliced

24 fresh tender spinach leaves

2 tablespoons bottled fat-free red wine vinaigrette salad dressing

12 thin slices tomato

$^1\!/_4$ cup plus 2 tablespoons chopped black olives

2 thin slices red onion, separated into rings

$^1\!/_4$ cup plus 2 tablespoons crumbled nonfat or reduced-fat feta cheese

**1.** Place the cream cheese, garlic, and oregano in a medium-sized bowl, and stir until smooth.

**2.** Arrange the tortillas on a flat surface. Spread a quarter of the cream cheese mixture over each tortilla, extending the cheese to the outer edges. Arrange 2 ounces of the turkey or roast beef over the *bottom half only* of each tortilla, leaving a 1-inch margin on each outer edge. Arrange 6 spinach leaves over the turkey or roast beef, and drizzle 1$^1\!/_2$ teaspoons of the vinaigrette dressing over the spinach. Top with 3 tomato slices, 1$^1\!/_2$ tablespoons of olives, a few onion rings, and 1$^1\!/_2$ tablespoons of feta cheese.

**3.** Starting at the bottom, roll each tortilla up tightly. Cut a 1$^1\!/_4$-inch piece off each end, and discard. Slice the remainder of each tortilla into six 1$^1\!/_4$-inch pieces. Arrange the rolls on a platter, and serve.

## NUTRITIONAL FACTS
(Per Appetizer)

| | | | |
|---|---|---|---|
| Cal: 55 | Carbs: 6 g | Chol: 8 mg | Fat: 0.8 g |
| Fiber: 0.7 g | Protein: 5.4 g | Sodium: 165 mg | |

## Time-Saving Tip

To avoid a last-minute rush, make Athenos Roll-Ups as much as 24 hours before your party, cover with plastic wrap, and refrigerate. When guests arrive, simply remove the plastic wrap and serve.

# Mediterranean Meatballs

Yield: 48 appetizers

MEATBALLS
12 ounces 95% lean ground beef
1 1/2 teaspoons crushed fresh garlic
1 1/2 teaspoons dried oregano
1/4 teaspoon salt
1/4 teaspoon ground black pepper
1 package (10 ounces) frozen chopped
    spinach, thawed and squeezed dry
1 1/2 cups cooked brown rice or bulgur wheat
3/4 cup finely chopped onion
1/4 cup grated nonfat Parmesan cheese
1/4 cup fat-free egg substitute

SAUCE
2 cups bottled fat-free marinara sauce

1. Place the beef, garlic, oregano, salt, and pepper in a medium-sized bowl, and mix thoroughly. Add the remaining meatball ingredients, and mix well.

2. Coat a large baking sheet with nonstick cooking spray. Shape the meatball mixture into 48 (1-inch) balls, and arrange them in a single layer on the baking sheet. Bake at 350°F for about 25 minutes, or until nicely browned and no longer pink inside. Transfer the meatballs to a chafing dish or Crock-Pot heated casserole to keep warm.

3. Place the marinara sauce in a small pot, and cook over medium heat just until heated through. Pour the sauce over the meatballs, toss gently to mix, and serve.

## NUTRITIONAL FACTS
(Per Appetizer)

| | | | |
|---|---|---|---|
| Cal: 24 | Carbs: 2.7 g | Chol: 4 mg | Fat: 0.4 g |
| Fiber: 0.4 g | Protein: 2.3 g | Sodium: 62 mg | |

# Creamy Fruit Dip

Yield: 1 1/4 cups

1 cup plain nonfat yogurt cheese, nonfat sour
    cream, or nonfat cream cheese
1/4–1/3 cup apricot, strawberry, or cherry
    preserves

1. Place the yogurt cheese, sour cream, or cream cheese and the preserves in a small bowl, and stir to mix well.

2. Cover and chill for at least 2 hours. Serve with fresh fruit, bagel slices, and whole grain crackers.

## NUTRITIONAL FACTS
(Per Tablespoon)

| | | | |
|---|---|---|---|
| Cal: 18 | Carbs: 3.6 g | Chol: 0 mg | Fat: 0 g |
| Fiber: 0 g | Protein: 0.9 g | Sodium: 10 mg | |

# Sensational Strawberries

## Yield: 6 servings

6 cups fresh whole strawberries
¾ cup nonfat sour cream
¼ cup plus 2 tablespoons light brown sugar

1. Rinse the strawberries, and pat dry with paper towels. Leave the stems on.

2. Place the sour cream and brown sugar in separate small serving dishes, and place the dishes in the center of a large serving platter. Arrange the strawberries on the platter around the sour cream and brown sugar.

3. To eat, dip the end of a strawberry first in the sour cream, and then in the brown sugar.

### NUTRITIONAL FACTS
(Per Serving)

| Cal: 107 | Carbs: 23 g | Chol: 0 mg | Fat: 0.5 g |
|---|---|---|---|
| Fiber: 2.2 g | Protein: 3.2 g | Sodium: 33 mg | |

# Gorgonzola-Walnut Dip

## Yield: 2½ cups

2 cups nonfat sour cream
⅓ cup crumbled Gorgonzola or blue cheese
⅓ cup chopped walnuts
⅛ teaspoon dried thyme

1. Place all of the ingredients in a medium-sized bowl, and stir to mix well.

2. Cover and chill for at least 2 hours. Serve with fresh apple or pear slices (dip in pineapple juice to prevent browning), celery and carrot sticks, bagel slices, and whole grain crackers.

### NUTRITIONAL FACTS
(Per Tablespoon)

| Cal: 23 | Carbs: 2.2 g | Chol: 1 mg | Fat: 0.9 g |
|---|---|---|---|
| Fiber: 0 g | Protein: 1.2 g | Sodium: 24 mg | |

# Crab Louis Dip

## Yield: 2½ cups

½ cup plus 2 tablespoons nonfat or reduced-fat mayonnaise
½ cup plus 2 tablespoons nonfat or reduced-fat sour cream
¼ cup chili sauce
1 cup flaked cooked crab meat, or 1 can (6 ounces) crab meat, drained
⅓ cup chopped green or black olives
2 tablespoons finely chopped onion

1. Place the mayonnaise, sour cream, and chili sauce in a medium-sized bowl, and stir to mix well. Add the crab, olives, and onion, and stir to mix well.

2. Cover and chill for at least 2 hours. Serve with whole grain crackers, celery sticks, and carrot sticks.

### NUTRITIONAL FACTS
(Per Tablespoon)

| Cal: 12 | Carbs: 1.5 g | Chol: 2 mg | Fat: 0.2 g |
|---|---|---|---|
| Fiber: 0 g | Protein: 0.9 g | Sodium: 66 mg | |

## The Healing Power of Culinary Herbs

*Health-conscious cooks have long known that the liberal use of herbs and spices is one of the best ways to trim both fat and salt from your dishes. Why? These seasonings can add so much flavor that no one will notice that fat and salt were reduced. Now researchers are discovering that many culinary herbs and spices are also rich in health-promoting phytochemicals, providing an even better reason to expand your seasoning horizons. For instance, oregano, rosemary, sage, thyme, orange and lemon rinds, ginger, garlic, turmeric, celery seed, caraway, and many other common seasonings have been found to contain antioxidants, cancer-fighting compounds, and other beneficial chemicals. The compounds in ginger can soothe an upset stomach, prevent motion sickness, and help fight inflammation. And garlic can help fight cardiovascular disease, cancer, and infections. These are just a few examples of the healing powers of culinary herbs and spices.*

*So as you prepare your healthy low-fat dishes, experiment with herbs and spices. You will not only open up a whole new world of flavors, but you will also reap the many health benefits that these wonderful foods have to offer.*

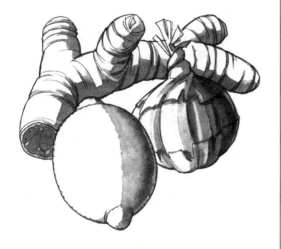

# Bueno Bean Dip

Yield: 8 servings

1 can (15 ounces) black or pinto beans, rinsed and drained
¼ cup bottled salsa
1 teaspoon chili powder
1 cup nonfat sour cream
1 cup finely shredded romaine or iceberg lettuce
½ cup finely chopped tomato
¾ cup finely shredded nonfat Cheddar cheese
⅓ cup chopped black olives

**1.** Place the beans, salsa, and chili powder in a medium-sized bowl. Using a potato masher or a fork, mash until the ingredients are well mixed and the mixture is smooth or slightly chunky, depending on your personal preference.

**2.** Spread the bean mixture over the bottom of a 9-inch glass pie pan. Spread the sour cream in an even layer over the bean mixture. Top the sour cream layer with the lettuce, tomatoes, Cheddar, and, finally, the olives. Serve immediately with baked tortilla chips, or cover with plastic wrap and chill for up to 2 hours before serving.

### NUTRITIONAL FACTS
(Per Serving)

Cal: 101   Carbs: 15 g   Chol: 1 mg   Fat: 0.8 g
Fiber: 3.3 g   Protein: 8.1 g   Sodium: 225 mg

# Baked Artichoke Dip

### Yield: 2½ cups

2 packages (9 ounces each) frozen artichoke
 hearts, thawed, drained, and chopped, or
 2 cans (14 ounces each) artichoke hearts,
 drained and chopped

⅔ cup nonfat or reduced-fat mayonnaise

1 tablespoon Dijon or spicy mustard

½ cup grated Parmesan cheese, divided*

\* In this recipe, use regular Parmesan cheese, not a
 fat-free product.

**1.** Place the artichokes, mayonnaise, mustard,
 and ¼ cup plus 2 tablespoons of the Parmesan in a food processor, and process for
 about 20 seconds, or until the mixture is
 well blended but still slightly chunky.

**2.** Coat a 1-quart casserole dish with nonstick
 cooking spray, and spread the mixture
 evenly in the dish. Sprinkle the remaining 2
 tablespoons of Parmesan over the top.

**3.** Cover with aluminum foil, and bake at
 350°F for 25 minutes, or until the mixture is
 heated through. Remove the foil, and bake
 for 10 additional minutes, or until the top is
 lightly browned. Serve hot, accompanied
 by whole grain crackers.

### NUTRITIONAL FACTS
#### (Per Tablespoon)

| | | | |
|---|---|---|---|
| Cal: 14 | Carbs: 1.6 g | Chol: 0 mg | Fat: 0.5 g |
| Fiber: 0.8 g | Protein: 0.8 g | Sodium: 62 mg | |

# Honey-Mustard Dip

### Yield: 1⅛ cups

½ cup nonfat sour cream

½ cup nonfat or low-fat mayonnaise

2 tablespoons Dijon mustard

2 tablespoons honey

**1.** Place the sour cream and mayonnaise in a
 medium-sized bowl, and stir to mix well. Add
 the mustard and honey, and stir to mix well.

**2.** Serve immediately, or cover and chill until
 ready to serve. Serve with fresh vegetables
 such as broccoli and cauliflower florets, carrot and celery sticks, red and green bell pepper strips, and blanched asparagus and
 snow peas. This dip is also delicious with
 cubes or rolled-up slices of lean turkey or
 ham, and cubes of low-fat Swiss cheese.

### NUTRITIONAL FACTS
#### (Per Tablespoon)

| | | | |
|---|---|---|---|
| Cal: 19 | Carbs: 4 g | Chol: 0 mg | Fat: 0.1 g |
| Fiber: 0.1 g | Protein: 0.5 g | Sodium: 73 mg | |

# Healthy Hummus

### Yield: 1¾ cups

1 can (19 ounces) chickpeas, rinsed and
 drained, or 2 cups cooked chickpeas

¼ cup plus 2 tablespoons plain nonfat yogurt

3–4 tablespoons toasted sesame tahini

3 tablespoons lemon juice

½ teaspoon ground cumin

1 teaspoon crushed fresh garlic

3 tablespoons chopped fresh parsley

1. Place the chickpeas, yogurt, tahini, lemon juice, cumin, and garlic in a food processor, and process until smooth. Add the parsley, and process until the ingredients are well mixed and the parsley is finely chopped.

2. Transfer the mixture to a covered container, and chill for several hours. Serve with wedges of pita bread or whole grain crackers, or use as a sandwich filling.

**NUTRITIONAL FACTS**
(Per Tablespoon)

| | | | |
|---|---|---|---|
| Cal: 29 | Carbs: 3.4 g | Chol: 0 mg | Fat: 1.2 g |
| Fiber: 1.2 g | Protein: 1.2 g | Sodium: 28 mg | |

# Spiced Lentil and Split Pea Pâté

### Yield: 2 cups

$\frac{1}{2}$ cup dried brown lentils, cleaned (page 102)

$\frac{1}{2}$ cup dried green or yellow split peas, cleaned (page 102)

$2\frac{1}{2}$ cups water

2 teaspoons instant vegetable or chicken bouillon granules

1–2 tablespoons extra virgin olive oil

$\frac{1}{2}$ cup chopped red or yellow onion

1 tablespoon crushed fresh garlic

1 teaspoon ground turmeric

1 teaspoon ground cumin

$\frac{1}{2}$ teaspoon chili powder

$\frac{1}{4}$ teaspoon ground black pepper

$\frac{1}{4}$ cup (packed) chopped fresh cilantro or parsley

1. Place the lentils, split peas, water, and bouillon granules in a $2\frac{1}{2}$-quart pot, and bring to a boil over high heat. Reduce the heat to low, cover, and simmer, stirring occasionally, for about 45 minutes, or until the lentils and peas are very soft and all of the liquid has been absorbed. Remove the pot from the heat, and set aside.

2. Place the olive oil in a small nonstick skillet, and preheat over medium heat. Add the onion and garlic, and cook, stirring often, for about 3 minutes, or until the onion is translucent. Add the turmeric, cumin, chili powder, and pepper, and cook for another 30 seconds. Remove the skillet from the heat, and set aside.

3. Place the lentil-split pea mixture, onion mixture, and cilantro or parsley in a food processor, and process until smooth. Transfer the mixture to a serving dish, and serve at room temperature with wedges of pita bread and whole wheat crackers.

**NUTRITIONAL FACTS**
(Per Tablespoon)

| | | | |
|---|---|---|---|
| Cal: 26 | Carbs: 4 g | Chol: 0 mg | Fat: 0.5 g |
| Fiber: 1.8 g | Protein: 1.7 g | Sodium: 36 mg | |

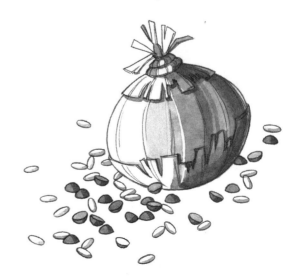

# Spicy Garbanzo Spread

## Yield: 1⅓ cups

¼ cup plus 2 tablespoons chopped green bell pepper

¼ cup plus 2 tablespoons chopped red bell pepper

¼ cup plus 2 tablespoons chopped onion

2 teaspoons crushed fresh garlic

½ teaspoon whole cumin seeds

1 can (15 ounces) chickpeas, rinsed and drained

¼ cup plain nonfat yogurt

¼ teaspoon cayenne pepper

1. Coat a medium-sized nonstick skillet with nonstick cooking spray, and preheat over medium heat. Add the green pepper, red pepper, onion, garlic, and cumin. Cover and cook, stirring often, for about 3 minutes, or until the vegetables start to soften. Add a little broth or water to the skillet if it becomes too dry.

2. Place the chickpeas, yogurt, and pepper in a food processor. Add the vegetable mixture, and process until smooth. Serve at room temperature as a dip with whole grain crackers, baked tortilla chips, and cut raw vegetables, or use as a filling for sandwiches.

## NUTRITIONAL FACTS
### (Per Tablespoon)

| | | | |
|---|---|---|---|
| Cal: 16 | Carbs: 3.3 g | Chol: 0 mg | Fat: 0.3 g |
| Fiber: 1 g | Protein: 1 g | Sodium: 25 mg | |

# Lentil and Walnut Pâté

## Yield: 2¼ cups

1 cup dried brown or red lentils, cleaned (page 102)

2½ cups water

2 teaspoons instant vegetable or chicken bouillon granules

½ cup plus 2 tablespoons chopped onion

2 teaspoons crushed fresh garlic

1 teaspoon ground cumin

½ teaspoon dried thyme or oregano

¼ teaspoon ground allspice

¼ teaspoon coarsely ground black pepper

⅓ cup chopped walnuts

1. Place the lentils, water, and bouillon granules in a 2½-quart pot, and bring to a boil over high heat. Reduce the heat to low, cover, and simmer, stirring occasionally, for about 35 minutes, or until the lentils are very soft and all of the liquid has been absorbed. Remove the pot from the heat, and set aside.

2. Coat a small nonstick skillet with olive oil cooking spray, and preheat over medium heat. Add the onion and garlic, cover, and cook, stirring frequently, for about 3 minutes, or until the onion is translucent. Add a little water if the skillet seems too dry. Remove the skillet from the heat, and set aside.

3. Place the lentil mixture, onion mixture, spices, and walnuts in a food processor, and process until smooth. Transfer the mixture to a serving dish, and serve at room temperature with wedges of pita bread and whole wheat crackers.

**NUTRITIONAL FACTS**
(Per Tablespoon)

| Cal: 25 | Carbs: 3.5 g | Chol: 0 mg | Fat: 0.7 g |
|---|---|---|---|
| Fiber: 1.8 g | Protein: 1.8 g | Sodium: 32 mg | |

# Chutney Chicken Spread

Yield: 2¼ cups

1 block (8 ounces) nonfat cream cheese,
  softened to room temperature
¼ cup plus 2 tablespoons finely chopped onion
¼ cup plus 2 tablespoons finely chopped celery
¼ cup mango chutney
¾ cup finely chopped cooked chicken or turkey
  breast, or 1 can (6 ounces) white meat
  chicken or turkey, drained
3 tablespoons toasted sliced almonds or
  chopped roasted peanuts

1. Place the cream cheese, onion, celery, and chutney in a medium-sized bowl, and stir to mix well. Add the chicken or turkey, and stir to mix well.

2. Spread the mixture in a small bowl, and sprinkle the almonds or peanuts over the top. Cover and chill for at least 2 hours. Serve with whole grain crackers, carrot sticks, and celery sticks, or use as a filling for finger sandwiches.

**NUTRITIONAL FACTS**
(Per Tablespoon)

| Cal: 18 | Carbs: 1 g | Chol: 3 mg | Fat: 0.4 g |
|---|---|---|---|
| Fiber: 0.1 g | Protein: 2.2 g | Sodium: 38 mg | |

# Dilled Chicken Spread

*For variety, substitute ¾ cup canned, drained salmon or ¾ cup flaked cooked crab meat for the chicken.*

Yield: 2 cups

1 block (8 ounces) nonfat cream cheese,
  softened to room temperature
¼ cup nonfat sour cream
¼ cup plus 2 tablespoons finely chopped onion
¼ cup plus 2 tablespoons finely chopped celery
3–4 teaspoons finely chopped fresh dill, or
  1–1¼ teaspoons dried
¾ cup finely chopped cooked chicken or turkey
  breast, or 1 can (6 ounces) white meat
  chicken or turkey, drained
¼ cup plus 2 tablespoons toasted finely
  chopped almonds or walnuts

1. Place the cream cheese, sour cream, onion, celery, and dill in a medium-sized bowl, and stir to mix well. Add the chicken or turkey, and stir to mix well.

2. Shape the mixture into an 8-inch-long log, and roll in the almonds or walnuts, turning to coat all sides. Cover and chill for at least 2 hours. Serve with whole grain crackers, or use as a filling for finger sandwiches.

**NUTRITIONAL FACTS**
(Per Tablespoon)

| Cal: 21 | Carbs: 1.2 g | Chol: 3 mg | Fat: 0.8 g |
|---|---|---|---|
| Fiber: 0.2 g | Protein: 2.7 g | Sodium: 40 mg | |

# Mandarin Cream Cheese Spread

### Yield: 1¾ cups

1 block (8 ounces) nonfat cream cheese, softened to room temperature

½ cup canned mandarin oranges, well drained

1 can (8 ounces) crushed pineapple, well drained

½ cup golden raisins

¼ cup toasted sliced almonds or toasted chopped pecans

1. Place the cream cheese in a medium-sized bowl, and beat with an electric mixer until smooth. Add the drained mandarin oranges, and beat until the oranges are broken down and mixed throughout. Stir in first the drained pineapple, and then the raisins and nuts.

2. Cover and chill for 8 hours or overnight, or until the raisins are plumped and the spread has thickened. Stir the mixture, and serve with whole grain crackers or bagel slices.

### NUTRITIONAL FACTS
#### (Per Tablespoon)

| | | | |
|---|---|---|---|
| Cal: 26 | Carbs: 3.6 g | Chol: 0 mg | Fat: 0.8 g |
| Fiber: 0.3 g | Protein: 1.4 g | Sodium: 39 mg | |

# 6.

# Soups That Satisfy

There's nothing quite as warming and comforting as a steaming bowl of homemade soup. And soups are naturals for healthy low-fat cooking. Lean meats and poultry, whole grains, pasta, beans, and fresh vegetables can be combined to produce a variety of culinary creations that are satisfying without being fattening.

Watching your weight? Soups can help. Soups take a longer time to eat than most foods, so that less food and fewer calories are consumed in the twenty minutes or so it takes for the brain to realize that the stomach is full. This helps to prevent overeating.

Soups are perhaps the most versatile of foods, and so are as much a boon to the menu planner as they are to the calorie counter. A light soup is the perfect introduction to a full meal. A more substantial soup needs only crusty whole grain bread and a salad to make a satisfying lunch or light supper. Grabbing your lunches away from home? Take along a thermos of hot soup, and you'll have a nourishing meal on hand whenever you get hungry.

Of course, homemade soups have more than one advantage over commercial brews. Made from fresh, wholesome ingredients, homemade soups are bursting with nutrients and garden-fresh flavor. Just as important, while most commercially prepared soups are loaded with fat and salt, your soups can easily be made low in sodium and, of course, practically fat-free. Will your low-salt soups taste flat? Absolutely not! Herbs like oregano, marjoram, thyme, and bay leaf; lots of celery and onion; a clove or two of fresh garlic; a splash of wine vinegar; and plenty of other flavorful ingredients will make your soups so savory, no one will miss the salt.

This chapter presents a variety of delectable low-fat, low-salt, high-nutrient soups. Whether you are looking for a golden broth floating with tender noodles and chunks of chicken, a hearty bean soup, a spicy tomato-dill soup, or a cool and colorful gazpacho, there's a dish that will meet your needs deliciously. So take out your kettle, and get ready to make soups a healthful part of your menus.

# Red Bean and Sausage Soup

## Yield: 7 servings

1½ cups dried red kidney beans, cleaned and soaked (page 102)

6 cups water or unsalted chicken broth

¼ teaspoon salt

2 cups sliced smoked turkey sausage, at least 97% lean (about 10 ounces)

1 cup chopped yellow onion

¾ cup chopped celery (include the leaves)

2 bay leaves

1 tablespoon ground paprika

1 tablespoon dark brown sugar or molasses

2 teaspoons crushed fresh garlic

1½ teaspoons dried thyme

¼ teaspoon ground black pepper

1. Place the beans, water or broth, and salt in a 3-quart pot, and bring to a boil over high heat. Reduce the heat to low, cover, and simmer, stirring occasionally, for 45 minutes.

2. Add all of the remaining ingredients to the pot, increase the heat to medium-high, and allow the mixture to come to a boil. Reduce the heat to low, cover, and simmer, stirring occasionally, for 45 to 60 additional minutes, or until the beans are soft and the liquid is thick. Periodically check the pot during cooking, and add a little more water or broth if needed. Remove the bay leaves, and serve hot. If desired, serve over brown rice.

## NUTRITIONAL FACTS
### (Per 1-Cup Serving)

| Cal: 202 | Carbs: 32 g | Chol: 18 mg | Fat: 1.7 g |
|---|---|---|---|
| Fiber: 8.3 g | Protein: 16 g | Sodium: 446 mg | |

# Cauliflower-Cheese Soup

## Yield: 7 cups

1 large head cauliflower (about 1¾ pounds)

2 cups chicken or vegetable broth

1 medium yellow onion, chopped

1 teaspoon dry mustard

¼ teaspoon salt

⅛ teaspoon ground white pepper

2 cups skim or 1% low-fat milk, divided

3 tablespoons toasted garbanzo flour or unbleached flour

4 ounces nonfat or reduced-fat process Cheddar cheese or reduced-fat Cheddar cheese, shredded or diced (about 1 cup)

¼ cup thinly sliced scallions (garnish)

1. Trim the leaves from the cauliflower, rinse well, and separate into small florets.

2. Place the cauliflower florets, broth, onion, dry mustard, salt, and pepper in a 3-quart pot, and bring to a boil over high heat. Reduce the heat to low, cover, and simmer for 10 minutes, or until the cauliflower is tender.

3. Remove the pot from the heat, and, using a slotted spoon, transfer half of the cauliflower to a blender. Add 1½ cups of the milk to the blender and cover, leaving the lid slightly ajar to allow steam to escape. Carefully process at low speed until smooth.

4. Return the puréed cauliflower mixture to the pot, increase the heat to medium, and allow the mixture to come to a boil, stirring frequently. Place the remaining ½ cup of milk and the flour in the blender, and process until the flour is dissolved. Slowly stir the flour mixture into the soup. Cook

and stir for a minute or 2, or until the mixture thickens slightly.

5. Add the cheese to the pot, and cook, stirring constantly, until the cheese is melted. Serve hot, topping each serving with a sprinkling of scallions.

## NUTRITIONAL FACTS
(Per 1-Cup Serving)

| Cal: 86 | Carbs: 12 g | Chol: 1 mg | Fat: 0.4 g |
|---|---|---|---|
| Fiber: 2.2 g | Protein: 9.6 g | Sodium: 398 mg | |

# Dahl (Indian Lentil) Soup

Yield: 7 cups

1½ cups dried red lentils, cleaned (page 102)

6 cups water or unsalted chicken broth

1 cup chopped tomato (about 1 medium-large)

1¼ cups diced peeled potato (about 1 medium-large)

1 medium yellow onion, chopped

2–3 teaspoons curry paste

1 tablespoon instant chicken or vegetable bouillon granules

2 teaspoons crushed fresh garlic

¼ teaspoon ground black pepper

1. Place all of the ingredients in a 3-quart pot, and bring to a boil over high heat.

2. Reduce the heat to low, cover, and simmer, stirring occasionally, for about 30 minutes, or until the lentils are soft and the liquid is thick. Serve hot.

## NUTRITIONAL FACTS
(Per 1-Cup Serving)

| Cal: 183 | Carbs: 30 g | Chol: 0 mg | Fat: 1.4 g |
|---|---|---|---|
| Fiber: 6.6 g | Protein: 12.5 g | Sodium: 297 mg | |

# Golden Grains Soup

Yield: 7 cups

4½ cups unsalted vegetable or chicken broth or water

2 cups diced peeled sweet potato (about 1 medium-large)

½ cup chopped yellow onion

1 stalk celery, sliced (include the leaves)

1 tablespoon instant chicken or vegetable bouillon granules

¼ teaspoon ground ginger

¼ teaspoon dried thyme

⅛ teaspoon ground white pepper

¾ cup quick-cooking barley or quick-cooking brown rice

1 cup fresh or frozen whole kernel corn

1. Place the broth or water, sweet potato, onion, celery, bouillon granules, ginger, thyme, and pepper in a 3-quart pot, and bring to a boil over high heat. Reduce the heat to low, cover, and simmer for 10 minutes, or until the sweet potatoes are tender.

2. Using a slotted spoon, transfer the sweet potatoes and vegetables to a blender. Add 2 cups of the broth to the blender and cover, leaving the lid slightly ajar to allow steam to escape. Carefully process at low speed until smooth.

3. Return the puréed mixture to the pot, along with the barley or brown rice. Increase the heat to high, and allow the mixture to come to a boil. Reduce the heat to low, cover, and simmer for 5 minutes.

4. Add the corn to the pot, cover, and simmer for 5 additional minutes, or until the barley or rice is tender. Add a little more broth if the soup seems too thick, and serve hot.

## NUTRITIONAL FACTS
### (Per 1-Cup Serving)

| | | | |
|---|---|---|---|
| Cal: 125 | Carbs: 29 g | Chol: 0 mg | Fat: 0.4 g |
| Fiber: 3.8 g | Protein: 3.2 g | Sodium: 298 mg | |

# Roasted Onion Soup

### Yield: 4 servings

3 cups unsalted beef broth

1½ teaspoons instant beef bouillon granules

Four ¾-inch-thick slices French bread, toasted

2 tablespoons grated nonfat or regular Parmesan cheese

¾ cup shredded nonfat or regular mozzarella, provolone, or Swiss cheese

ROASTED ONION MIXTURE

1 pound sweet onions (about 3 medium)

6 cloves garlic, peeled

1 tablespoon plus 1 teaspoon balsamic vinegar

1 teaspoon dried thyme

¼ teaspoon coarsely ground black pepper

Nonstick olive oil cooking spray

1. To make the roasted onion mixture, peel the onions, trim the ends off, and cut into ¼-inch-thick wedges. Place the onions in a large bowl, add the garlic cloves, vinegar, thyme, and pepper, and toss to mix well.

2. Coat an 8-inch nonstick pan with nonstick olive oil cooking spray, and spread the onion mixture over the bottom of the pan. Spray the tops of the onions lightly with the cooking spray, and bake at 450°F for 20 minutes. Turn the onions over, and bake for 20 additional minutes, or until tender and nicely browned.

3. Place the roasted onion mixture in a 2-quart pot. Remove the garlic cloves from the mixture, and smash with the blade of a large knife. Return the garlic to the pot.

4. Use 1 cup of the broth to "rinse out" the pan used for roasting the onions. Add this liquid, the remaining broth, and the bouillon granules to the pot. Bring the mixture to a boil over high heat. Reduce the heat to low, cover, and simmer for 10 minutes, or just until the flavors are blended.

5. Place 1 cup of the onion soup in each of four 12-ounce oven-proof bowls. Float a piece of French bread on top of each serving, and sprinkle the bread first with 1½ teaspoons of Parmesan, and then with 3 tablespoons of the mozzarella, provolone, or Swiss.

6. Place the soup bowls under a preheated broiler for about 1 minute, or just until the cheese is melted. Serve immediately.

## NUTRITIONAL FACTS
### (Per Serving)

| | | | |
|---|---|---|---|
| Cal: 160 | Carbs: 24 g | Chol: 4 mg | Fat: 0.8 g |
| Fiber: 2.2 g | Protein: 14.4 g | Sodium: 564 mg | |

# Bean and Barley Soup

### Yield: 7 servings

1 cup dried 15-bean mixture, cleaned and soaked (page 102)

6 cups water or unsalted chicken broth

½ cup hulled or pearled barley

1 cup sliced fresh mushrooms

1 cup sliced carrots

1 cup chopped yellow onion

1 cup sliced celery (include the leaves)

2 teaspoons dried thyme

2 teaspoons crushed fresh garlic

1 tablespoon instant chicken bouillon granules

¼ teaspoon ground black pepper

**1.** Place the beans and the water or broth in a 3-quart pot, and bring to a boil over high heat. Reduce the heat under the pot to low, cover, and simmer, stirring occasionally, for 45 minutes.

**2.** Add all of the remaining ingredients to the pot, increase the heat to medium-high, and allow the mixture to come to a boil. Reduce the heat to low, cover, and simmer, stirring occasionally, for 45 to 60 additional minutes, or until the beans are soft, the barley is tender, and the liquid is thick. Periodically check the pot during cooking, and add a little more water or broth if needed. Serve hot.

## NUTRITIONAL FACTS
### (Per 1-Cup Serving)

Cal: 178    Carbs: 36 g    Chol: 0 mg    Fat: 0.7 g
Fiber: 9.1 g    Protein: 8.7 g    Sodium: 272 mg

# French Market Soup

### Yield: 7 servings

1½ cups dried 15-bean mixture, cleaned and soaked (page 102)

5½ cups water or unsalted chicken broth

1½ teaspoons instant chicken or vegetable bouillon granules

1½ cups sliced smoked turkey sausage or kielbasa, at least 97% lean (about 8 ounces)

1¼ cups diced unpeeled potato (about 1 medium-large)

¾ cup chopped yellow onion

1 medium carrot, peeled and sliced

1 stalk celery, sliced (include the leaves)

2 teaspoons crushed fresh garlic

2 teaspoons ground paprika

2 bay leaves

1½ teaspoons dried savory

¼ teaspoon ground black pepper

**1.** Place the beans, water or broth, and bouillon in a 3-quart pot, and bring to a boil over high heat. Reduce the heat to low, cover, and simmer, stirring occasionally, for 45 minutes.

**2.** Add all of the remaining ingredients to the pot, increase the heat to medium-high, and allow the mixture to come to a boil. Reduce the heat to low, cover, and simmer, stirring occasionally, for 45 to 60 additional minutes, or until the beans are soft and the liquid is thick. Periodically check the pot during cooking, and add a little more water or broth if needed. Remove the bay leaves, and serve hot.

## NUTRITIONAL FACTS
### (Per 1-Cup Serving)

Cal: 219    Carbs: 37 g    Chol: 14 mg    Fat: 1.5 g
Fiber: 8.7 g    Protein: 16 g    Sodium: 421 mg

# Bean Basics

*Beans have proven to have so many health benefits that they are clearly a must for anyone who wants to promote optimal health and longevity. To start with, beans are both fat- and cholesterol-free. Add to this the fact that they are nutritional powerhouses, providing generous amounts of protein, complex carbohydrates, B vitamins, iron, zinc, copper, and potassium. As for fiber, no food surpasses beans. Just a half cup of cooked beans provides 4 to 8 grams of fiber—up to four times the amount found in most other plant foods. But the benefits of beans don't stop here. Like oats, beans contain fiber that helps lower cholesterol, thus reducing the risk for heart disease. And as a bonus, beans help stabilize blood sugar levels, making you feel full and satisfied long after the meal is over—a definite benefit if you're watching your weight. In fact, it's a good idea to include some beans in your diet every day. Fortunately, this is easy to do, as beans can star in a variety of delicious dishes, from appetizers and salads to soups and entrées. The recipes in this book will show you how to make good use of these tasty morsels.*

*Some people avoid eating beans because of "bean bloat." What causes this problem? The complex sugars in beans, called oligosaccharides, sometimes form gas when broken down in the lower intestine. This side effect usually subsides when beans are made a regular part of the diet, and the body becomes more*

*efficient at digesting them. In addition, the proper cleaning, soaking, and cooking of dried beans can help prevent bean bloat. The following techniques will help you make beans a delicious and healthful part of your diet.*

## Cleaning

*Because beans are a natural product, packages of dried beans sometimes contain shriveled or discolored beans, as well as small twigs and other items. Before cooking, sort through your beans and discard any discolored or blemished legumes. Rinse the beans well, cover them with water, and discard any that float to the top.*

## Soaking

*There are two methods used to soak beans in preparation for cooking. If you have time—if you intend to cook your dish the next day, for instance—you may want to use the long method, as this technique is best for reducing the gas-producing oligosaccharides. If dinner is just a couple of hours away, though, the quick method is your best bet. Keep in mind that not all beans must be soaked before cooking. Black-eyed peas, brown and red lentils, and split peas do not require soaking.*

# Spanish Black Bean Soup

### Yield: 8 cups

2 cups dried black beans, cleaned and soaked (page 102)

5 cups water or unsalted chicken broth

1 cup chopped yellow onion

1 cup chopped celery (include the leaves)

1 tablespoon crushed fresh garlic

2 teaspoons ground paprika

1½ teaspoons dried oregano

½ teaspoon ground cumin

¼ teaspoon ground black pepper

1 tablespoon plus 1 teaspoon instant chicken bouillon granules

1 can (14½ ounces) unsalted stewed tomatoes, crushed

⅓ cup finely chopped red onion (garnish)

⅓ cup finely chopped green bell pepper (garnish)

## The Long Method

*After cleaning the beans, place them in a large bowl or pot, and cover them with four times as much water. Soak the beans for at least four hours, and for as long as twelve hours. If soaking them for more than four, place the bowl or pot in the refrigerator. After soaking, discard the water and replace with fresh water before cooking.*

## The Quick Method

*After cleaning the beans, place them in a large pot, and cover them with four times as much water. Bring the pot to a boil over high heat, and continue to boil for two minutes. Remove the pot from the heat, cover, and let stand for one hour. After soaking, discard the water and replace with fresh water before cooking.*

## Cooking

*To cook beans for use in salads, casseroles, and other dishes that contain little or no liquid, clean and soak as described above, discard the soaking water, and replace with two cups of water for each cup of dried beans. When beans are to be cooked in soups or stews that include acidic ingredients—lemon juice, vinegar, or tomatoes, for instance—add these ingredients at the end of the cooking time. Acidic foods can toughen the*

*beans' outer layer, slowing the rate at which the beans cook. You'll know that the beans are done when you can mash them easily with a fork. Keep in mind that old beans may take longer to cook. During long cooking times, periodically check the pot, and add more liquid if necessary.*

*The following table gives approximate cooking times for several different beans. Need a meal in a hurry? Lentils, split peas, and black-eyed peas require no soaking and cook quickly. Lentils are the fastest cooking of all the legumes; they can be ready in less than thirty minutes. Split peas cook in less than an hour, and black-eyed peas, in about an hour.*

### Cooking Times for Dried Beans and Legumes

| Bean or Legume | Cooking Time |
|---|---|
| Black, garbanzo, great northern, kidney, navy, pinto, and white beans | $1^1/_2$–2 hours |
| Black-eyed peas* | 1–$1^1/_4$ hours |
| Lentils, brown* | 20–30 minutes |
| Lentils, red* | 15–20 minutes |
| Lima beans, baby | 45 minutes–$1^1/_4$ hours |
| Lima beans, large | 1–$1^1/_2$ hours |
| Split peas* | 45–50 minutes |

*\* These beans do not require soaking.*

1. Place the beans, water or broth, onion, and celery in a 4-quart pot, and bring to a boil over high heat. Reduce the heat to low, cover, and simmer, stirring occasionally, for $1^1/_4$ to $1^1/_2$ hours, or until the beans are soft.

2. Add all of the remaining ingredients except for the garnishes to the pot, increase the heat to medium-high, and allow the mixture to come to a boil. Reduce the heat to low, cover, and simmer, stirring occasionally, for 30 additional minutes, or until the beans are soft and the liquid is thick. Periodically check the pot during cooking, and add a little more water or broth if needed.

3. Transfer 2 cups of the soup to a blender and cover, leaving the lid slightly ajar to allow steam to escape. Carefully process at low speed until the beans are smooth.

4. Return puréed beans to pot, and simmer for 5 additional minutes. Serve hot, topping each serving with some of the onions and green peppers. If desired, serve over brown rice.

### NUTRITIONAL FACTS
#### (Per 1-Cup Serving)

Cal: 187    Carbs: 35 g    Chol: 0 mg    Fat: 0.8 g
Fiber: 12 g    Protein: 11.6 g    Sodium: 308 mg

# Hearty Chicken and Barley Soup

## Yield: 8 cups

2 bone-in skinless chicken breast halves (about 8 ounces each)

5 cups water or unsalted chicken broth

½ cup hulled or pearled barley

1 tablespoon plus 1 teaspoon instant chicken bouillon granules

1½ teaspoons crushed fresh garlic

1 teaspoon poultry seasoning

¼ teaspoon ground black pepper

2 cups sliced fresh mushrooms

2 cups diced unpeeled potatoes (about 2 medium)

¾ cup chopped yellow onion

¾ cup sliced carrots

¾ cup sliced celery (include the leaves)

1. Rinse the chicken, and place the chicken, water or broth, barley, bouillon granules, garlic, poultry seasoning, and pepper in a 3-quart pot, and bring to a boil over medium-high heat. Reduce the heat to low, cover, and simmer for about 30 minutes, or until the chicken is tender and no longer pink inside.

2. Remove the chicken from the pot, and set aside. Add the mushrooms, potatoes, onion, carrots, and celery to the pot, and increase the heat to return the mixture to a boil. Reduce the heat to low, cover, and simmer, stirring occasionally, for 25 additional minutes, or until the barley and vegetables are tender and the flavors are well blended.

3. Pull the chicken meat from the bones, and tear it into bite-sized pieces. Add the chicken to the soup, and simmer for 5 minutes more. Serve hot.

## NUTRITIONAL FACTS
(Per 1-Cup Serving)

| | | | |
|---|---|---|---|
| Cal: 130 | Carbs: 21 g | Chol: 18 mg | Fat: 0.7 g |
| Fiber: 3.4 g | Protein: 9 g | Sodium: 332 mg | |

# Country Vegetable Soup

## Yield: 8 cups

3 cups water, unsalted vegetable broth, or unsalted beef broth

1 cup diced unpeeled potato (about 1 medium)

1 cup chopped yellow onion

1 medium-large carrot, peeled, halved lengthwise, and sliced

2 stalks celery, thinly sliced (include the leaves)

1 tablespoon instant vegetable or beef bouillon granules

1½ teaspoons dried thyme

2 bay leaves

¼ teaspoon ground black pepper

1 can (14½ ounces) unsalted tomatoes, crushed

1 can (15 ounces) red kidney beans, drained

1½ cups coarsely chopped cabbage

1 cup fresh or frozen whole kernel corn

1. Place the water or broth, potato, onion, carrot, celery, bouillon granules, thyme, bay leaves, and pepper in a 4-quart pot, and bring to a boil over high heat. Reduce the heat to low, cover, and simmer, stirring occasionally, for 15 minutes, or until the vegetables are tender.

2. Add all of the remaining ingredients to the pot, and increase the heat to return the mixture to a boil. Reduce the heat to low, cover,

and simmer, stirring occasionally, for 15 additional minutes, or until the cabbage is tender and the flavors are well blended. Serve hot.

## NUTRITIONAL FACTS
### (Per 1-Cup Serving)

Cal: 126   Carbs: 26 g   Chol: 0 mg   Fat: 0.5 g
Fiber: 7.6 g   Protein: 6 g   Sodium: 242 mg

# Savory Vegetable-Beef Soup

## Yield: 11 cups

1¼ pounds beef top round, trimmed of visible fat and cut into ½-inch pieces

4 cups water

3 cups canned vegetable juice, like V-8 vegetable juice

1 tablespoon instant beef bouillon granules

1½ teaspoons dried oregano

1 teaspoon chili powder

2 bay leaves

¼ teaspoon ground black pepper

1½ cups diced unpeeled potatoes (about 1½ medium)

1½ cups sliced carrots

1 medium-large yellow onion, cut into thin wedges

1½ cups fresh cut green beans

1½ cups fresh or frozen whole kernel corn

1. Coat a 4-quart pot with nonstick cooking spray, and preheat over medium-high heat. Add the meat, and stir-fry for about 4 minutes, or until nicely browned.

2. Add the water, vegetable juice, bouillon granules, oregano, chili powder, bay leaves, and pepper to the pot, and bring the mixture to a boil. Reduce the heat to low, cover, and simmer, stirring occasionally, for 30 minutes.

3. Add the potatoes, carrots, onion, and green beans to the pot, and increase the heat slightly to return the mixture to a boil. Reduce the heat to low, cover, and simmer, stirring occasionally, for 20 additional minutes, or until the vegetables are tender.

4. Add the corn to the pot, and increase the heat slightly to return the mixture to a boil. Reduce the heat to low, cover, and simmer for 10 minutes, or until the vegetables are tender. Serve hot.

## NUTRITIONAL FACTS
### (Per 1-Cup Serving)

Cal: 128   Carbs: 14 g   Chol: 32 mg   Fat: 2.1 g
Fiber: 2.8 g   Protein: 14 g   Sodium: 389 mg

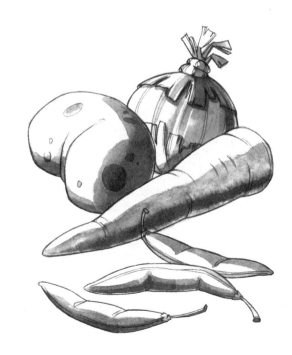

# Tomato-Dill Soup

### Yield: 5 cups

2 cans (14½ ounces each) unsalted tomatoes, crushed

2½ cups vegetable or chicken broth

1 cup chopped yellow onion

¼ cup finely chopped celery (include the leaves)

2 teaspoons crushed fresh garlic

2 teaspoons dried thyme, or 2 tablespoons finely chopped fresh

2 teaspoons light brown sugar

½ teaspoon dried dill, or 1½ teaspoons finely chopped fresh

⅛ teaspoon ground black pepper

1 teaspoon dried dill, or 1 tablespoon finely chopped fresh (garnish)

**1.** Place all of the ingredients except for the dill garnish in a 3-quart pot, and bring to a boil over high heat. Reduce the heat to low, cover, and simmer, stirring occasionally, for about 30 minutes, or until the onion and celery are soft.

**2.** Transfer 2 cups of the soup to a blender and cover, leaving the lid slightly ajar to allow steam to escape. Carefully process the mixture at low speed until smooth. Repeat this procedure until all of the soup has been blended.

**3.** Return all of the puréed soup to the pot, and cook over medium heat for a couple of minutes to reheat. Add a little more broth if the soup seems too thick. Serve hot, topping each serving with a sprinkling of dill.

### NUTRITIONAL FACTS
#### (Per 1-Cup Serving)

| | | | |
|---|---|---|---|
| Cal: 54 | Carbs: 11.9 g | Chol: 0 mg | Fat: 0.4 g |
| Fiber: 3.5 g | Protein: 1.9 g | Sodium: 304 mg | |

## *Glorious Garlic*

*Used for thousands of years to treat a variety of conditions, garlic has quite a reputation in medicinal folklore. However, only in the past few decades have scientists begun to unravel the mysteries of this pungent herb. If you are a garlic lover, you will be pleased to know that research is providing plenty of reasons to eat more of this versatile ingredient. First, studies show that including one clove of fresh garlic in your daily diet can lower blood cholesterol by as much as 9 percent. Garlic has also been shown to reduce blood triglycerides and blood pressure, and to make your blood less likely to form dangerous clots. And researchers have also discovered that garlic eaters have less stomach cancer than those who eat little garlic. Furthermore, there is growing evidence*
*that garlic can fight the bacteria that causes ulcers.*

*So don't shy away from garlic. Instead, aim for one or two cloves per day as part of a well-balanced diet. Is raw garlic better than cooked? Fresh uncooked garlic seems to be best for fighting cardiovascular disease. However, lightly sautéed garlic also retains much of its phytonutrient powers. And cooked garlic still has many of its cancer-fighting properties. So enjoy garlic in a variety of different ways. Use it raw in pestos and salad dressings, lightly sauté it with vegetables, cook it in soups and sauces, or roast whole cloves and squeeze the pulp onto bread instead of butter. You will find that it's easy to enjoy the flavor—and the health benefits—of garlic each and every day.*

# Country Bean Soup With Ham

### Yield: 9 cups

2 cups dried navy beans, cleaned and soaked (page 102)

7 cups water or unsalted chicken broth

2 medium yellow onions, diced

1 stalk celery, finely chopped (include the leaves)

2 teaspoons instant chicken bouillon granules

¼ teaspoon ground black pepper

2 cups diced ham, at least 97% lean (about 10 ounces)

1 teaspoon dried sage

1 teaspoon dry mustard

2 bay leaves

1. Place the beans, water or broth, onions, celery, bouillon granules, and pepper in a 4-quart pot, and bring to a boil over high heat. Reduce the heat to low, cover, and simmer, stirring occasionally, for 45 minutes.

2. Add all of the remaining ingredients to the pot, increase the heat to medium-high, and allow the mixture to come to a boil. Reduce the heat to low, cover, and simmer, stirring occasionally, for 45 to 60 additional minutes, or until the beans are soft and the liquid is thick. Periodically check the pot during cooking, and add a little more water or broth if needed. Remove the bay leaves, and serve hot.

### NUTRITIONAL FACTS
(Per 1-Cup Serving)

| | | | |
|---|---|---|---|
| Cal: 187 | Carbs: 30 g | Chol: 11 mg | Fat: 1.1 g |
| Fiber: 9 g | Protein: 14.7 g | Sodium: 419 mg | |

# Chunky Chicken Noodle Soup

### Yield: 7 cups

2 bone-in skinless chicken breast halves (about 8 ounces each)

6½ cups water or unsalted chicken broth

1 tablespoon plus 1½ teaspoons instant chicken bouillon granules

¾ cup thinly sliced celery (include the leaves)

¾ cup sliced carrots

1 cup sliced fresh mushrooms

1 medium yellow onion, chopped

1 teaspoon dried savory

½ teaspoon dried thyme

⅛ teaspoon ground white pepper

3 ounces medium no-yolk egg noodles (about 1½ cups)

2 tablespoons chopped fresh parsley

1. Rinse the chicken, and place the chicken, water or broth, and bouillon granules in a 3-quart pot, and bring to a boil over high heat. Reduce the heat to low, cover, and simmer for about 30 minutes, or until the chicken is tender and no longer pink inside.

2. Remove the chicken from the pot, and set aside. Add the celery, carrots, mushrooms, onion, savory, thyme, and pepper to the pot, and bring the mixture to a boil over high heat. Reduce the heat to low, cover, and simmer, stirring occasionally, for 15 additional minutes, or until the vegetables are tender.

3. Pull the chicken meat from the bones, and tear or dice it into bite-sized pieces. Add it to the soup along with the noodles.

**4.** Increase the heat slightly to return the mixture to a boil. Then reduce the heat to medium-low, cover, and simmer for about 5 minutes, or until the noodles are al dente. (Be careful not to overcook, as the noodles will continue to soften as long as they remain in the hot broth.) Stir the parsley into the soup, and serve hot.

## NUTRITIONAL FACTS
### (Per 1-Cup Serving)

| | | | |
|---|---|---|---|
| Cal: 115 | Carbs: 15 g | Chol: 23 mg | Fat: 0.8 g |
| Fiber: 1.2 g | Protein: 11.8 g | Sodium: 463 mg | |

# Cool Gazpacho

### Yield: 5 cups

3 cups diced tomatoes (about 4 medium)

1 cup diced peeled and seeded cucumber (about 1 medium)

1 cup diced green bell pepper (about 1 medium)

½ cup plus 2 tablespoons chopped onion

⅓ cup sliced black olives

1 cup canned vegetable juice, like V-8 vegetable juice

3–4 tablespoons red wine vinegar

1 teaspoon chili powder

¾ teaspoon dried oregano

1½ teaspoons crushed fresh garlic

1 teaspoon sugar

¼ teaspoon salt

TOPPINGS

½ cup nonfat sour cream (optional)

½ cup plus 2 tablespoons ready-made fat-free or low-fat croutons (optional)

**1.** Place all of the vegetables and the olives in a large bowl. Stir to mix, and set aside.

**2.** Place the vegetable juice, vinegar, and seasonings in a medium-sized bowl, and stir to mix well. Pour the vegetable juice mixture over the vegetables, and toss to mix.

**3.** Transfer the vegetable mixture to a blender or food processor, and, working in batches as necessary, process for a few seconds, or just until the vegetables are finely chopped. Transfer the soup to a covered container, and chill for 2 to 6 hours.

**4.** When ready to serve, place 1 cup of the gazpacho in each of 5 serving bowls. Top each serving with a rounded tablespoon of the sour cream and 2 tablespoons of the croutons, if desired, and serve immediately.

## NUTRITIONAL FACTS
### (Per 1-Cup Serving)

| | | | |
|---|---|---|---|
| Cal: 62 | Carbs: 12 g | Chol: 0 mg | Fat: 1.4 g |
| Fiber: 3 g | Protein: 2 g | Sodium: 321 mg | |

# 7.

# Salads for All Seasons

Salads are among the most versatile of dishes. Depending on their ingredients, they can be light or substantial; sweet or savory; a protein-packed entrée, or a refreshing side dish. Because most salads can be made ahead of time, they are great for entertaining. And because they are portable, they are as much at home at picnics and pot-luck suppers as they are on your own dining room table.

If you're watching your weight, though, beware. Despite the salad's reputation for being a "diet" food, many have no place in either a fat- or a calorie-controlled menu. Consider your typical chef's salad, for instance. A pile of fresh greens topped with strips of full-fat cheese and meat, a hard-boiled egg, and two tablespoons of regular salad dressing can easily deliver 650 calories and 50 grams of fat. And that's if you stop at just two tablespoons of dressing!

The truth is that the calories and fat you consume from salads can have a big impact on your overall health. This is especially true when you consider that the average woman gets more fat from salad dressing than from any other food!

Made properly, though, salads are just what the doctor ordered. Ingredients like non-fat and reduced-fat mayonnaise, oil-free salad dressings, nonfat sour cream, nonfat and reduced-fat cheeses, and ultra-lean meats make it possible to create a dazzling array of salads with little or no fat, and with much fewer calories than traditional versions. The recipes in this chapter combine these ingredients with crisp vegetables, ripe fruits, satisfying pastas, and nutritious whole grains to create a variety of fresh salads that will help you get your five-a-day of fruits and veggies in the most healthful and enjoyable way possible.

So whether you're looking for a main dish grilled-chicken salad, a berry-studded spinach salad, a temptingly sweet fruit salad, or a hearty pasta or bean salad, you need look no further. You'll find that—without sacrificing the flavors you love—you can create a salad that minimizes fat and calories, while maximizing the nutrients that promote health and longevity.

# *Greens, Glorious Greens*

*Fresh and crisp, salad greens are rich in folate, carotenoids, phytochemicals, and many other nutrients. And these days, grocery stores offer a lot more than just iceberg lettuce, allowing you to create exciting salads that are as beautiful as they are delicious. Following are descriptions of some of the different greens you are likely to find in your local grocery store.*

***Arugula.*** *Also known as rocket and Italian cress, arugula is a popular Mediterranean salad green that is often mixed with other greens. Its tender, narrow, dark green leaves have a peppery flavor.*

***Belgian Endive.*** *These small, oblong heads feature long, pale leaves that have a pleasant bitter flavor.*

*Scoop-shaped, endive leaves can also be stuffed with a filling and served as appetizers.*

***Butterhead Lettuce.*** *These small heads feature loosely packed leaves with a subtly sweet, buttery flavor. Boston and Bibb lettuce are varieties of butterhead.*

***Curly Endive.*** *Also known as chicory, these pleasantly bitter greens form a loose head, with frilly narrow leaves that are dark green on the edges and lighter toward the center.*

***Escarole.*** *A member of the chicory family, escarole forms a loose head with broad green leaves. It has a mildly bitter, nutty flavor.*

# Mediterranean Chef's Salad

### Yield: 4 servings

10 cups torn romaine lettuce or mixed salad greens

1 medium cucumber, peeled and sliced

8 cherry tomatoes, halved

1 can (12 ounces) water-packed albacore tuna, drained

1 can (15 ounces) white beans, rinsed and drained

½ cup crumbled nonfat or reduced-fat feta cheese

¼ cup sliced black olives

4 slices red onion, separated into rings

½ cup bottled nonfat or low-fat Italian or Caesar salad dressing

1. Arrange a quarter of the lettuce over the bottom of each of 4 large plates. Arrange a quarter of the cucumber slices and 4 cherry tomato halves around the edges of each plate.

2. Top the greens on each plate with ⅓ cup of the tuna; then scatter ⅓ cup of the beans over the tuna. Sprinkle with 2 tablespoons of feta and a tablespoon of olives. Top with some of the onion rings.

3. Drizzle 2 tablespoons of the dressing over each salad, and serve immediately.

## NUTRITIONAL FACTS
### (Per Serving)

Cal: 224     Carbs: 27 g     Chol: 28 mg     Fat: 1.9 g
Fiber: 4.2 g     Protein: 25 g     Sodium: 676 mg

*Iceberg.* This crisp, tight, pale green head has a mild flavor, and is the least nutritious of all the salad greens. (In general, the darker the green, the more nutritious the vegetable.)

*Leaf Lettuce.* These large, sprawling, mild-flavored leaves form loose heads that may be green or green with reddish tips.

*Mesclun.* This mixture of delicate baby lettuces offers a variety of flavors, textures, and colors. Sometimes referred to as spring salad mix, mesclun has become increasingly popular in grocery stores and restaurants.

*Radicchio.* Resembling a small head of purple cabbage, radicchio is frequently mixed with other salad greens, such as arugula and romaine. In these mixtures, radicchio adds a beautiful contrasting color and a slightly bitter, peppery flavor.

*Romaine.* With long, dark, narrow leaves and a crisp texture, romaine has a mild flavor. It is best known as the main ingredient in Caesar salads.

*Sorrel.* These smooth, oblong leaves look similar to spinach. Sorrel can be mixed with other greens to add a sharp, lemony tang.

*Spinach.* This earthy-flavored green may have either smooth or crinkled leaves, and forms a nutritious and delicious base for salads.

*Watercress.* The small round leaves on edible stems have a dark green color. Watercress is frequently mixed with other salad greens or used instead of lettuce to add a peppery taste to sandwiches.

# Berry Delicious Spinach Salad

### Yield: 4 servings

4 cups fresh spinach

1 1/2 cups sliced fresh strawberries

1/2 cup diced nonfat or reduced-fat mozzarella cheese

4 thin slices red onion, separated into rings

1/4 cup diagonally sliced celery

1/2 cup bottled nonfat or low-fat raspberry vinaigrette salad dressing

1/4 cup golden raisins

1/4 cup toasted chopped pecans or almonds (optional)

1. Place the spinach, strawberries, cheese, onion rings, and celery in a large bowl, and toss to mix well. Pour the dressing over the salad, and toss to mix well.

2. Divide the salad among 4 salad bowls. Top each serving with a tablespoon of the raisins and, if desired, a tablespoon of the pecans. Serve immediately.

## NUTRITIONAL FACTS
(Per 1 3/4-Cup Serving)

| | | | |
|---|---|---|---|
| Cal: 124 | Carbs: 28 g | Chol: 1 mg | Fat: 0.5 g |
| Fiber: 3.3 g | Protein: 7 g | Sodium: 183 mg | |

# Roasted Vegetable Salad

## Yield: 4 servings

8 cups mixed baby salad greens (mesclun)

1 cup canned chickpeas, rinsed and drained

3/4 cup crumbled nonfat or reduced-fat feta cheese

1 cup ready-made herb-flavored fat-free or low-fat croutons

1/2 cup bottled nonfat or low-fat red wine or balsamic vinaigrette salad dressing

ROASTED VEGETABLE MIXTURE

20 fresh asparagus spears

4 slices (1/2-inch thick) red onion

12 large fresh mushrooms, sliced 1/2-inch thick

1 large red bell pepper, cut into 1/2-inch-thick strips

1 teaspoon dried fines herbes*

1/4 teaspoon ground black pepper

1/4 teaspoon salt (optional)

Nonstick olive oil cooking spray

* A blend of thyme, oregano, sage, rosemary, marjoram, and basil, fines herbes can be found in the dried spice section of most grocery stores.

**1.** To prepare the roasted vegetable mixture, coat a large baking sheet with nonstick cooking spray. Arrange all of the vegetables in a single layer on the sheet, and sprinkle with the herbs, pepper, and, if desired, the salt. Spray the tops of the vegetables lightly with the cooking spray.

**2.** Bake at 450°F for 10 minutes, or until the asparagus are tender. Remove the asparagus, and set aside. Using a spatula, turn the remaining vegetables over and bake for 5 to 7 additional minutes, or until tender and nicely browned. Remove the vegetables from the oven, and allow to cool to room temperature.

**3.** When the vegetables have cooled, cut the asparagus into 1-inch pieces, and separate the onion slices into rings. Place the asparagus and onions in a medium-sized bowl, add the remaining vegetables, and toss to mix well. Cover the mixture, and chill for at least 2 hours before assembling the salad. (Note that you can prepare the roasted vegetable mixture the day before, and refrigerate until ready to assemble the salad.)

**4.** To assemble the salads, arrange 2 cups of salad greens over the bottom of each of 4 large serving plates. Top the greens on each plate with 1/4 cup of chickpeas, a quarter of the roasted vegetable mixture, 3 tablespoons of feta cheese, and 1/4 cup of croutons. Serve immediately, accompanied by the dressing.

## NUTRITIONAL FACTS
### (Per Serving)

| | | | |
|---|---|---|---|
| Cal: 250 | Carbs: 43 g | Chol: 2 mg | Fat: 2.8 g |
| Fiber: 9.8 g | Protein: 14.6 g | Sodium: 814 mg | |

# Rocket Salad

## Yield: 4 servings

6 cups arugula

12 cherry tomatoes, halved

3/4 cup shredded nonfat or reduced-fat mozzarella cheese

3/4 cup ready-made herb-flavored fat-free or low-fat croutons

1/2 cup bottled nonfat or low-fat balsamic vinaigrette salad dressing

1. Arrange $1^1/_2$ cups of arugula over the bottom of each of 4 salad plates. Top the arugula with 6 cherry tomato halves, 3 tablespoons of mozzarella, and 3 tablespoons of croutons.
2. Drizzle 2 tablespoons of the salad dressing over each salad, and serve immediately.

### NUTRITIONAL FACTS
(Per Serving)

| | | | |
|---|---|---|---|
| Cal: 116 | Carbs: 16 g | Chol: 2 mg | Fat: 0.7 g |
| Fiber: 2.4 g | Protein: 8.8 g | Sodium: 450 mg | |

## Cabbage-Apple Salad

### Yield: 8 servings

4 cups coarsely shredded cabbage (about $1/_2$ medium head)

2 cups $1/_2$-inch pieces of unpeeled red Delicious apples (about 2 medium)

$3/_4$ cup chopped celery

$1/_4$ cup plus 2 tablespoons dark raisins

DRESSING

$1/_2$ cup nonfat or reduced-fat mayonnaise

2–3 tablespoons frozen apple juice concentrate, thawed

1. Place the cabbage, apples, celery, and raisins in a large bowl, and toss to mix well. Place the dressing ingredients in a small bowl, and whisk until smooth.
2. Pour the dressing over the salad, and toss to mix well. Add a little more mayonnaise if the salad seems too dry. Cover the salad and chill for 8 hours or overnight before serving.

### NUTRITIONAL FACTS
(Per $3/_4$-Cup Serving)

| | | | |
|---|---|---|---|
| Cal: 71 | Carbs: 16 g | Chol: 0 mg | Fat: 0.3 g |
| Fiber: 2 g | Protein: 0.9 g | Sodium: 123 mg | |

## Sesame Slaw

### Yield: 6 servings

4 cups coarsely shredded cabbage (about $1/_2$ medium head)

1 can (8 ounces) sliced water chestnuts, drained

$1/_2$ cup finely chopped celery

$1/_2$ cup finely chopped red bell pepper

DRESSING

$1/_4$ cup plus 2 tablespoons seasoned rice vinegar

1 tablespoon sesame oil

1 tablespoon honey

$1/_4$ teaspoon salt

$1/_8$ teaspoon ground white pepper

1. Place the cabbage, water chestnuts, celery, and bell pepper in a large bowl, and toss to mix well. Place all of the dressing ingredients in a small bowl, and stir to mix well.
2. Pour the dressing over the cabbage mixture, and toss to mix well. Cover the salad and chill for several hours or overnight before serving.

### NUTRITIONAL FACTS
(Per $2/_3$-Cup Serving)

| | | | |
|---|---|---|---|
| Cal: 65 | Carbs: 11 g | Chol: 0 mg | Fat: 2.4 g |
| Fiber: 2.2 g | Protein: 1.2 g | Sodium: 110 mg | |

# Florentine Pasta Salad

## Yield: 5 servings

½ cup chopped sun-dried tomatoes (not packed in oil)

8 ounces bow tie or rigatoni pasta (about 3¼ cups)

4 cups chopped fresh spinach

¼ cup finely chopped red onion

1 can (15 ounces) white beans, rinsed and drained, or 1 can (12 ounces) water-packed albacore tuna, drained

½ cup crumbled nonfat or reduced-fat feta cheese

DRESSING

½ cup bottled nonfat or low-fat red wine vinaigrette or Italian salad dressing

1½ teaspoons crushed fresh garlic

½ teaspoon dried oregano

1. Place the tomatoes in a heatproof bowl, and add boiling water just to cover. Set aside for 10 minutes, or until the tomatoes have plumped. Drain well, and set aside.

2. Cook the pasta al dente according to package directions. Drain well, rinse with cool water, and drain again.

3. Place the pasta, drained tomatoes, spinach, onion, and beans or tuna in a large bowl, and toss to mix well.

4. To make the dressing, place all of the dressing ingredients in a small bowl, and stir to mix well. Pour the dressing over the salad, and toss to mix well.

5. Cover the salad and chill for 2 to 4 hours. Divide among individual serving plates, and top each serving with a rounded tablespoon of the cheese. Serve chilled.

## NUTRITIONAL FACTS
### (Per 1½-Cup Serving)

| | | | |
|---|---|---|---|
| Cal: 310 | Carbs: 60 g | Chol: 2 mg | Fat: 1.1 g |
| Fiber: 5.9 g | Protein: 15.3 g | Sodium: 611 mg | |

# Brown Rice and Lentil Salad

## Yield: 6 servings

2 cups cooked brown rice

1 cup cooked brown lentils (page 102)

¾ cup chopped seeded plum tomatoes (about 3 medium)

¼ cup thinly sliced scallions

DRESSING

1 tablespoon balsamic vinegar

1 tablespoon extra virgin olive oil

1 teaspoon Dijon mustard

½ teaspoon dried oregano

¼ teaspoon salt

1. Place the rice, lentils, tomatoes, and scallions in a medium-sized bowl, and toss to mix well. Add the salad dressing, oregano, and, if desired, the olive oil, and toss to mix well.

2. Place the dressing ingredients in a small bowl, and stir to mix. Pour the dressing over the salad, and toss to mix.

3. Cover the salad and chill for 2 to 5 hours before serving.

## NUTRITIONAL FACTS
### (Per ⅔-Cup Serving)

| | | | |
|---|---|---|---|
| Cal: 141 | Carbs: 23 g | Chol: 0 mg | Fat: 3.2 g |
| Fiber: 4.6 g | Protein: 5 g | Sodium: 126 mg | |

# Mediterranean White Bean Salad

## Yield: 6 servings

²/₃ cup bulgur wheat

1¹/₃ cups boiling water

1 can white beans (15 ounces), rinsed and drained

¹/₂ cup thinly sliced celery

¹/₂ cup chopped red onion

¹/₄ cup finely chopped fresh parsley

DRESSING

3 tablespoons lemon juice

1 tablespoon extra virgin olive oil

2 teaspoons Dijon mustard

1 teaspoon sugar

1 teaspoon crushed fresh garlic

¹/₄ teaspoon ground cumin

1 pinch ground black pepper

**1.** Place the bulgur wheat in a large heatproof bowl, and pour the boiling water over the wheat. Stir to mix, cover, and set aside for 30 to 45 minutes, or until most of the liquid is absorbed. Drain off any excess liquid. (Alternatively, prepare according to package directions.)

**2.** Add the beans, celery, onion, and parsley to the bulgur, and toss to mix well. Place all of the dressing ingredients in a small bowl, and stir to mix well.

**3.** Pour the dressing over the salad, and toss to mix well. Cover the salad and chill for at least 2 hours before serving.

## NUTRITIONAL FACTS
### (Per ²/₃-Cup Serving)

Cal: 172    Carbs: 30 g    Chol: 0 mg    Fat: 2.8 g
Fiber: 7.4 g    Protein: 8 g    Sodium: 212 mg

# Gorgonzola Garden Salad

## Yield: 4 servings

8 cups mixed salad greens or torn butter crunch or romaine lettuce

1 can (10 ounces) mandarin oranges, well drained

¹/₂ cup diagonally sliced celery

4 thin slices red or sweet white onion, separated into rings

¹/₄ cup crumbled Gorgonzola or blue cheese

¹/₄ cup dark raisins

¹/₄ cup chopped walnuts (optional)

¹/₂ cup bottled nonfat or low-fat raspberry or balsamic vinaigrette salad dressing

**1.** Arrange 2 cups of the salad greens over the bottom of each of 4 salad plates. Top the lettuce on each plate with a quarter of the mandarin oranges, 2 tablespoons of celery, and a quarter of the onion rings. Sprinkle with 1 tablespoon each of cheese, raisins, and, if desired, walnuts.

**2.** Serve immediately, topping each salad with 2 tablespoons of the dressing.

## NUTRITIONAL FACTS
### (Per 2¹/₂-Cup Serving)

Cal: 141    Carbs: 26.5 g    Chol: 6 mg    Fat: 2.7 g
Fiber: 4.3 g    Protein: 4.7 g    Sodium: 222 mg

# Greek Couscous Salad

## Yield: 7 servings

1½ cups water

1 cup whole wheat couscous

1¼ cups peeled, seeded, chopped cucumber (about 1 large)

1 cup chopped seeded plum tomato (3–4 medium)

½ cup chopped red onion

½ cup chopped black olives

2 tablespoons finely chopped fresh mint

½ cup crumbled nonfat feta cheese

DRESSING

3 tablespoons lemon juice

2 teaspoons Dijon mustard

2 teaspoons sugar

¼ teaspoon salt

¼ teaspoon ground black pepper

1 tablespoon extra virgin olive oil

1. Place the water and couscous in a medium-sized pot, and bring to a boil over high heat. Cover the pot, remove from the heat, and allow to stand for 5 minutes, or until all of the water is absorbed.

2. Place the couscous, cucumber, tomato, onion, olives, mint, and feta cheese in a large bowl, and toss to mix well. Place all of the dressing ingredients in a small bowl, and stir to mix well.

3. Pour the dressing over the salad, and toss to mix well. Cover the salad and chill for at least 2 hours before serving.

## NUTRITIONAL FACTS
### (Per ¾-Cup Serving)

| | | | |
|---|---|---|---|
| Cal: 145 | Carbs: 24 g | Chol: 1 mg | Fat: 3.3 g |
| Fiber: 4.8 g | Protein: 5.7 g | Sodium: 332 mg | |

# Primavera Pasta Salad

## Yield: 7 servings

8 ounces tricolor rotini pasta (about 3 cups)

2 cups fresh broccoli florets

1 cup frozen whole kernel corn, thawed

¾ cup diced red bell pepper

½ cup bottled nonfat or low-fat Italian or red wine vinaigrette salad dressing

1. Cook the pasta al dente according to package directions. About 1 minute before the pasta is done, add the broccoli, and cook for 1 minute more, or until the pasta is al dente and the broccoli turns bright green and is crisp-tender. Drain the pasta and broccoli, rinse with cool water, and drain again.

2. Place the pasta and broccoli in a large bowl, add the corn and red pepper, and toss to mix well. Pour the dressing over the salad, and toss to mix well.

3. Cover the salad and chill for at least 2 hours before serving. Toss in a little more dressing just before serving if the mixture seems too dry.

## NUTRITIONAL FACTS
### (Per 1-Cup Serving)

| | | | |
|---|---|---|---|
| Cal: 171 | Carbs: 37 g | Chol: 0 mg | Fat: 0.6 g |
| Fiber: 2.3 g | Protein: 5.7 g | Sodium: 182 mg | |

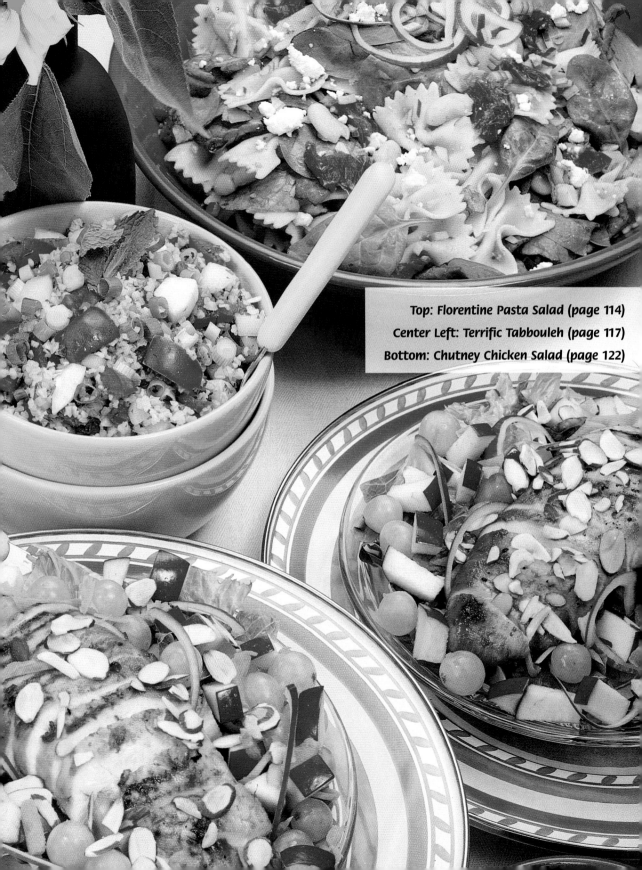

**Top:** Florentine Pasta Salad (page 114)

**Center Left:** Terrific Tabbouleh (page 117)

**Bottom:** Chutney Chicken Salad (page 122)

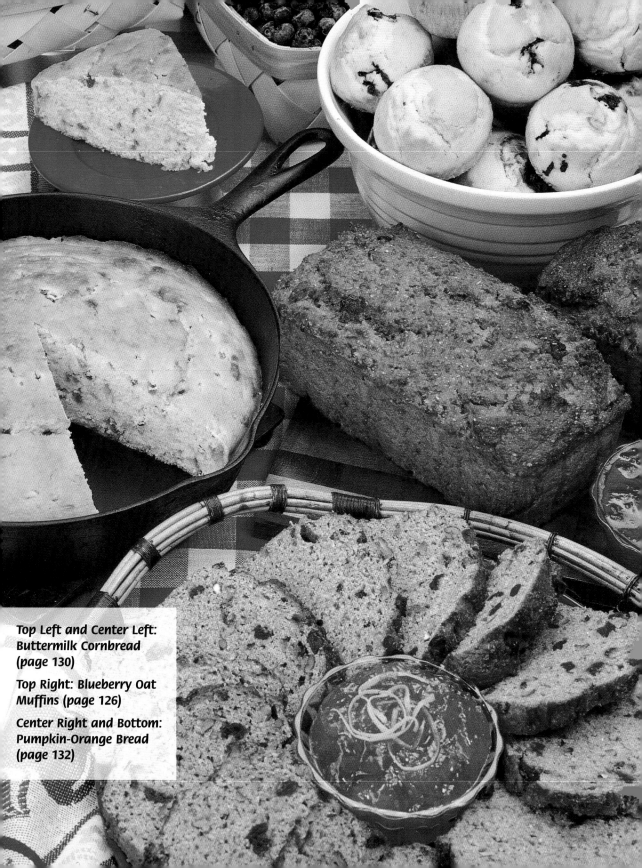

**Top Left and Center Left:**
**Buttermilk Cornbread**
**(page 130)**

**Top Right: Blueberry Oat**
**Muffins (page 126)**

**Center Right and Bottom:**
**Pumpkin-Orange Bread**
**(page 132)**

# Terrific Tabbouleh

## Yield: 8 servings

1 cup bulgur wheat
2 cups boiling water
1 cup chopped tomatoes (about 2 medium)
1 cup peeled, seeded, chopped cucumber
 (about 1 large)
½ cup (packed) chopped fresh parsley
½ cup thinly sliced scallions
1–2 tablespoons finely chopped fresh mint

DRESSING
¼ cup lemon juice
1–2 tablespoons extra virgin olive oil
1 teaspoon crushed fresh garlic
¼ teaspoon salt
¼ teaspoon ground black pepper

1. Place the bulgur wheat in a large heatproof bowl, and pour the boiling water over the wheat. Stir to mix, cover, and set aside for 30 to 45 minutes, or until most of the liquid is absorbed. Drain off any excess liquid. (Alternatively, prepare according to package directions.)

2. Add the tomatoes, cucumber, parsley, scallions, and mint to the bulgur, and toss to mix well. Place all of the dressing ingredients in a small bowl, and stir to mix well.

3. Pour the dressing over the salad, and toss to mix well. Cover the salad and chill for at least 3 hours before serving.

## NUTRITIONAL FACTS
### (Per ⅔-Cup Serving)

| | | | |
|---|---|---|---|
| Cal: 86 | Carbs: 16 g | Chol: 0 mg | Fat: 2 g |
| Fiber: 3.9 g | Protein: 2.7 g | Sodium: 75 mg | |

# Rice-Almond Salad

## Yield: 6 servings

2½ cups cooked brown rice
½ cup finely chopped celery
½ cup finely chopped carrot
¼ cup toasted slivered almonds
¼ cup golden raisins

DRESSING
¼ cup plus 2 tablespoons nonfat or reduced-fat mayonnaise
1 tablespoon mango chutney
½ teaspoon ground ginger
½ teaspoon curry paste

1. Place the rice, celery, carrot, almonds, and raisins in a large bowl, and toss to mix well. Place all of the dressing ingredients in a small bowl, and stir to mix well.

2. Add the dressing to the rice mixture, and toss to mix well, adding a little more mayonnaise if the mixture seems too dry. Cover the salad and chill for at least 2 hours before serving.

## NUTRITIONAL FACTS
### (Per ⅔-Cup Serving)

| | | | |
|---|---|---|---|
| Cal: 142 | Carbs: 25 g | Chol: 0 mg | Fat: 3.7 g |
| Fiber: 2.3 g | Protein: 3.1 g | Sodium: 139 mg | |

# Sweet Potato Salad

## Yield: 6 servings

1 pound sweet potatoes (about 2 medium)

1 can (8 ounces) crushed pineapple in juice, well drained

¼ cup diced celery

¼ cup plus 2 tablespoons golden raisins

¼ cup toasted chopped pecans

3 tablespoons shredded sweetened coconut

DRESSING

¼ cup nonfat sour cream

¼ cup nonfat or reduced-fat mayonnaise

⅛ teaspoon ground ginger

1. Peel the potatoes, and cut into ⅝-inch cubes. Measure the potatoes. There should be 3 cups. Adjust the amount if necessary.

2. Place the potatoes in a 2-quart pot. Add enough water to barely cover the potatoes.

3. Bring the potatoes to a boil over high heat. Reduce the heat to medium, cover, and cook for 5 minutes, or just until the potatoes are tender. Drain the potatoes, rinse with cool water, and drain again.

4. Place the potatoes in a large bowl. Add the drained pineapple and the celery, raisins, pecans, and coconut, and toss to mix well.

5. Place all of the dressing ingredients in a small bowl, and stir to mix well. Add the dressing to the salad, and toss to mix well. Cover the salad and chill for at least 3 hours before serving.

## NUTRITIONAL FACTS
### (Per ⅔-Cup Serving)

Cal: 137     Carbs: 24 g     Chol: 0 mg     Fat: 4.6 g
Fiber: 2.5 g   Protein: 1.7 g   Sodium: 19 mg

# Picnic Potato Salad

## Yield: 8 servings

5 cups ¾-inch chunks of unpeeled white or red potato (about 1½ pounds)

3 eggs

¼ teaspoon salt

½ cup finely chopped celery

½ cup finely chopped red bell pepper

½ cup finely chopped onion

¼ cup plus 2 tablespoons chopped drained sweet or dill pickles

Paprika (garnish)

DRESSING

½ cup nonfat or reduced-fat mayonnaise

¼ cup plus 2 tablespoons nonfat cottage cheese

2 tablespoons yellow mustard

⅛ teaspoon ground black pepper

1. Place the potatoes and eggs in a 3-quart pot, cover with water, and add the salt. Bring to a boil over high heat. Reduce the heat to medium-low, cover, and cook for about 10 minutes, or until the potatoes are tender.

2. Drain the potatoes and eggs, and rinse with cool water. Place the potatoes in a large bowl.

3. Peel the eggs, cut in half, and discard all or part of the yolks. Chop the remaining eggs, and add to the potatoes.

4. Add the celery, red pepper, onion, and pickles to the potato mixture, and toss to mix well. Set aside.

5. Place all of the dressing ingredients in a mini-food processor or mini-blender, and process until smooth and creamy. Add the dressing to the potato mixture, and toss to mix well.

# The Benefits of Organic Produce

*Eating your five-a-day of fruits and vegetables is a simple yet effective way to insure health and longevity. And while all fruits and vegetables supply essential nutrients, one type—which is now increasingly available at grocery and health foods stores—surpasses others in its longevity-promoting qualities. What is this gold mine of good health? Organic produce.*

*Grown without chemical fertilizers or pesticides, organic produce reduces your exposure to a variety of harmful substances. But its benefits don't stop there. Some studies indicate that organic produce also is more nutritious than its commercially grown counterpart. Researchers analyzed the mineral content of apples, pears, potatoes, corn, and wheat purchased in Chicago-area supermarkets over a two-year period,*

*and found that organic foods contained about twice as many beneficial minerals as commercial produce. On average, the organic produce contained close to four times as much selenium; over twice as much magnesium, potassium, manganese, and strontium; and 50 to 80 percent more boron, calcium, copper, chromium, and zinc. These researchers also found that organic produce has about a third fewer toxic metals such as aluminum, cadmium, lead, and mercury.*

*So, by all means, enjoy your five-a-day—or even six-a-day or seven-a-day, if you can. And to make those veggies and fruits really count, buy organic produce whenever possible. Your body will appreciate the difference.*

---

**6.** Cover the salad and chill for at least 3 hours. Sprinkle with paprika just before serving.

## NUTRITIONAL FACTS
### (Per ¾-Cup Serving)

| | | | |
|---|---|---|---|
| Cal: 115 | Carbs: 23.5 g | Chol: 1 mg | Fat: 0.3 g |
| Fiber: 1.7 g | Protein: 4.6 g | Sodium: 295 mg | |

---

# Eggless Egg Salad

### Yield: 6 servings

1 pound light silken firm, light silken extra firm, or regular firm tofu

1 large stalk celery, finely chopped

⅓ cup finely chopped onion

3 tablespoons sweet pickle relish

DRESSING

⅓ cup nonfat or reduced-fat mayonnaise

3 tablespoons mustard

½ teaspoon ground turmeric

¼ teaspoon ground black pepper

**1.** Place the tofu in a medium-sized bowl, and, using a fork, mash the tofu until it is crumbly. Add the celery, onion, and relish, and toss to mix well.

**2.** Place all of the dressing ingredients in a small bowl, and stir to mix well. Add the dressing to the tofu mixture, and stir to mix well. Cover the salad and chill for at least 2 hours before serving. Serve over a bed of lettuce or use as a sandwich filling.

## NUTRITIONAL FACTS
### (Per ½-Cup Serving)

| | | | |
|---|---|---|---|
| Cal: 61 | Carbs: 7 g | Chol: 0 mg | Fat: 1.3 g |
| Fiber: 0.6 g | Protein: 5.1 g | Sodium: 313 mg | |

# Autumn Fruit Salad

## Yield: 4 servings

1 cup bulgur wheat

2 cups boiling water

2 cups diced golden Delicious or Granny Smith apples

1 cup seedless red grapes

¼ cup chopped dates

¼ cup toasted chopped almonds (optional)

4 cups torn romaine lettuce

1 cup shredded nonfat or reduced-fat Swiss, mozzarella, or Monterey jack cheese

DRESSING
¾ cup plain nonfat yogurt

2 tablespoons plus 2 teaspoons honey

1 tablespoon plus 1 teaspoon lemon juice

1. Place the bulgur wheat in a large heatproof bowl, and pour the boiling water over the wheat. Stir to mix, cover, and set aside for 30 to 45 minutes, or until most of the liquid is absorbed. Drain off any excess liquid. (Alternatively, prepare according to package directions.) Cover and refrigerate until well chilled.

2. Place all of the dressing ingredients in a small bowl, and stir to mix well. Set aside.

3. Place the apples, grapes, dates, and if desired, the almonds in a medium-sized bowl, and toss to mix well. Set aside.

4. Arrange 1 cup of the romaine over the bottom of each of 4 serving plates. Top the lettuce with ³/₄ cup of the chilled bulgur, a quarter of the fruit mixture, and ¹/₄ cup of cheese. Serve immediately, accompanied by the dressing.

## NUTRITIONAL FACTS
### (Per Serving)

| | | | |
|---|---|---|---|
| Cal: 371 | Carbs: 79 g | Chol: 3 mg | Fat: 1.3 g |
| Fiber: 11 g | Protein: 18 g | Sodium: 266 mg | |

# Cranberry-Apple Salad

## Yield: 6 servings

3 cups diced unpeeled red Delicious apples (about 4 medium)

1 cup sliced celery

¼ cup plus 2 tablespoons dried cranberries

⅓ cup toasted chopped pecans (optional)

DRESSING
¼ cup nonfat or reduced-fat mayonnaise

¼ cup nonfat sour cream

1. Place the apples, celery, cranberries, and, if desired, the pecans in a medium-sized bowl, and stir to mix well. Place the dressing ingredients in a small bowl, and stir to mix well.

2. Add the dressing to the apple mixture, and toss to mix well. Cover the salad and chill for at least 2 hours before serving.

## NUTRITIONAL FACTS
### (Per ³/₄-Cup Serving)

| | | | |
|---|---|---|---|
| Cal: 80 | Carbs: 19.4 g | Chol: 0 mg | Fat: 0.3 g |
| Fiber: 1.7 g | Protein: 1.1 g | Sodium: 96 mg | |

# Thai Shrimp and Noodle Salad

*For variety, substitute shredded turkey or chicken for the shrimp.*

## Yield: 5 servings

8 ounces fettuccine pasta

2 cups 1-inch pieces young fresh green beans or asparagus (about 8 ounces)

2 cups cooked shrimp (about 10 ounces)

1 cup matchstick-sized pieces red bell pepper (about 1 medium)

½ cup plus 2 tablespoons sliced scallions

1 can (8 ounces) bamboo shoots, drained

DRESSING

¼ cup plus 1 tablespoon chicken broth

¼ cup plus 1 tablespoon seasoned rice vinegar

2 tablespoons reduced-sodium soy sauce

2 tablespoons peanut butter

1 tablespoon light brown sugar or honey

1 teaspoon crushed fresh garlic

½ teaspoon ground ginger, or 1½ teaspoons freshly grated ginger root

1. Cook the pasta al dente according to package directions. About 4 minutes before the pasta is done, add the green beans, and continue to cook until the pasta is al dente and the green beans are tender. (If you are using asparagus, add the vegetables 2 minutes before the pasta is done.) Drain the pasta and green beans, rinse with cool water, and drain again. Place in a large bowl.

2. Add the shrimp, red pepper, scallions, and bamboo shoots to the pasta mixture, and toss to mix well.

3. Place all of the dressing ingredients in a blender, and process until smooth. Pour the dressing over the pasta mixture, and toss to mix well. Cover the salad and chill for at least 2 hours before serving.

## NUTRITIONAL FACTS
(Per 1¾-Cup Serving)

| | | | |
|---|---|---|---|
| Cal: 317 | Carb: 47 g | Chol: 110 mg | Fat: 4.8 g |
| Fiber: 4 g | Protein: 21 g | Sodium: 556 mg | |

# Sicilian Grilled Chicken and Pasta Salad

## Yield: 5 servings

1 pound boneless skinless chicken breasts

⅓ cup chopped sun-dried tomatoes (not packed in oil)

⅓ cup boiling water

10 ounces rigatoni pasta (about 4 cups)

¾ cup chopped frozen (thawed) or canned (drained) artichoke hearts

⅓ cup sliced black olives

¼ cup thinly sliced scallions

⅓ cup chopped walnuts (optional)

¼ cup plus 2 tablespoons bottled nonfat Italian salad dressing

10 cups mixed salad greens or torn romaine lettuce

MARINADE

¼ cup plus 3 tablespoons nonfat Italian salad dressing

1 tablespoon plus 1 teaspoon balsamic vinegar

1. Place the marinade ingredients in a small bowl, and stir to mix well. Set aside.

2. Rinse the chicken, and pat it dry with paper towels. Place the chicken in a shallow non-metal container. Pour $1/4$ cup plus 1 tablespoon of the marinade over the chicken, lifting the chicken to allow some of the dressing to flow underneath. Cover and refrigerate for 6 to 24 hours, turning occasionally. Place the remaining marinade mixture in the refrigerator until ready to make the salad.

3. When ready to prepare the salad, place the dried tomatoes in a small heatproof bowl, and cover with the boiling water. Allow to sit for at least 10 minutes, or until the tomatoes are plumped.

4. Remove the chicken from the marinade, and discard the marinade. Turning occasionally, cook the chicken over medium coals or broil 6 inches under a preheated broiler for 12 to 15 minutes, or until the meat is nicely browned and no longer pink inside. During the last half of the cooking time, baste the chicken with the reserved marinade. Set the chicken aside to cool.

5. While the chicken is cooking, cook the pasta al dente according to package directions. Drain the pasta, rinse with cool water, drain again, and set aside.

6. Slice the chicken thinly across the grain. Set aside. (Note that the chicken can be cooked the day before, refrigerated, and sliced just before assembling the salad.)

7. Place the pasta, artichoke hearts, olives, scallions, and, if desired, the walnuts in a large bowl. Drain the tomatoes, and add to the pasta mixture. Add the chicken, and toss to mix well. Pour the Italian dressing over the salad, and toss to mix well.

8. Cover the salad and chill for at least 2 hours before serving. Toss in a little more Italian dressing just before serving if the mixture seems too dry.

9. To serve, arrange 2 cups of the salad greens over the bottom of each of 5 serving plates. Top with $1 2/3$ cups of the pasta salad, and serve.

## NUTRITIONAL FACTS
### (Per Serving)

| | | | |
|---|---|---|---|
| Cal: 382 | Carbs: 58 g | Chol: 43 mg | Fat: 4.2 g |
| Fiber: 5.4 g | Protein: 26.4 g | Sodium: 497 mg | |

# Chutney Chicken Salad

*For variety, substitute fresh tuna steaks for the chicken breasts.*

### Yield: 4 servings

4 boneless skinless chicken breast halves (about 5 ounces each)

Nonstick cooking spray

10 cups torn romaine lettuce

1 medium carrot, peeled and coarsely shredded with a potato peeler

4 thin slices red onion, separated into rings

1 cup seedless grapes or pineapple chunks

1 cup diced unpeeled red or golden Delicious apples

$1/4$ cup dark raisins, toasted sliced almonds, or toasted chopped pecans

### MARINADE

$1/4$ cup plus 2 tablespoons unsweetened pineapple juice

$1/4$ cup mango chutney

2 tablespoons reduced-sodium soy sauce

$1 1/2$ teaspoons crushed fresh garlic

DRESSING

¼ cup plus 2 tablespoons mango chutney

¼ cup plus 2 tablespoons nonfat or reduced-fat mayonnaise

¼ cup plus 2 tablespoons nonfat sour cream

1. Rinse the chicken, and pat it dry with paper towels. Place the chicken in a shallow non-metal container. Place the marinade ingredients in a blender, and process until smooth. Pour the marinade over the chicken, cover, and refrigerate for 6 to 24 hours, turning occasionally.

2. To make the dressing, place all of the dressing ingredients in a small bowl, and stir to mix well. Cover and chill for at least 2 hours, or until ready to serve the salad.

3. When ready to prepare the salad, remove the chicken from the marinade, and discard the marinade. Spray the tops of the chicken breasts lightly with cooking spray, and, turning occasionally, cook over medium coals or broil 6 inches under a preheated broiler for 12 to 15 minutes, or until the meat is nicely browned and no longer pink inside. Set the chicken aside to cool for 15 minutes.

4. Slice the chicken thinly across the grain. Set aside. (Note that the chicken can be cooked the day before, refrigerated, and sliced just before you assemble the salads.)

5. To serve, place the lettuce, carrots, and onions in a large bowl, and toss to mix well. Spread a quarter of the lettuce mixture over the bottom of each of 4 large plates. Arrange a sliced chicken breast over the lettuce mixture. Then arrange some of the grapes and apples around the outer edge of each plate, and sprinkle with the raisins, almonds, or pecans. Serve immediately, accompanied by some of the dressing.

## NUTRITIONAL FACTS
### (Per Serving)

| | | | |
|---|---|---|---|
| Cal: 335 | Carbs: 40 g | Chol: 82 mg | Fat: 2.6 g |
| Fiber: 3.5 g | Protein: 37.2 g | Sodium: 679 mg | |

# Crunchy Chicken and Rice Salad

### Yield 5 servings

1 cup wild rice

2½ cups water

2 cups diced cooked chicken or turkey breast (about 10 ounces)

1½ cups halved seedless green grapes or diced peeled apples

1 can (8 ounces) water chestnuts, drained and coarsely chopped

½ cup chopped celery

½ cup toasted slivered almonds, cashews, or pecans (optional)

DRESSING

½ cup nonfat or reduced-fat mayonnaise

½ cup nonfat sour cream

⅛ teaspoon ground ginger

1. Place the rice and water in a 2-quart pot, and bring to a boil over high heat. Reduce the heat to low, cover, and simmer without stirring for 50 to 60 minutes, or until the water is absorbed and the rice is tender. Allow the rice to cool to room temperature, or transfer to a covered container and chill until ready to assemble the salad.

2. Place the cooled rice, chicken or turkey, grapes or apples, water chestnuts, celery, and, if desired, the nuts in a large bowl, and

toss to mix well. Place all of the dressing ingredients in a small bowl, and stir to mix well.

**3.** Add the dressing to the salad, and toss to mix well. Cover the salad and chill for at least 2 hours before serving.

## NUTRITIONAL FACTS
### (Per 1⅔-Cup Serving)

---

Cal: 283    Carbs: 40 g    Chol: 48 mg    Fat: 2.6 g
Fiber: 2.4 g    Protein: 23 g    Sodium: 254 mg

---

# Greek Grilled Chicken Salad

### Yield: 4 servings

4 boneless skinless chicken breast halves (about 5 ounces each)

2–3 tablespoons Lemon Herb Rub (page 163)

Nonstick olive oil cooking spray

10 cups torn romaine lettuce or mixed salad greens

1 medium cucumber, peeled, quartered lengthwise, and sliced

12 cherry tomatoes, halved

¼ cup sliced black olives

4 thin slices red onion, separated into rings

½ cup crumbled nonfat or reduced-fat feta cheese

8 Greek salad peppers (optional)

¾ cup bottled nonfat red wine vinaigrette, Caesar, or balsamic vinaigrette salad dressing

**1.** Rinse the chicken, and pat it dry with paper towels. Using your fingers, rub both sides of each piece of chicken with some of the rub. If you have time, set aside for 15 to 30 minutes. (This will allow the flavors to better penetrate the meat.)

**2.** Coat a broiler pan with nonstick cooking spray, and arrange the chicken on the pan. Spray the tops of the chicken breasts lightly with the cooking spray, and, turning occasionally, cook over medium coals or broil 6 inches under a preheated broiler for 12 to 15 minutes, or until the meat is nicely browned and no longer pink inside. Set the chicken aside to cool.

**3.** Slice the chicken thinly across the grain. Set aside. (Note that the chicken can be cooked the day before, refrigerated, and sliced just before assembling the salads.)

**4.** To serve, arrange 2½ cups of lettuce over the bottom of each of 4 plates. Arrange some of the cucumber, tomatoes, and olives around the outer edges of the lettuce on each plate. Top the lettuce with some of the onion rings. Arrange a sliced chicken breast over the lettuce, sprinkle with some of the feta, and garnish with 2 Greek salad peppers, if desired. Serve immediately, accompanied by some of the dressing and, if desired, wedges of warm pita bread.

## NUTRITIONAL FACTS
### (Per Serving)

---

Cal: 302    Carbs: 28 g    Chol: 82 mg    Fat: 3.2 g
Fiber: 3.9 g    Protein: 39 g    Sodium: 988 mg

---

# 8.

# Bountiful Breads

Bread is often called the staff of life. Acknowledging the goodness of this highly revered food, the creators of the USDA Food Guide Pyramid have made breads and other grain products the base of this guide to healthful eating, recommending six to eleven servings daily. But, unfortunately, until very recently, most muffins, quick breads, and other baked goods were made with large amounts of butter, margarine, oil, and other high-fat ingredients—ingredients that must be kept to a minimum in a healthy diet. Just as bad, most breads and muffins contained only nutrient-poor refined flours. The good news is that times have changed, and we now know that delicious baked goods can be made with little or no fat, and with a wide range of wholesome, high-nutrient ingredients.

As the recipes in this chapter show, it is a simple matter to boost the nutritional value of your muffins, quick breads, biscuits, and other treats by using a variety of whole grain flours, and by reducing the amount of sugar used. In fact, the baked goods recipes in this book contain 25 to 50 percent less sugar than traditional recipes. Naturally sweet and flavorful ingredients like fruit juices, fruit purées, and oats reduce the need for sugar while enhancing the taste and aroma of your home-baked treats.

Will your baked goods be dry if you leave out all that oil and butter? Not if you replace the usual fat with fruit juices, fruit purées, nonfat buttermilk, and other healthful fat substitutes. The recipes in this chapter artfully combine these naturally flavorful substitutes with a variety of whole grain flours, fresh and dried fruits, fresh veggies, nutrient-packed nuts, and other wholesome ingredients to produce an array of super-moist, super-tempting breads.

From Pumpkin-Orange Bread to Blueberry Oat Muffins to Buttermilk Cornbread to flaky Buttermilk Drop Biscuits, you'll find breads for every meal of the day.

So take out your baking pans, preheat your oven, and get ready to create some of the healthiest, most flavorful breads you've ever tasted! It's easy, once you know the secrets of cooking for long life.

# Blueberry Oat Muffins

## Yield: 12 muffins

1 cup unbleached flour
1 cup oat flour or barley flour
¼ cup plus 3 tablespoons sugar, divided
2 teaspoons baking powder
¼ teaspoon baking soda
1 cup nonfat or low-fat vanilla yogurt
3 tablespoons fat-free egg substitute
¼ cup reduced-fat margarine or light butter, melted
¾ cup fresh or frozen (unthawed) blueberries

1. Place the flours, 6 tablespoons of the sugar, and all of the baking powder and baking soda in a large bowl, and stir to mix well. Add the yogurt, egg substitute, and margarine or butter, and stir just until the dry ingredients are moistened. Fold in the blueberries.

2. Coat muffin cups with nonstick cooking spray, and fill three-fourths full with the batter. Sprinkle ¼ teaspoon of the remaining sugar over the top of each muffin, and bake at 350°F for about 15 minutes, or just until a wooden toothpick inserted in the center of a muffin comes out clean. Be careful not to overbake.

3. Remove the muffin tin from the oven, and allow it to sit for 5 minutes before removing the muffins. Serve warm, refrigerating any leftovers not eaten within 24 hours.

## NUTRITIONAL FACTS
### (Per Muffin)

Cal: 133   Carbs: 24 g   Chol: 1 mg   Fat: 2.4 g
Fiber: 1.5 g   Protein: 3.7 g   Sodium: 150 mg

# Honey Oat Bran Muffins

## Yield: 12 muffins

2½ cups oat bran
2 teaspoons baking powder
¼ teaspoon baking soda
1½ cups nonfat or low-fat buttermilk
½ cup honey
2 egg whites, lightly beaten, or ¼ cup fat-free egg substitute
1 teaspoon vanilla extract
½ cup dark raisins, walnuts, or toasted pecans, or ¾ cup fresh or frozen (unthawed) blueberries (optional)

1. Place the oat bran, baking powder, and baking soda in a large bowl, and stir to mix well. Add the buttermilk, honey, egg whites or egg substitute, and vanilla extract to the oat bran mixture, and stir just until the dry ingredients are moistened. Fold in the raisins, nuts, or blueberries, if desired.

2. Coat muffin cups with nonstick cooking spray, and fill three-fourths full with the batter. Bake at 350°F for about 14 minutes, or just until a wooden toothpick inserted in the center of a muffin comes out clean. Be careful not to overbake.

3. Remove the muffin tin from the oven, and allow it to sit for 5 minutes before removing the muffins. Serve warm or at room temperature, refrigerating any leftovers not eaten within 24 hours.

## NUTRITIONAL FACTS
### (Per Muffin)

Cal: 107   Carbs: 18 g   Chol: 1 mg   Fat: 1.6 g
Fiber: 3.1 g   Protein: 5.1 g   Sodium: 150 mg

## Variation

To make Applesauce Oat Bran Muffins, substitute unsweetened applesauce for $1/2$ cup of the buttermilk, and add $1/2$ to 1 teaspoon ground cinnamon to the dry ingredients.

## NUTRITIONAL FACTS
### (Per Muffin)

| Cal: 107 | Carbs: 18.5 g | Chol: 0 mg | Fat: 1.5 g |
|---|---|---|---|
| Fiber: 3.2 g | Protein: 4.8 g | Sodium: 140 mg | |

## Variation

To make Banana Oat Bran Muffins, substitute $1/2$ cup of very ripe mashed banana (about 1 large) for $1/2$ cup of the buttermilk, and add $1/4$ teaspoon of ground nutmeg to the dry ingredients.

## NUTRITIONAL FACTS
### (Per Muffin)

| Cal: 111 | Carbs: 19.5 g | Chol: 0 mg | Fat: 1.6 g |
|---|---|---|---|
| Fiber: 3.3 g | Protein: 4.8 g | Sodium: 139 mg | |

# Zucchini-Spice Muffins

### Yield: 12 muffins

1 cup whole wheat pastry flour or unbleached flour

1 cup oat bran

$1 1/2$ teaspoons ground cinnamon

2 teaspoons baking powder

$3/4$ teaspoon baking soda

$3/4$ cup nonfat buttermilk

$1/2$ cup dark brown sugar

2 egg whites, or $1/4$ cup fat-free egg substitute

2 tablespoons vegetable oil

1 cup (packed) shredded zucchini (about 1 medium-large)

$1/2$ cup dark raisins

$1/3$ cup chopped walnuts (optional)

1. Place the flour, oat bran, cinnamon, baking powder, and baking soda in a large bowl, and stir to mix well.

2. Place the buttermilk, brown sugar, egg whites or egg substitute, and oil in a small bowl, and whisk until smooth.

3. Add the buttermilk mixture and the zucchini to the flour mixture, and stir just until the dry ingredients are moistened. Fold in the raisins, and if desired, the walnuts.

4. Coat muffin cups with nonstick cooking spray, and fill three-fourths full with the batter. Bake at 350°F for about 16 minutes, or just until a wooden toothpick inserted in the center of a muffin comes out clean. Be careful not to overbake.

5. Remove the muffin tin from the oven, and allow it to sit for 10 minutes before removing the muffins. Serve warm or at room temperature, refrigerating any leftovers not eaten within 24 hours.

## NUTRITIONAL FACTS
### (Per Muffin)

| Cal: 132 | Carbs: 24 g | Chol: 0 mg | Fat: 2.9 g |
|---|---|---|---|
| Fiber: 2.6 g | Protein: 3.9 g | Sodium: 168 mg | |

# Alternatives to Eggs in Baked Goods

Eggs are standard ingredients in muffins, quick breads, and other baked goods, where they add richness and texture to the finished product. But, as everyone knows, eggs also add cholesterol and fat. Fortunately, this problem is easily solved by substituting egg whites or a fat-free egg substitute for whole eggs. There are also plenty of other less well-known options for replacing eggs in baked goods. If you are allergic to eggs or simply prefer not to use them, experiment with some of the following alternatives.

❑ **Liquids.** Replace each whole egg with 2 tablespoons of water, fruit purée, applesauce, or another liquid. Or replace each egg white with $1\frac{1}{2}$ tablespoons of liquid. This simple substitution works especially well in fat-free quick breads. In fact, all of the quick bread recipes in this book use this substitution.

❑ **Flaxseeds.** When ground and mixed with water, flaxseeds develop a texture and binding capacity similar to that of egg whites. Simply place $1\frac{1}{2}$ tablespoons of

flaxseeds in a mini-blender, and blend until finely ground. Then add $\frac{1}{4}$ cup plus 2 tablespoons of water, and blend for another minute, or until the mixture has the consistency of raw egg whites. Use 3 tablespoons of this mixture to replace 1 whole egg, or use 2 tablespoons to replace 1 egg white. Since flaxseeds can turn rancid quickly once ground, this mixture should be freshly made for each use. Flaxseeds have a slightly sweet, nutty taste that enhances the flavors of muffins, breads, and other baked goods. Plus they contain fibers and gums that improve the texture and quality of baked goods.

❑ **Tofu.** Replace each whole egg with 3 tablespoons of blended soft tofu, or each egg white with 2 tablespoons of blended soft tofu.

❑ **ENER-G Egg Replacer.** Made from potato starch, tapioca flour, and vegetable gums, this product can be found in most health foods stores. Use according to package directions to replace eggs in baked goods as well as casseroles, quiches, and other dishes.

---

# Moist Cornmeal Muffins

*Be sure to use only finely ground cornmeal for the lightest and most tender texture.*

## Yield: 12 muffins

2 cups finely ground yellow or white cornmeal

2 teaspoons baking powder

$\frac{1}{2}$ teaspoon baking soda

2 cups nonfat or low-fat buttermilk

$\frac{1}{4}$ cup plus 2 tablespoons fat-free egg substitute

2–3 tablespoons honey

**1.** Place the cornmeal, baking powder, and baking soda in a large bowl, and stir to mix well. Add the buttermilk, egg substitute,

and honey, and stir just until the dry ingredients are moistened.

**2.** Coat muffin cups with nonstick cooking spray, and fill three-fourths full with the batter. Bake at 350°F for 15 to 18 minutes, or just until a wooden toothpick inserted in the center of a muffin comes out clean. Be careful not to overbake.

**3.** Remove the muffin tin from the oven, and allow it to sit for 5 minutes before removing the muffins. Serve warm, refrigerating any leftovers not eaten within 24 hours.

## NUTRITIONAL FACTS
### (Per Muffin)

| | | | |
|---|---|---|---|
| Cal: 115 | Carbs: 22 g | Chol: 1 mg | Fat: 0.9 g |
| | Fiber: 2 g | Protein: 4 g | Sodium: 189 mg |

# Molasses Bran Muffins

## Yield: 12 muffins

1¼ cups whole wheat pastry flour

1½ cups wheat bran

1 teaspoon baking soda

¾ cup nonfat or low-fat buttermilk

½ cup plus 2 tablespoons applesauce

¼ cup plus 2 tablespoons molasses

¼ cup fat-free egg substitute, or 2 egg whites, lightly beaten

2 tablespoons vegetable oil

½ cup dark raisins, chopped prunes, or chopped dried apricots

¼ cup chopped walnuts (optional)

1. Place the flour, bran, and baking soda in a large bowl, and stir to mix well. Add the buttermilk, applesauce, molasses, egg substitute or egg whites, and vegetable oil, and stir just until the dry ingredients are moistened. Fold in the raisins, prunes, or apricots, and, if desired, the walnuts.

2. Coat muffin cups with nonstick cooking spray, and fill three-fourths full with the batter. Bake at 350°F for about 16 minutes, or just until a wooden toothpick inserted in the center of a muffin comes out clean. Be careful not to overbake.

3. Remove the muffin tin from the oven, and allow it to sit for 5 minutes before removing the muffins. Serve warm or at room temperature, refrigerating any leftovers not eaten within 24 hours.

## NUTRITIONAL FACTS
### (Per Muffin)

Cal: 131    Carbs: 26 g    Chol: 0 mg    Fat: 2.9 g
Fiber: 4 g    Protein: 3.6 g    Sodium: 135 mg

# Pumpkin-Spice Bread

## Yield: 16 slices

2 cups whole wheat pastry flour

½ cup plus 2 tablespoons sugar

2 teaspoons baking powder

¾ teaspoon baking soda

2 teaspoons pumpkin pie spice

1¼ cups mashed cooked or canned pumpkin

¾ cup apple juice

1½ teaspoons vanilla extract

½ cup chopped walnuts or toasted pecans

1. Place the flour, sugar, baking powder, baking soda, and pumpkin pie spice in a large bowl, and stir to mix well. Add the pumpkin, apple juice, and vanilla extract, and stir just until the dry ingredients are moistened. Fold in the nuts.

2. Coat an 8-x-4-inch loaf pan with nonstick cooking spray, and spread the mixture evenly in the pan. Bake at 325°F for about 55 minutes, or just until a wooden toothpick inserted in the center of the loaf comes out clean. Be careful not to overbake.

3. Remove the loaf from the oven, and let sit for 10 minutes. Invert the loaf onto a wire rack, turn right side up, and cool to room temperature. Wrap the loaf in plastic wrap or aluminum foil, and allow to sit for 8 hours or overnight before slicing and serving. (Overnight storage will give the loaf a softer, moister crust.) Refrigerate any leftovers not eaten within 24 hours.

## NUTRITIONAL FACTS
### (Per Slice)

Cal: 117    Carb: 22 g    Chol: 0 mg    Fat: 2.6 g
Fiber: 2.6 g    Protein: 3.2 g    Sodium: 122 mg

# Boston Brown Bread

### Yield: 32 slices

2 cups whole wheat pastry flour
1 cup yellow cornmeal
1 teaspoon baking soda
2 cups nonfat or low-fat buttermilk
¾ cup molasses
1 cup dark raisins

**1.** Place the flour, cornmeal, and baking soda in a large bowl, and stir to mix well. Add the buttermilk and molasses, and stir just until the dry ingredients are moistened. Fold in the raisins.

**2.** Coat four 1-pound cans with nonstick cooking spray. Divide the batter evenly among the cans, and bake at 300°F for about 45 minutes, or just until a wooden toothpick inserted in the center of the loaf comes out clean. Be careful not to overbake.

**3.** Remove the bread from the oven, and let sit for 10 minutes. Invert the loaves onto a wire rack, and cool to room temperature. Wrap the loaves in aluminum foil or plastic wrap, and allow to sit overnight before slicing and serving. (Overnight storage will give the loaves a softer, moister crust.) Refrigerate any leftovers not eaten within 24 hours.

## NUTRITIONAL FACTS
### (Per Slice)

Cal: 80      Carbs: 18 g     Chol: 0 mg      Fat: 0.4 g
Fiber: 1.7 g    Protein: 2 g    Sodium: 60 mg

# Buttermilk Cornbread

*Be sure to use only finely ground cornmeal for the lightest, most tender texture.*

### Yield: 12 servings

2 cups finely ground yellow or white cornmeal
2 tablespoons sugar
2 teaspoons baking powder
½ teaspoon baking soda
2 cups nonfat or low-fat buttermilk
¼ cup plus 2 tablespoons fat-free egg substitute

**1.** Place the cornmeal, sugar, baking powder, and baking soda in a medium-sized bowl, and stir to mix well. Add the buttermilk and egg substitute, and stir with a wire whisk to mix well.

**2.** Coat a 10-inch cast iron skillet with nonstick cooking spray, and spread the batter evenly in the pan. Bake at 375°F for 25 to 28 minutes, or just until a wooden toothpick inserted in the center of the bread comes out clean. Be careful not to overbake. Cut into wedges, and serve hot, refrigerating any leftovers not eaten within 24 hours.

## NUTRITIONAL FACTS
### (Per Serving)

Cal: 102      Carbs: 19 g     Chol: 1 mg      Fat: 0.9 g
Fiber: 1.5 g    Protein: 3.8 g    Sodium: 195 mg

## Variations

For a change of pace, after whisking in the buttermilk and egg substitute, fold one or more of the following ingredients into the batter:

- ❐ ¾ to 1 cup frozen (thawed) whole kernel corn, drained, or 1 can (8 ounces) whole kernel corn, drained
- ❐ ¾ cup to 1 cup shredded nonfat or reduced-fat Cheddar cheese
- ❐ 2 to 4 tablespoons finely chopped seeded fresh jalapeño peppers, or 2 to 4 tablespoons finely chopped pickled jalapeño peppers
- ❐ 1 can (4 ounces) chopped green chilies, drained
- ❐ ¼ cup cooked crumbled turkey bacon

# Applesauce-Bran Bread

## Yield: 16 slices

1¾ cups whole wheat pastry flour

½ cup wheat bran or apple fiber*

2 teaspoons baking powder

¾ teaspoon baking soda

¾ teaspoon ground cinnamon

1½ cups unsweetened applesauce

½ cup maple syrup or molasses

1 teaspoon vanilla extract

½ cup dark raisins, dried cranberries, or chopped prunes

½ cup chopped walnuts or pecans (optional)

\* Apple fiber is a fiber-rich product extracted from apples. Look for brands like Good Shepherd in health foods stores and many grocery stores.

**1.** Place the flour, wheat bran or apple fiber, baking powder, baking soda, and cinnamon in a large bowl, and stir to mix well. Add the applesauce, maple syrup or molasses, and vanilla extract, and stir just until the dry ingredients are moistened. Fold in the dried fruits, and, if desired, the nuts.

**2.** Coat an 8-x-4-inch loaf pan with nonstick cooking spray, and spread the mixture evenly in the pan. Bake at 325°F for about 50 minutes, or just until a wooden toothpick inserted in the center of the loaf comes out clean. Be careful not to overbake.

**3.** Remove the loaf from the oven, and let sit for 10 minutes. Invert the loaf onto a wire rack, turn right side up, and cool to room temperature. Wrap the loaf in plastic wrap or aluminum foil, and allow to sit for 8 hours or overnight before slicing and serving. (Overnight storage will give the loaf a softer, moister crust.) Refrigerate any leftovers not eaten within 24 hours.

### NUTRITIONAL FACTS
(Per Slice)

| | | | |
|---|---|---|---|
| Cal: 100 | Carbs: 24 g | Chol: 0 mg | Fat: 0.4 g |
| Fiber: 2.8 g | Protein: 2.3 g | Sodium: 104 mg | |

# Carrot Spice Bread

## Yield: 16 slices

2 cups whole wheat pastry flour

2 teaspoons baking powder

¾ teaspoon baking soda

½ teaspoon ground cinnamon

¼ teaspoon ground nutmeg

1 cup apple juice

⅓ cup honey

1 cup (packed) grated carrots (about 2 medium)

⅓ cup golden raisins

⅓ cup honey crunch wheat germ

⅓ cup toasted chopped pecans

1. Place the flour, baking powder, baking soda, cinnamon, and nutmeg in a large bowl, and stir to mix well. Add the apple juice, honey, and carrots, and stir just until the dry ingredients are moistened. Fold in the raisins, wheat germ, and pecans.

2. Coat an 8-x-4-inch loaf pan with nonstick cooking spray, and spread the mixture evenly in the pan. Bake at 325°F for about 45 minutes, or just until a wooden toothpick inserted in the center of the loaf comes out clean. Be careful not to overbake.

3. Remove the loaf from the oven, and let sit for 10 minutes. Invert the loaf onto a wire rack, turn right side up, and cool to room temperature. Wrap the loaf in plastic wrap or aluminum foil, and allow to sit for 8 hours or overnight before slicing and serving. (Overnight storage will give the loaf a softer, moister crust.) Refrigerate any leftovers not eaten within 24 hours.

### NUTRITIONAL FACTS
#### (Per Slice)

| | | | |
|---|---|---|---|
| Cal: 118 | Carbs: 22 g | Chol: 0 mg | Fat: 2.2 g |
| Fiber: 2.5 g | Protein: 3.8 g | Sodium: 105 mg | |

# Pumpkin-Orange Bread

## Yield: 16 slices

2 cups whole wheat pastry flour

1/3 cup sugar

2 teaspoons baking powder

3/4 teaspoon baking soda

3/4 cup mashed cooked or canned pumpkin

3/4 cup orange juice

1/3 cup orange marmalade

1 teaspoon vanilla extract

1/2 cup chopped dates, golden raisins, or dried cranberries

1/3 cup honey crunch wheat germ or toasted chopped pecans

1. Place flour, sugar, baking powder, and baking soda in a large bowl, and stir to mix well.

2. Place the pumpkin, orange juice, marmalade, and vanilla extract in a small bowl, and stir to mix well.

3. Add the pumpkin mixture to the flour mixture, and stir just until the dry ingredients are moistened. Fold in the dates, raisins, or cranberries and the wheat germ or pecans.

---

## *Bread Boosters*

*Although the breads in this chapter are already rich in nutrients and fiber, you can easily give them a further nutritional boost by adding ingredients such as soy flour, flaxseeds, and wheat germ to the batter before baking. Here are some ideas:*

❏ *Substitute soy flour for 10 to 15 percent of the whole wheat flour in muffin and quick bread recipes using the guidelines on page 56.*

❏ *Substitute flax meal (page 63) for 1/4 to 1/3 cup of the whole wheat flour in muffin and quick bread recipes. Or add a few tablespoons of flaxseeds to muffin and quick bread batters.*

❏ *Substitute toasted wheat germ for 1/4 to 1/3 cup of the whole wheat flour in muffin and quick bread recipes. This will add a nutty taste to the baked goods —with only a fraction of the fat found in nuts.*

4. Coat an 8-x-4-inch loaf pan with nonstick cooking spray, and spread the mixture evenly in the pan. Bake at 325°F for about 50 minutes, or just until a wooden toothpick inserted in the center of the loaf comes out clean. Be careful not to overbake.

5. Remove the loaf from the oven, and let sit for 10 minutes. Invert the loaf onto a wire rack, turn right side up, and cool to room temperature. Wrap the loaf in plastic wrap or aluminum foil, and allow to sit for 8 hours or overnight before slicing and serving. (Overnight storage will give the loaf a softer, moister crust.) Refrigerate any leftovers not eaten within 24 hours.

## NUTRITIONAL FACTS
### (Per Slice)

Cal: 116    Carbs: 27 g    Chol: 0 mg    Fat: 0.6 g
Fiber: 2.7 g    Protein: 2.9 g    Sodium: 106 mg

# Apricot-Pecan Bread

*For variety, substitute prunes for the apricots, and walnuts for the pecans.*

## Yield: 16 slices

1 cup chopped dried apricots

1 teaspoon baking soda

¾ cup boiling water

2 cups whole wheat pastry flour

½ cup sugar

¼ cup instant nonfat dry milk powder

1 teaspoon baking powder

½ cup plus 1 tablespoon applesauce

2 teaspoons vanilla extract

¾ cup toasted chopped pecans

1. Place the apricots in a medium-sized bowl. Stir the baking soda into the boiling water; then pour the water over the apricots. Set aside to cool to lukewarm temperature.

2. Place the flour, sugar, milk powder, and baking powder in a large bowl, and stir to mix well. Add the applesauce, vanilla extract, and undrained cooled apricots, and stir just until the dry ingredients are moistened. Fold in the pecans.

3. Coat an 8-x-4-inch loaf pan with nonstick cooking spray, and spread the mixture evenly in the pan. Bake at 300°F for about 1 hour, or just until a wooden toothpick inserted in the center of the loaf comes out clean. Be careful not to overbake.

4. Remove the loaf from the oven, and let sit for 10 minutes. Invert the loaf onto a wire rack, turn right side up, and cool to room temperature. Wrap the loaf in plastic wrap or aluminum foil, and store for 8 hours or overnight before slicing and serving. (Overnight storage will give the loaf a softer, moister crust.) Refrigerate any leftovers not eaten within 24 hours.

## NUTRITIONAL FACTS
### (Per Slice)

Cal: 139    Carbs: 23 g    Chol: 0 mg    Fat: 3.9 g
Fiber: 3 g    Protein: 3.2 g    Sodium: 117 mg

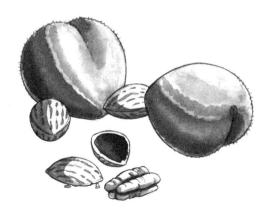

# Whole Wheat Banana-Nut Bread

### Yield: 16 slices

2 cups whole wheat pastry flour
$\frac{1}{2}$ cup sugar
2 teaspoons baking powder
$\frac{3}{4}$ teaspoon baking soda
$\frac{1}{4}$ teaspoon ground nutmeg
2 cups mashed very ripe banana (about 4 large)
1 teaspoon vanilla extract
$\frac{1}{2}$ cup chopped walnuts

1. Place the flour, sugar, baking powder, baking soda, and nutmeg in a large bowl, and stir to mix well. Add the banana and vanilla extract, and stir just until the dry ingredients are moistened. Fold in the walnuts.

2. Coat an 8-x-4-inch loaf pan with nonstick cooking spray, and spread the mixture evenly in the pan. Bake at 325°F for about 55 minutes, or just until a wooden toothpick inserted in the center of the loaf comes out clean. Be careful not to overbake.

3. Remove the loaf from the oven, and let sit for 15 minutes. Invert the loaf onto a wire rack, turn right side up, and cool to room temperature. Wrap the loaf in plastic wrap or aluminum foil, and allow to sit for 8 hours or overnight before slicing and serving. (Overnight storage will give the loaf a softer, moister crust.) Refrigerate any leftovers not eaten within 24 hours.

## NUTRITIONAL FACTS
### (Per Slice)

| | | | |
|---|---|---|---|
| Cal: 124 | Carbs: 24 g | Chol: 0 mg | Fat: 2.6 g |
| Fiber: 2.6 g | Protein: 3.3 g | Sodium: 121 mg | |

# Buttermilk Drop Biscuits

### Yield: 12 biscuits

1$\frac{1}{2}$ cups unbleached flour
$\frac{1}{4}$ cup plus 2 tablespoons oat bran
1 tablespoon plus 1$\frac{1}{2}$ teaspoons sugar
2$\frac{1}{2}$ teaspoons baking powder
$\frac{1}{4}$ cup ($\frac{1}{2}$ stick) chilled reduced-fat margarine or light butter, cut into pieces
1 cup nonfat or low-fat buttermilk

1. Place the flour, oat bran, sugar, and baking powder in a medium-sized bowl, and stir to mix well.

2. Add the margarine or butter to the flour mixture, and, using a pastry cutter or two knives, cut the margarine or butter into the flour mixture until the mixture resembles coarse crumbs.

3. Add the buttermilk to the flour mixture, and stir just until the dry ingredients are moistened. Add a little more buttermilk if needed to form a moderately thick batter.

4. Coat a baking sheet with nonstick cooking spray, and drop rounded tablespoonfuls of the batter onto the sheet. For crusty biscuits, space the biscuits 1 inch apart. For soft biscuits, space the biscuits so that they are barely touching.

5. Bake at 400°F for about 16 minutes, or just until the tops are lightly browned. Be careful not to overbake. Serve hot, refrigerating any leftovers not eaten within 24 hours.

## NUTRITIONAL FACTS
### (Per Biscuit)

| | | | |
|---|---|---|---|
| Cal: 89 | Carbs: 15 g | Chol: 1 mg | Fat: 2.2 g |
| Fiber: 0.8 g | Protein: 2.7 g | Sodium: 146 mg | |

# Hearty Oatmeal Bread

## Yield: 16 slices

1 can (1 pound) pear halves in juice, undrained

1½ cups whole wheat pastry flour

½ cup quick-cooking oats

½ cup dark brown sugar

¼ cup wheat bran or flax meal (page 63)

2 teaspoons baking powder

¾ teaspoon baking soda

1 teaspoon vanilla extract

½ cup chopped dried apricots, prunes, or dark raisins

⅓ cup chopped walnuts or toasted pecans

1. Drain the pears, reserving the juice. Place the pears in a blender, and process until smooth. Pour the puréed pears into a 2-cup measure, and add enough of the reserved juice to bring the volume up to 1½ cups. Set aside.

2. Place the flour, oats, brown sugar, and wheat bran or flax meal in a large bowl, and stir to mix well. Use the back of a spoon to press out any lumps in the brown sugar. Add the baking powder and baking soda, and stir to mix well.

3. Add the pears and vanilla extract to the flour mixture, and stir just until the dry ingredients are moistened. Fold in the apricots, prunes, or raisins and the walnuts or pecans.

4. Coat an 8-x-4-inch loaf pan with nonstick cooking spray, and spread the mixture evenly in the pan. Bake at 325°F for about 45 minutes, or just until a wooden toothpick inserted in the center of the loaf comes out clean. Be careful not to overbake.

5. Remove the loaf from the oven, and let sit for 10 minutes. Invert the loaf onto a wire rack, turn right side up, and cool to room temperature. Wrap the loaf in plastic wrap or aluminum foil, and allow to sit for 8 hours or overnight before slicing and serving. (Overnight storage will give the loaf a softer, moister crust.) Refrigerate any leftovers not eaten within 24 hours.

## NUTRITIONAL FACTS
### (Per Slice)

| | | | |
|---|---|---|---|
| Cal: 103 | Carbs: 20 g | Chol: 0 mg | Fat: 1.9 g |
| Fiber: 2.8 g | Protein: 2.9 g | Sodium: 105 mg | |

# Prune and Walnut Bread

## Yield: 16 slices

2 cups whole wheat pastry flour

½ cup sugar

2 teaspoons baking powder

¾ teaspoon baking soda

½ teaspoon ground cinnamon

1¼ cups unsweetened applesauce

¼ cup evaporated skim milk

1 teaspoon vanilla extract

1 cup chopped prunes

½ cup chopped walnuts

1. Place the flour, sugar, baking powder, baking soda, and cinnamon in a large bowl, and stir to mix well. Add the applesauce, evaporated milk, and vanilla extract, and stir just until the dry ingredients are moistened. Fold in the prunes and walnuts.

**2.** Coat an 8-x-4-inch loaf pan with nonstick cooking spray, and spread the mixture evenly in the pan. Bake at 325°F for about 55 minutes, or just until a wooden toothpick inserted in the center of the loaf comes out clean. Be careful not to overbake.

**3.** Remove the loaf from the oven, and let sit for 10 minutes. Invert the loaf onto a wire rack, turn right side up, and cool to room temperature. Wrap the loaf in plastic wrap or aluminum foil, and allow to sit for 8 hours or overnight before slicing and serving. (Overnight storage will give the loaf a softer, moister crust.) Refrigerate any leftovers not eaten within 24 hours.

## NUTRITIONAL FACTS
### (Per Slice)

| | | | |
|---|---|---|---|
| Cal: 131 | Carbs: 25 g | Chol: 0 mg | Fat: 2.5 g |
| Fiber: 3.1 g | Protein: 3.6 g | Sodium: 115 mg | |

# 9.

# Pasta Perfection

Featured prominently in some of the world's most healthful cuisines, pasta is the perfect solution whenever you need a low-fat meal in a matter of minutes. And contrary to popular belief, pasta is not fattening. One cup of cooked pasta—about two ounces dry— has only about two hundred calories and one gram of fat. Pasta is also loaded with energizing complex carbohydrates, and is sodium-free. For the most nutrients, be sure to select whole grain pastas, like kamut, spelt, or whole wheat. Like whole grain breads, these pastas provide far more B vitamins, minerals, and fiber than do products made from refined white flour. As a bonus, whole grains lend pastas a nutty flavor that enhances any dish.

Why is pasta so often thought of as being fattening? The problem is not with the pasta— it's with what so often goes on top. Cream-enriched sauces, pools of olive oil or butter, gobs of high-fat cheese, and greasy sausages are just a few of the toppings that can turn a lean plate of pasta into a fat budget-busting nightmare. But can these fatty ingredients be eliminated without sacrificing flavor? Absolutely. This chapter will show you how.

As you will see, the recipes in this chapter require little or no added fat. Instead, they combine pasta with nonfat dairy products; ultra-lean meats; seafood; beans, tofu, and other meat alternatives; vegetables, herbs, and spices; and other wholesome ingredients. The result? Pasta creations that are every bit as tempting as their full-fat counterparts. And you'll be delighted to find that pasta is a snap to prepare. In fact, most of the dishes in this chapter can be whipped up in less than thirty minutes, making pasta a real boon to the busy cook.

This chapter presents a wide variety of pasta dishes that are sure to please. From Lasagna Siciliana and Capellini with Pesto Cheese Sauce to Bow Ties with Tuna and Tomatoes and Penne Primavera, you will find a wealth of ideas for preparing one of the most satisfying of comfort foods. So boil up some pasta, and get ready to enjoy the pleasures of healthful low-fat cooking.

# Penne California

### Yield: 4 servings

10 ounces penne pasta (about 3⅓ cups)

1 can (15 ounces) white beans, rinsed and drained, divided

1 tablespoon extra virgin olive oil (optional)

2–3 teaspoons crushed fresh garlic

¾ cup chopped sun-dried tomatoes (not packed in oil)

2 cups unsalted chicken or vegetable broth

1 teaspoon dried Italian seasoning

¼ teaspoon coarsely ground black pepper

½ cup sliced scallions

¼ cup sliced black olives

¼ cup grated nonfat or regular Parmesan cheese (optional)

1. Cook the pasta al dente according to package directions. Drain well, return to the pot, and cover to keep warm.

2. While the pasta is cooking, place ¼ cup of the beans in a small bowl. Mash with a fork until smooth, and set aside.

3. Coat a large nonstick skillet with olive oil cooking spray or with the olive oil, and preheat over medium-heat. Add the garlic, and sauté for about 30 seconds, or until the garlic just begins to turn color and smells fragrant.

4. Add the dried tomatoes, broth, Italian seasoning, and pepper to the skillet, and bring the mixture to a boil over medium-high heat. Reduce the heat to low, cover, and simmer for about 5 minutes, or until the tomatoes are soft. Add the mashed white beans to the skillet, and stir to mix well. (This will thicken the sauce slightly.)

5. Add the pasta, the remaining white beans, the scallions, and the olives to the skillet, and toss gently over low heat for a minute or 2, or until the beans are heated through and the flavors are well blended. Add a little more broth if the mixture seems too dry. Serve hot.

### NUTRITIONAL FACTS
(Per 2-Cup Serving)

| | | | |
|---|---|---|---|
| Cal: 408 | Carbs: 78 g | Chol: 0 mg | Fat: 2.6 g |
| Fiber: 8 g | Protein: 18 g | Sodium: 472 mg | |

# Savory Spaghetti With Lentils

### Yield: 4 servings

8 ounces plain or garlic-and-parsley-flavored spaghetti

1–2 tablespoons extra virgin olive oil

¾ cup finely chopped celery

¾ cup finely chopped onion

¾ cup finely chopped carrot

2 teaspoons crushed fresh garlic

2 teaspoons dried oregano

¼ teaspoon coarsely ground black pepper

¼ teaspoon salt

2 tablespoons lemon juice

1½ cups vegetable or chicken broth

2 cups cooked brown lentils (page 102)

¼ cup plus 2 tablespoons grated nonfat or regular Parmesan cheese (garnish)

1. Cook the spaghetti al dente according to package directions. Drain well, return to the pot, and cover to keep warm.

**2.** While the pasta is cooking, place the oil in a large nonstick skillet, and preheat over medium-high heat. Add the celery, onion, carrot, garlic, oregano, pepper, and salt, and sauté for a couple of minutes, or until the vegetables are crisp-tender. Cover the skillet periodically if it begins to dry out. (The steam from the cooking vegetables will moisten the skillet.) Add the vegetables to the pot containing the spaghetti, and set aside.

**3.** Add the lemon juice and broth to the skillet, and cook over medium-high heat for several minutes, or until the volume is reduced by half. Add the pasta mixture and the lentils to the skillet. Reduce the heat to medium, and toss for a minute or 2, or until heated through. Serve hot, topping each serving with a rounded tablespoon of the Parmesan.

### NUTRITIONAL FACTS
(Per 1⅔-Cup Serving)

| | | | |
|---|---|---|---|
| Cal: 403 | Carbs: 71 g | Chol: 7 mg | Fat: 4.7 g |
| Fiber: 12.1 g | Protein: 20 g | Sodium: 486 mg | |

# Rigatoni With Roasted Eggplant and Tomatoes

### Yield: 4 servings

10 ounces rigatoni pasta (about 4 cups)

¼ cup plus 2 tablespoons crumbled nonfat or reduced-fat feta cheese (garnish)

VEGETABLE MIXTURE

1½ pounds fresh plum tomatoes (about 10 medium), cut lengthwise into 1-inch wedges

3 cups ¾-inch cubes peeled eggplant (about 1 medium)

1 small yellow onion, cut into thin wedges

1 cup sliced fresh mushrooms

1 tablespoon crushed fresh garlic

1 tablespoon plus 1½ teaspoons balsamic vinegar

1½ teaspoons dried oregano

½ teaspoon salt

¼ teaspoon coarsely ground black pepper

1 tablespoon extra virgin olive oil (optional)

Nonstick olive oil cooking spray

**1.** To make the vegetable mixture, place the tomatoes, eggplant, onion, mushrooms, garlic, vinegar, oregano, salt, pepper, and, if desired, the olive oil in a large bowl, and toss to mix well.

**2.** Coat a 9-x-13-inch roasting pan with olive oil cooking spray, and spread the mixture evenly in the pan. If you did not use the olive oil, spray the vegetables lightly with the cooking spray.

**3.** Cover the pan with aluminum foil, and bake at 450°F for 20 minutes. Remove the foil, and bake for 15 additional minutes. Turn with a spatula, and bake for 10 to 15 minutes more, or until the tomatoes are soft and the vegetables are nicely browned.

**4.** While the vegetables are cooking, cook the rigatoni al dente according to package directions. Drain well, return to the pot, and cover to keep warm.

**5.** When the vegetables are done, add them to the rigatoni, and toss to mix well. Serve hot, topping each serving a rounded tablespoon of the feta cheese.

### NUTRITIONAL FACTS
(Per 2-Cup Serving)

| | | | |
|---|---|---|---|
| Cal: 353 | Carbs: 69 g | Chol: 2 mg | Fat: 2.1 g |
| Fiber: 5.5 g | Protein: 14.2 g | Sodium: 483 mg | |

# Capellini With Pesto Cheese Sauce

## Yield: 4 servings

10 ounces capellini (angel hair) pasta

1 block (8 ounces) nonfat cream cheese, or 8 ounces soft curd farmer cheese

$\frac{3}{4}$ cup skim or 1% low fat milk

1 cup chopped fresh plum tomatoes (about 3 medium) (garnish)

$\frac{1}{4}$ cup pine nuts (garnish)

### PESTO

$\frac{1}{2}$ cup (packed) fresh basil

$\frac{1}{2}$ cup (packed) fresh parsley

$\frac{1}{4}$ cup plus 2 tablespoons grated nonfat or regular Parmesan cheese

2 teaspoons crushed fresh garlic

1. Cook the pasta al dente according to package directions. Drain well, return to the pot, and cover to keep warm.

2. While the pasta is cooking, place all of the pesto ingredients in a food processor, and process until the herbs are very finely chopped. Transfer the mixture to a small bowl, and set aside.

3. Place the cream cheese or farmer cheese and the milk in the food processor, and process until smooth. Set aside.

4. Add the cheese mixture to the pasta, and toss over low heat for a minute or 2, or just until the sauce is warmed through. (Do not let the sauce boil.) Add a little more milk if the sauce seems too thick. Remove the pot from the heat, add the pesto, and toss to mix well.

5. Serve immediately, topping each serving with $\frac{1}{4}$ cup of the chopped tomatoes and a tablespoon of the pine nuts.

## NUTRITIONAL FACTS
(Per 1¾-Cup Serving)

Cal: 398    Carbs: 65 g    Chol: 12 mg    Fat: 5 g
Fiber: 2.8 g    Protein: 24.7 g    Sodium: 378 mg

# Tofu Lo Mein

## Yield: 5 servings

1 pound reduced-fat firm or extra-firm tofu, frozen and thawed (page 182)

Nonstick cooking spray

10 ounces linguine pasta

1$\frac{1}{2}$ teaspoons crushed fresh garlic

2 cups small broccoli florets

1 cup sliced fresh mushrooms

1 medium red bell pepper, cut into thin strips

$\frac{1}{2}$ cup sliced scallions

### SAUCE

1 cup vegetable or chicken broth

$\frac{1}{4}$ cup reduced-sodium soy sauce

$\frac{1}{4}$ cup dry sherry

2 tablespoons dark brown sugar

2–3 teaspoons sesame oil

1 teaspoon ground ginger

2 teaspoons cornstarch

1. To make the sauce, place all of the sauce ingredients except for the cornstarch in a small bowl, and stir to mix well. Cut the tofu into $\frac{1}{2}$-inch cubes, and place the cubes in a shallow nonmetal container. Pour $\frac{1}{4}$ cup of the sauce mixture over the tofu, toss to mix, and set aside for 10 minutes. Add the cornstarch to the remaining sauce, stir to dissolve the cornstarch, and set aside.

# The Mighty Tomato

*Numerous studies have linked diets high in fruits and vegetables with a reduced risk of cancer. But if you're a lover of Italian food, you'll be interested to learn that one form of produce appears to be especially protective against prostate cancer. What is this mighty miracle food? The tomato!*

*Researchers have found that men who eat tomato-based products at least ten times a week—products such as tomato sauce, fresh tomatoes, and even pizza—reduce their risk of developing prostate cancer by a third compared with men who eat these products less than twice a week. Of these foods, tomato sauce seems to offer the strongest protection against cancer.*

*What's in tomatoes that wards off prostate cancer? Scientists believe that lycopene, a carotenoid that gives tomatoes their red color, is responsible. This nutrient seems to be an even more potent antioxidant than beta-carotene. Why does tomato sauce offer more protection against cancer than fresh tomatoes? Chopping and cooking breaks down the cell walls of vegetables and fruits, which makes carotenoids like lycopene more available for absorption. In addition, tomato sauce usually contains a small amount of vegetable oil, which aids the absorption of this fat-soluble nutrient. Does this mean you should make a conscious effort to add fat to your food? No. Most people already get plenty of fat. And if you eat a diet rich in whole natural foods, there is no need to add oil, butter, or other fats to foods. However, if you want to use a little olive oil for cooking or in salads, feel free to do so, using your fat budget as a guide.*

2. Coat a large nonstick baking sheet with nonstick cooking spray. Drain off any sauce that the tofu has not soaked up, and spread the tofu cubes in a single layer on the sheet. Spray the tops of the cubes lightly with nonstick cooking spray. Bake at 375°F for 10 minutes, turn the cubes, and bake for 10 additional minutes, or until the cubes are nicely browned, crisp on the outside, and chewy on the inside. Remove the tofu from the oven, and set aside.

3. While the tofu is cooking, cook the pasta al dente according to package directions. Drain well, return to the pot, and cover to keep warm.

4. Coat a large nonstick skillet with nonstick cooking spray. Place the skillet over medium-high heat, and add the garlic, broccoli, mushrooms, red pepper, and scallions. Stir-fry the vegetables for about 4 minutes, or until crisp-tender, covering the skillet periodically if it begins to dry out. (The steam from the cooking vegetables will moisten the skillet.) Add a few teaspoons of water or broth to the skillet only if necessary. Add the tofu, and toss to mix well. Add the pasta, and toss to mix well.

5. Stir the reserved sauce, and add it to the skillet. Toss the mixture for a minute or 2, or just until the sauce thickens slightly. Serve hot.

## NUTRITIONAL FACTS
(Per 2-Cup Serving)

Cal: 356    Carbs: 55 g    Chol: 0 mg    Fat: 5.9 g
Fiber: 3.2 g    Protein: 18 g    Sodium: 546 mg

# Penne Primavera

## Yield: 4 servings

10 ounces penne pasta (about 3⅓ cups)

2 medium yellow squash, halved lengthwise and sliced (about 1⅓ cups)

1⅓ cups broccoli florets

1⅓ cups sliced fresh mushrooms

1⅓ cups sliced carrots or red bell pepper strips

2⅔ cups Chunky Garden Marinara Sauce (page 143) or bottled fat-free marinara sauce, heated

¼ cup grated nonfat or regular Parmesan cheese (garnish)

1. Cook the pasta al dente according to package directions. Drain well, return to the pot, and cover to keep warm.

2. While the pasta is cooking, coat a large nonstick skillet with nonstick olive oil cooking spray, and preheat over medium-high heat. Add the squash, broccoli, mushrooms, and carrots or red pepper, and stir-fry for about 4 minutes, or until crisp-tender. Cover the skillet periodically if it begins to dry out. (The steam from the cooking vegetables will moisten the skillet). Add a few teaspoons of water to the skillet if needed.

3. Spread ⅔ cup of sauce over the bottom of each of 4 serving plates. Top the sauce on each plate with a quarter of the pasta, leaving a 1-inch border of sauce showing under the pasta. Spoon a quarter of the vegetable mixture over the pasta, and sprinkle with a tablespoon of Parmesan. Serve hot.

## NUTRITIONAL FACTS
### (Per Serving)

Cal: 364    Carb: 71 g    Chol: 0 mg    Fat: 1.5 g
Fiber: 7.1 g    Protein: 15.9 g    Sodium: 362 mg

# Penne With Roasted Red Pepper Sauce

## Yield: 4 servings

12 ounces penne pasta (about 4 cups)

¼ cup grated nonfat Parmesan cheese (garnish)

¾ teaspoon dried basil, or 2¼ teaspoons finely chopped fresh basil (garnish)

SAUCE

1 jar (7 ounces) roasted red peppers, drained and chopped

1 cup evaporated skim milk

⅓ cup grated nonfat Parmesan cheese

1 tablespoon finely chopped fresh basil, or 1 teaspoon dried

1 teaspoon crushed fresh garlic

¼ teaspoon ground black pepper

1. Cook the pasta al dente according to package directions. Drain well, return to the pot, and cover to keep warm.

2. While the pasta is cooking, place all of the sauce ingredients in a blender, and process for about 1 minute, or until smooth.

3. Place the pot containing the pasta over low heat, and pour the sauce over the pasta. Cook and stir for a minute or 2, or until the sauce is warmed through. Add a little more evaporated milk if the sauce seems too dry. Serve hot, topping each serving with a tablespoon of the Parmesan and a sprinkling of basil.

## NUTRITIONAL FACTS
### (Per 1½-Cup Serving)

Cal: 416    Carbs: 78 g    Chol: 14 mg    Fat: 1.8 g
Fiber: 2.4 g    Protein: 21 g    Sodium: 364 mg

# *Perfect Pasta Sauces*

*This chapter demonstrates just how easy it is to make a wide variety of pasta sauces that are both rich in nutrients and absolutely irresistible. Need more pasta ideas? Following are two wonderfully versatile, easy-to-make—and easy-to-love—sauces that can be used on the pasta of your choice. If you like, prepare them whenever you have the time, and freeze them in serving-size containers for later use. Then heat them up and toss them with linguine, use them as a pizza sauce, or spoon them over baked chicken and top with mozzarella for a fast entrée. Who knew that perfect pasta sauces could be so healthy and so good?*

## Chunky Garden Marinara Sauce

Yield: 3$\frac{1}{2}$ cups

1 tablespoon extra virgin olive oil (optional)

2 teaspoons crushed fresh garlic

1 cup chopped fresh mushrooms

$\frac{3}{4}$ cup chopped red or green bell pepper

$\frac{1}{2}$ cup chopped onion

1 can (28 ounces) crushed tomatoes

2 tablespoons tomato paste

2 teaspoons instant vegetable or beef bouillon granules

1$\frac{1}{2}$ teaspoons dried Italian seasoning

1$\frac{1}{2}$ teaspoons sugar (optional)

$\frac{1}{4}$ teaspoon crushed red pepper

1. Coat a large nonstick skillet with nonstick cooking spray or with the olive oil, and preheat over medium heat. Add the garlic, mushrooms, bell pepper, and onion. Cover, and cook, stirring occasionally, for about 5 minutes, or until the vegetables start to soften and release their juices.

2. Add all of the remaining ingredients to the pan, and stir to mix. Increase the heat to medium-high, and bring the mixture to a boil. Reduce the heat to low, cover, and simmer, stirring occasionally, for about 20 minutes, or until the sauce is thick and the flavors are well blended. Serve hot over your choice of pasta.

### NUTRITIONAL FACTS

(Per $\frac{1}{2}$-Cup Serving)

| Cal: 48 | Carbs: 10 g | Chol: 0 mg | Fat: 0.1 g |
|---|---|---|---|
| | Fiber: 2.7 g   Protein: 2.5 g   Sodium: 228 mg | | |

## Savory Meat Sauce

Yield: 5$\frac{1}{3}$ cups

12 ounces 95% lean ground beef

1 medium yellow onion, chopped

1$\frac{1}{2}$ cups sliced fresh mushrooms

$\frac{1}{2}$ cup chopped green bell pepper

$\frac{1}{2}$ cup finely chopped celery (include the leaves)

2 teaspoons crushed fresh garlic

2$\frac{1}{2}$ teaspoons dried Italian seasoning

2 teaspoons instant beef bouillon granules

2 teaspoons sugar (optional)

1 can (28 ounces) crushed tomatoes

1. Coat a large nonstick skillet with nonstick cooking spray, and preheat over medium heat. Add the ground beef, and cook, stirring to crumble, until the meat is no longer pink.

2. Add all of the remaining ingredients to the pan except for the tomatoes, and stir to mix. Cover and cook, stirring occasionally, for about 5 minutes, or until the vegetables start to soften and release their juices.

3. Add the tomatoes to the pan, and stir to mix. Increase the heat to medium-high, and bring the mixture to a boil. Reduce the heat to low, cover, and simmer, stirring occasionally, for 20 to 25 minutes, or until the sauce is thick and the flavors are well blended. Serve hot over your choice of pasta.

### NUTRITIONAL FACTS

(Per $\frac{2}{3}$-Cup Serving)

| Cal: 97 | Carbs: 9.2 g | Chol: 26 mg | Fat: 2 g |
|---|---|---|---|
| | Fiber: 2.2 g   Protein: 10.5 g   Sodium: 225 mg | | |

# Penne With Walnut Pesto

*For a creamy pesto sauce with a calcium and protein boost, substitute evaporated skim milk for the broth.*

## Yield: 4 servings

10 ounces penne pasta (about $3\frac{1}{3}$ cups) or rigatoni pasta (about 4 cups)

1 cup warm chicken or vegetable broth

$\frac{3}{4}$ cup chopped seeded fresh plum tomatoes (about $2\frac{1}{2}$ medium) (garnish)

PESTO SAUCE

$\frac{2}{3}$ cup (tightly packed) fresh basil

$\frac{2}{3}$ cup (tightly packed) fresh spinach

$\frac{1}{2}$ cup plus 2 tablespoons grated nonfat or regular Parmesan cheese

$\frac{1}{3}$–$\frac{1}{2}$ cup chopped walnuts

4 cloves garlic, crushed

$\frac{1}{4}$ teaspoon ground white pepper

1. Cook the pasta al dente according to package directions. Drain well, return to the pot, and cover to keep warm.

2. While the pasta is cooking, place all of the pesto ingredients in a food processor, and process until finely ground. Add the pesto mixture to the pasta, and toss to mix well. Add the broth, and toss to mix well. Add a little more broth if the sauce seems too dry.

3. Serve hot, topping each serving with 3 tablespoons of the chopped tomatoes.

### NUTRITIONAL FACTS
(Per $1\frac{1}{2}$-Cup Serving)

| | | | |
|---|---|---|---|
| Cal: 379 | Carbs: 62 g | Chol: 12 mg | Fat: 7 g |
| Fiber: 3.2 g | Protein: 17.6 g | Sodium: 270 mg | |

# Mediterranean Linguine

## Yield: 4 servings

8 ounces linguine pasta

$1\frac{3}{4}$ cups unsalted chicken or vegetable broth

1 can (15 ounces) chickpeas, drained, divided

$1\frac{1}{2}$ teaspoons crushed fresh garlic

$\frac{1}{2}$ cup chopped sun-dried tomatoes (not packed in oil)

1 teaspoon dried oregano

$\frac{1}{2}$ teaspoon coarsely ground black pepper

3 cups (packed) chopped fresh spinach

$\frac{1}{4}$ cup plus 2 tablespoons crumbled nonfat or reduced-fat feta cheese (garnish)

1. Cook the pasta al dente according to package directions. Drain well, return to the pot, and cover to keep warm.

2. While the pasta is cooking, place all of the broth and $\frac{1}{4}$ cup plus 2 tablespoons of the chickpeas in a blender, and process until the mixture is smooth. Set aside.

3. Coat a large nonstick skillet with nonstick olive oil cooking spray, and preheat over medium-high heat. Add the garlic, and sauté for about 30 seconds, or just until the garlic begins to turn color and smells fragrant.

4. Add the broth mixture, dried tomatoes, oregano, and pepper to the skillet, and bring to a boil over high heat. Reduce the heat to low, cover, and simmer for 5 minutes, or until the tomatoes are soft.

5. Add the spinach to the skillet. Cook and stir for a minute or 2, or just until the spinach is wilted. Add the remaining chickpeas and the pasta to the skillet, and toss for a minute or 2, or until the mixture is thoroughly heated and the flavors are well blended. Serve hot, topping each serving with a rounded tablespoon of the feta cheese.

## NUTRITIONAL FACTS
### (Per 1¾-Cup Serving)

| | | | |
|---|---|---|---|
| Cal: 387 | Carbs: 72 g | Chol: 2 mg | Fat: 2.4 g |
| Fiber: 7.4 g | Protein: 17.5 g | Sodium: 562 mg | |

# Mega Macaroni and Cheese

### Yield: 6 servings

8 ounces ziti pasta (about 3 cups)

2½ cups skim or 1% low-fat milk, divided

3 tablespoons unbleached flour

1½ teaspoons dry mustard

⅛ teaspoon ground black pepper

¼ cup finely chopped onion

1 tablespoon water

8 ounces nonfat or reduced-fat process Cheddar cheese or reduced-fat Cheddar cheese, shredded or diced (about 2 cups)

1 jar (2 ounces) chopped pimento, drained

2 tablespoons Italian-style seasoned dried bread crumbs

Butter-flavored nonstick cooking spray

**1.** Cook the pasta al dente according to package directions. Drain well, return to the pot, and cover to keep warm.

**2.** While the pasta is cooking, place ½ cup of the milk and all of the flour, mustard, and pepper in a jar with a tight-fitting lid. Shake until smooth, and set aside.

**3.** Place the onion and water in a 2-quart nonstick pot. Cover and cook over medium heat, stirring occasionally, for about 3 minutes, or until the onions are soft.

**4.** Add the remaining 2 cups of milk to the pot, and bring to a boil over medium heat, stirring constantly. Add the flour mixture, and cook, still stirring, for about 1 minute, or just until the mixture begins to boil and thickens slightly. Reduce the heat to medium-low, add the cheese, and stir just until the cheese melts.

**5.** Pour the cheese sauce over the pasta. Add the pimento, and toss to mix well. Coat a 2½-quart casserole dish with nonstick cooking spray, and spread the pasta mixture evenly in the dish. Sprinkle the crumbs over the top, and spray the top with the cooking spray.

**6.** Bake at 350°F for about 30 minutes, or until hot and bubbly around the edges. Remove the dish from the oven, and let sit for 10 minutes before serving.

## NUTRITIONAL FACTS
### (Per 1-Cup Serving)

| | | | |
|---|---|---|---|
| Cal: 255 | Carbs: 38 g | Chol: 2 mg | Fat: 1.4 g |
| Fiber: 1.5 g | Protein: 20 g | Sodium: 322 mg | |

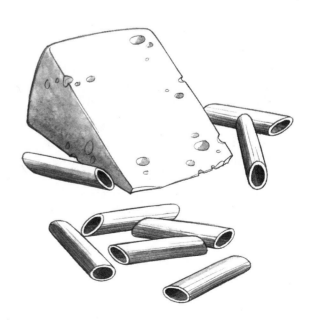

# Manicotti Florentine

## Yield: 7 servings

14 manicotti tubes (about 8 ounces)

1 recipe Chunky Garden Marinara Sauce (page 143), or $3\frac{1}{2}$ cups bottled fat-free marinara sauce

1 cup shredded nonfat or reduced-fat mozzarella cheese

FILLING

$3\frac{1}{2}$ cups nonfat ricotta cheese

1 package (10 ounces) frozen chopped spinach, thawed and squeezed dry

$\frac{1}{4}$ cup fat-free egg substitute

$\frac{1}{2}$ cup grated nonfat or regular Parmesan cheese

1. Cook the manicotti al dente according to package directions. Drain well, and set aside.

2. To make the filling, place all of the filling ingredients in a large bowl, and stir to mix well. Using a small spoon, stuff about $\frac{1}{3}$ cup of the filling mixture into each tube.

3. Spoon a thin layer of the sauce over the bottom of a large baking pan, and arrange the filled pasta in the pan. Pour the remaining sauce evenly over the manicotti.

4. Bake uncovered at 350°F for about 30 minutes, or until heated through. Sprinkle the mozzarella over the top, and bake for 10 additional minutes, or until the cheese has melted. Remove the dish from the oven, and let sit for 10 minutes before serving.

## NUTRITIONAL FACTS
### (Per Serving)

Cal: 327    Carbs: 47 g    Chol: 10 mg    Fat: 0.7 g
Fiber: 4.4 g    Protein: 33.5 g    Sodium: 547 mg

# Bow Ties With Tuna and Tomatoes

## Yield: 4 servings

$1\frac{1}{2}$ cups chopped fresh plum tomatoes (about 5 medium)

1 can (9 ounces) water-packed albacore tuna, drained

5 thin slices red onion

$\frac{1}{3}$ cup chopped fresh basil

$\frac{1}{4}$ cup chopped black olives

$\frac{1}{4}$ cup bottled nonfat Italian salad dressing

$1\frac{1}{2}$ teaspoons crushed fresh garlic

$\frac{1}{8}$ teaspoon coarsely ground black pepper

10 ounces bow tie pasta (about 5 cups) or rigatoni pasta (about 4 cups)

$\frac{1}{4}$ cup grated nonfat or regular Parmesan cheese (optional)

1. Place the tomatoes, tuna, onion, basil, olives, salad dressing, garlic, and pepper in a large bowl, and toss gently to mix well. Set aside for 30 minutes.

2. Cook the pasta al dente according to package directions. Drain well, and return to the pot.

3. Add the tomato-tuna mixture to the pasta, and toss gently to mix well. Serve immediately, topping each serving with a tablespoon of Parmesan, if desired.

## NUTRITIONAL FACTS
### (Per 2-Cup Serving)

Cal: 375    Carbs: 61 g    Chol: 17 mg    Fat: 2.8 g
Fiber: 3 g    Protein: 25 g    Sodium: 462 mg

## Spicy Spaghetti and Shrimp

### Yield: 4 servings

8 ounces thin spaghetti

1 1/2 teaspoons crushed fresh garlic

12 ounces cleaned raw shrimp

1 can (14 1/2 ounces) unsalted stewed tomatoes, crushed

1/4 cup coarsely chopped black olives

1 tablespoon plus 1 teaspoon small capers*

3/4 teaspoon dried oregano or basil

1/4 teaspoon crushed red pepper

1/4 cup grated nonfat or regular Parmesan cheese (garnish)

* If only large capers are available, coarsely chop them before using.

1. Cook the pasta according to package directions. Drain well, return to the pot, and cover to keep warm.

2. While the pasta is cooking, coat a large nonstick skillet with nonstick olive oil cooking spray, and preheat over medium-high heat. Add the garlic and shrimp, and stir-fry for about 4 minutes, or until the shrimp turn pink.

3. Add the undrained tomatoes, olives, capers, oregano or basil, and crushed red pepper to the shrimp mixture, and bring to a boil over medium-high heat. Reduce the heat to low, cover, and simmer, stirring occasionally, for about 5 minutes, or until the flavors are well blended.

4. Add the pasta to the skillet, and toss to mix well. Serve hot, topping each serving with a tablespoon of the Parmesan.

### NUTRITIONAL FACTS
(Per 1 1/2-Cup Serving)

| | | | |
|---|---|---|---|
| Cal: 323 | Carbs: 51 g | Chol: 126 mg | Fat: 2.6 g |
| Fiber: 3.2 g | Protein: 23 g | Sodium: 382 mg | |

## The Truth About Shrimp

One of the most popular seafood choices in the United States, shrimp is also well known for its high cholesterol content. How much cholesterol does shrimp contain? A 3 1/2-ounce serving of cooked shrimp contains 195 milligrams of cholesterol—which means that it consumes at least two-thirds of your daily cholesterol budget of 300 milligrams or less. Why can shrimp still be included in a healthy diet? Shrimp is exceptionally low in fat. In fact, a 3 1/2-ounce serving contains a mere gram of fat. Furthermore, the fat in shrimp contains a significant amount of heart-healthy omega-3 fat, and very little artery-clogging saturated fat.

A 1996 study showed that a diet containing as much as 10 ounces of shrimp per day—about 590 milligrams of cholesterol—does not worsen the cholesterol profile of a healthy individual. People who followed this diet for three weeks did experience a rise in their blood cholesterol. However, their HDL, or "good" cholesterol, rose more than did their LDL, or "bad" cholesterol. And because the increase in LDL (7 percent) was less than the increase in HDL (12 percent), the shrimp diet did not worsen the risk of heart disease.

Does this mean you can eat unlimited amounts of shrimp? In the interest of leaving room in your diet for nutrient-rich vegetables, fruits, legumes, and whole grains, it's a good idea to limit all meats, seafood, and poultry to 6 ounces or less per day. Furthermore, the subjects in this study all had normal blood cholesterol levels to begin with, and researchers are not sure whether people with high blood cholesterol levels would respond in the same way. However, if you enjoy shrimp, substituting it for high-fat meat is a good idea, and will probably reduce your risk of developing heart disease.

# Lasagna Siciliana

## Yield: 10 servings

12 lasagna noodles (about 9 ounces)

2¾ cups shredded nonfat mozzarella cheese

1 tablespoon grated nonfat or regular Parmesan cheese

### FILLING

15 ounces nonfat ricotta cheese

1½ cups nonfat or low-fat cottage cheese

½ cup grated nonfat or regular Parmesan cheese

3 tablespoons finely chopped fresh parsley

### SAUCE

12 ounces 95% lean ground beef

1 can (28 ounces) crushed tomatoes

1 can (6 ounces) Italian-style tomato paste

2 cups ½-inch cubes peeled eggplant (about 1 small)

1 cup chopped fresh mushrooms

1 cup chopped onion

1 large red bell pepper, diced

2 teaspoons crushed fresh garlic

2½ teaspoons dried Italian seasoning

1. To make the sauce, coat a 3-quart pot with nonstick olive oil cooking spray, and preheat over medium heat. Add the ground beef, and cook, stirring to crumble, until the meat is no longer pink.

2. Add all of the remaining sauce ingredients to the pot, and bring the mixture to a boil over medium-high heat. Reduce the heat to low, cover, and simmer, stirring occasionally, for about 30 minutes, or until the vegetables are soft and the flavors are well blended. (Note that the sauce will be very thick at first, but will thin down a bit as the vegetables cook and release their juices.) Remove from the heat, and cover to keep warm.

3. To make the filling, place all of the filling ingredients in a medium-sized bowl, and stir to mix well. Set aside.

4. To assemble the lasagna, coat a 9-x-13-inch pan with nonstick cooking spray. Spoon 1 cup of the sauce over the bottom of the pan. Lay 4 of the *uncooked* lasagna noodles over the bottom of the pan, arranging 3 of the noodles lengthwise and 1 noodle crosswise. Allow a little space between the noodles for expansion. (You will have to break about 1 inch off the crosswise noodle to make it fit the pan.)

5. Top the noodles with half of the filling mixture, 1 cup of the mozzarella, and 1½ cups of the sauce. Repeat the noodle, filling, mozzarella, and sauce layers. Finally, top with the remaining noodles followed by the remaining sauce, and sprinkle with the Parmesan.

6. Spray the underside of a large rectangle of aluminum foil with nonstick cooking spray, cover the dish with the foil, and bake at 350°F for 45 minutes. Remove the foil, and sprinkle the remaining ¾ cup of mozzarella over the top. Return the dish to the oven, and bake for 15 additional minutes, or until the edges are bubbly and the top is browned. Remove the dish from the oven, and let sit for 15 minutes before cutting into squares and serving.

## NUTRITIONAL FACTS
### (Per Serving)

| | | | |
|---|---|---|---|
| Cal: 308 | Carbs: 38 g | Chol: 31 mg | Fat: 2.3 g |
| Fiber: 3.9 g | Protein: 35 g | Sodium: 555 mg | |

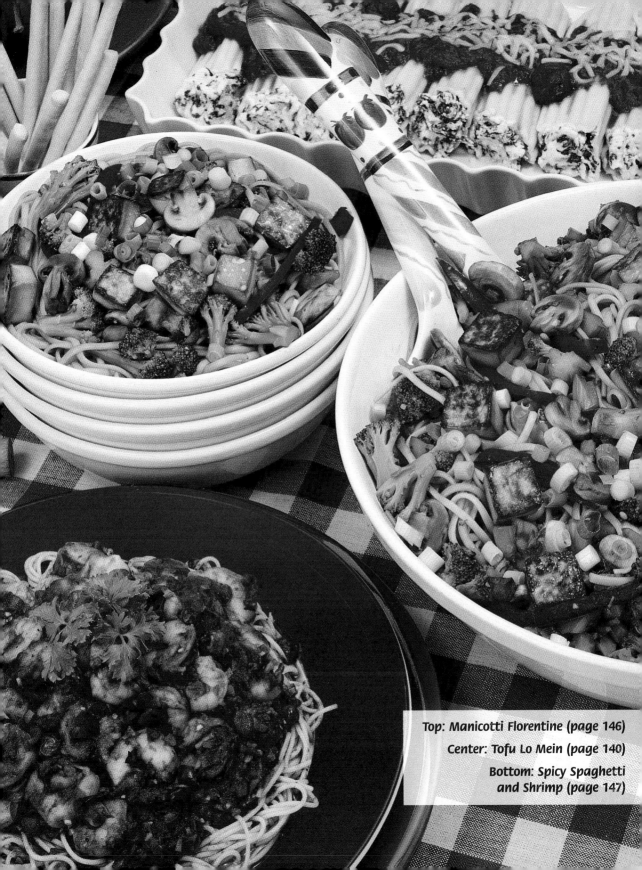

**Top: Manicotti Florentine (page 146)**

**Center: Tofu Lo Mein (page 140)**

**Bottom: Spicy Spaghetti and Shrimp (page 147)**

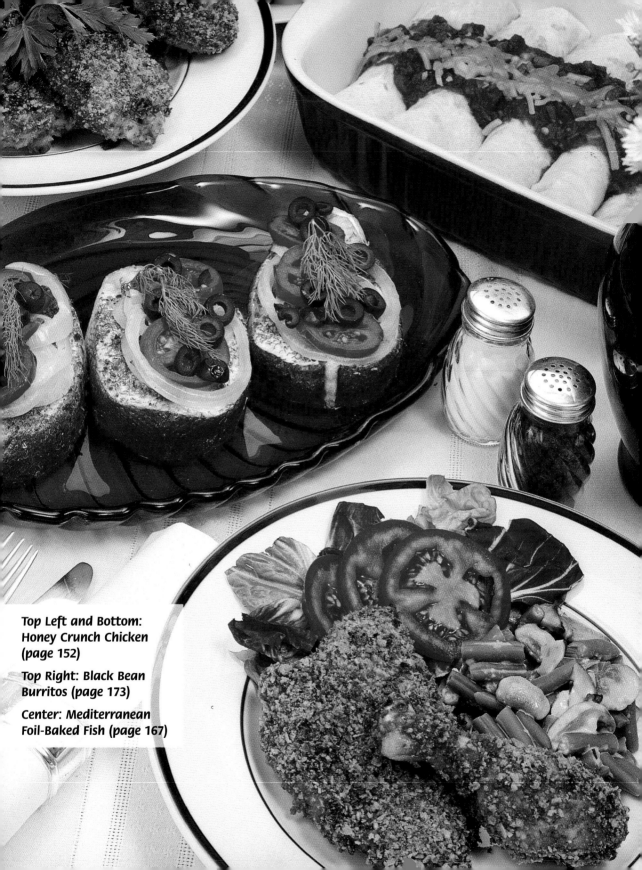

**Top Left and Bottom:
Honey Crunch Chicken
(page 152)**

**Top Right: Black Bean
Burritos (page 173)**

**Center: Mediterranean
Foil-Baked Fish (page 167)**

# Pasta Piselli

Yield: 4 servings

8 ounces thin spaghetti

¾ cup frozen (unthawed) green peas

1 cup plus 2 tablespoons evaporated skim milk

3 tablespoons fat-free egg substitute

3 tablespoons grated nonfat Parmesan cheese

1 teaspoon crushed fresh garlic

1 cup sliced fresh mushrooms

5 ounces ham, at least 97% lean, diced or cut into thin strips (about 1 cup)

1. Cook the pasta according to package directions. About 2 minutes before the pasta is done, add the peas, and cook for 2 minutes more, or until the peas are tender and the pasta is al dente. Drain well, return to the pot, and cover to keep warm.

2. Place the evaporated milk, egg substitute, and Parmesan cheese in a small bowl. Stir to mix well, and set aside.

3. Coat a large nonstick skillet with nonstick cooking spray, and preheat over medium-high heat. Add the garlic, mushrooms, and ham, and cook, stirring frequently, for about 4 minutes, or until the mushrooms and ham are nicely browned. Cover the skillet periodically if it begins to dry out. (The steam from the cooking vegetables will moisten the skillet.)

4. Reduce the heat under the skillet to medium-low, and add the pasta to the skillet mixture. Slowly pour the evaporated milk mixture over the pasta, and toss gently for a minute or 2, or until the sauce thickens slightly. Add a little more evaporated milk if the sauce seems too dry. Serve hot.

## NUTRITIONAL FACTS
(Per 1⅔-Cup Serving)

| | | | |
|---|---|---|---|
| Cal: 354 | Carbs: 58 g | Chol: 22 mg | Fat: 2.2 g |
| Fiber: 3.2 g | Protein: 25 g | Sodium: 533 mg | |

# Rigatoni and Sausage Primavera

Yield: 4 servings

8 ounces rigatoni pasta (about 3¼ cups) or rotini pasta (about 2¾ cups)

8 ounces sliced smoked turkey sausage or kielbasa, at least 97% lean (about 1¼ cups)

1 medium zucchini, halved lengthwise and sliced ¼-inch thick

1 cup sliced fresh mushrooms

¾ cup matchstick-sized pieces of red bell pepper

1 teaspoon crushed fresh garlic

1 cup chicken or vegetable broth

¾ teaspoon dried oregano

1 cup chopped fresh plum tomatoes (about 3 medium)

¼ cup grated nonfat or regular Parmesan cheese (optional)

1. Cook the pasta al dente according to package directions. Drain well, return to the pot, and cover to keep warm.

2. While the pasta is cooking, coat a large nonstick skillet with nonstick olive oil cooking spray, and preheat over medium-high heat. Add the sausage, zucchini, mushrooms, red pepper, and garlic, and stir-fry for about 3 minutes, or until the sausage is browned and the vegetables are crisp-tender. Cover the skillet periodically if it begins to dry out. (The

steam from the cooking vegetables will moisten the skillet.) Add a few teaspoons of water to the skillet if needed.

3. Transfer the sausage and vegetables to a large bowl, and cover to keep warm. Add the broth and oregano to the skillet, and cook uncovered over medium-high heat, stirring frequently, for a couple of minutes, or until the broth is reduced by half.

4. Add the tomatoes to the skillet, cover, and cook over medium-high heat for about 1 minute, or until the tomatoes are heated through and beginning to soften.

5. Reduce the heat to medium, and add the pasta and the sausage-vegetable mixture to the skillet. Toss for a minute or 2 to blend the flavors, adding a little more broth if the mixture seems too dry. Serve hot, topping each serving with a tablespoon of Parmesan, if desired.

## NUTRITIONAL FACTS
### (Per 2-Cup Serving)

Cal: 306    Carbs: 52 g    Chol: 25 mg    Fat: 2.7 g
Fiber: 2.8 g    Protein: 17.7 g    Sodium: 638 mg

# 10.

# Wholesome and Hearty Entrées

Many people believe that adopting a healthy, low-fat lifestyle means waving good-bye to the hearty home-style dishes they love so much. The truth is that you don't have to give up crispy fried chicken, hearty chili, savory meat loaf, home-style skillet dinners, or any of your other favorites just because you're cutting down on fat. Nor do you have to spend hours in specialty stores searching for exotic ingredients, or added time in the kitchen learning complicated cooking methods. By replacing common high-fat ingredients with low-fat or no-fat foods, and by using a few simple cooking techniques, you can enjoy just about all of your favorite foods and many new ones, as well. This chapter will show you how.

The entrées in this chapter begin with the freshest seafood or the leanest cuts of poultry, beef, or pork. Then fat is kept to an absolute minimum by using nonstick skillets and nonstick cooking sprays, and by replacing full-fat dairy products with their healthful nonfat and reduced-fat counterparts. Of course, fresh vegetables, hearty grains, and savory seasonings play an important role in these dishes by adding not only great flavors and textures, but also a wealth of nutrients. The result? Satisfying home-style entrées, most of which have a mere two to three grams of fat per serving!

As you glance through the pages of this chapter, remember that these are just some of the delicious low-fat entrées that are within your reach. Delicious pasta entrées are presented in Chapter 9, crowd-pleasing meatless main dishes can be found in Chapter 11, and a wide variety of hearty main-dish salads can be found in Chapter 7. And, of course, many of your own family favorites can very easily be "slimmed down" *and* given a nutritional boost with the help of the techniques and ingredients used within this chapter.

The following pages present a wide range of hearty home-style entrées guaranteed to provide a tempting answer to that age-old question, "What's for dinner?" So whether you're looking for a simple baked chicken dish, a spicy stir-fry, or a fast and easy skillet dish, you will be sure to find something to make any evening special.

# Honey Crunch Chicken

*For variety, substitute coarsely ground toasted pecans for half of the wheat germ.*

### Yield: 8 servings

3 pounds bone-in skinless chicken breast halves (about 6 ounces each), or 3 pounds bone-in skinless chicken breasts halves, legs, and thighs

1$\frac{1}{2}$ cups nonfat or low-fat buttermilk

Nonstick cooking spray

COATING

4 cups corn flakes

$\frac{1}{2}$ cup honey crunch wheat germ

1 teaspoon poultry seasoning

$\frac{1}{4}$ teaspoon ground black pepper

$\frac{1}{4}$ teaspoon salt

1. Rinse the chicken, and pat it dry with paper towels. Place the chicken in a shallow non-metal dish, and pour the buttermilk over the chicken. Turn the pieces to coat, cover, and refrigerate for 6 to 24 hours.

2. To make the coating, place the corn flakes in a food processor, and process into crumbs. Measure the crumbs; there should be 1 cup plus 2 tablespoons. Adjust the amount if necessary.

3. Place the corn flake crumbs and all of the remaining coating ingredients in a gallon-sized plastic bag. Close the bag, and shake well to mix.

4. Remove 2 pieces of chicken from the buttermilk, place in the coating bag, and shake to coat evenly. Repeat with the remaining chicken.

5. Coat a large baking sheet with nonstick cooking spray, and arrange the chicken on the pan. Spray each piece of chicken lightly with the nonstick cooking spray, and bake at 400°F for 50 minutes, or until the meat is tender and the chicken is no longer pink inside. Serve hot.

### NUTRITIONAL FACTS
#### (Per Serving)

| | | | |
|---|---|---|---|
| Cal: 224 | Carbs: 13 g | Chol: 83 mg | Fat: 2.5 g |
| Fiber: 1.1 g | Protein: 36 g | Sodium: 283 mg | |

# French Herb Chicken

### Yield: 4 servings

4 bone-in skinless chicken breast halves (about 6 ounces each)

$\frac{1}{2}$ teaspoon garlic powder

$\frac{1}{2}$ teaspoon coarsely ground black pepper

$\frac{1}{4}$ teaspoon salt

4 medium-small unpeeled potatoes, quartered (about 12 ounces)

2 small yellow onions, quartered

2 medium carrots, peeled, halved lengthwise, and cut into 2-inch pieces

1 large stalk celery, cut into 1-inch pieces (include the leaves)

8 whole mushrooms

2 teaspoons dried rosemary

$\frac{1}{2}$ cup dry white wine or sherry

$\frac{1}{2}$ cup chicken broth

GRAVY

$\frac{1}{2}$ cup skim or 1% low-fat milk

3 tablespoons unbleached flour

1$\frac{1}{2}$ teaspoons instant chicken bouillon granules

1. Rinse the chicken, and pat it dry with paper towels. Rub both sides of the chicken with the garlic, and sprinkle with the pepper and salt.

2. Coat a large oven-proof nonstick skillet with nonstick olive oil cooking spray, and preheat over medium-high heat. Add the chicken to the skillet, and cook for 2 to 3 minutes on each side, or until nicely browned. Remove the skillet from the heat.

3. Remove the chicken from the skillet, and set aside. Arrange the vegetables over the bottom of the skillet, and top with the chicken. Sprinkle with the rosemary, and pour the wine and broth over the top. Cover the skillet with aluminum foil, and bake at 350°F for about 55 minutes, or until the vegetables are tender and the chicken is no longer pink inside. Transfer the chicken and vegetables to a serving platter, and cover the dish to keep warm.

4. Place the milk and flour in a jar with a tight-fitting lid, and shake until smooth. Place the skillet containing the pan juices over medium heat, add the bouillon granules, and bring to a boil. Slowly whisk in the milk mixture. Cook and stir for a minute or 2, or until thickened and bubbly. Serve the chicken and vegetables hot, accompanied by the gravy.

### NUTRITIONAL FACTS
#### (Per Serving)

| | | | |
|---|---|---|---|
| Cal: 329 | Carbs: 33 g | Chol: 82 mg | Fat: 2.3 g |
| Fiber: 4.3 g | Protein: 37 g | Sodium: 504 mg | |

# Italian Baked Chicken

### Yield: 4 servings

4 boneless skinless chicken breast halves (about 5 ounces each)

3/4 teaspoon dried Italian seasoning

1/2 teaspoon garlic powder, or 2 teaspoons crushed fresh garlic

1/4 teaspoon coarsely ground black pepper

1/4 teaspoon salt

1 can (14 1/2 ounces) Italian-style stewed tomatoes, undrained

2 tablespoons tomato paste

1 medium zucchini, halved lengthwise and sliced 3/4-inch thick

2 cups halved fresh mushrooms

1 medium yellow onion cut into 1/2-inch-thick wedges

1. Rinse the chicken, and pat it dry with paper towels. Place the Italian seasoning, garlic powder or garlic, pepper, and salt in a small bowl, and stir to mix well. Rub both sides of the chicken with the spice mixture.

2. Coat a large oven-proof nonstick skillet with nonstick olive oil cooking spray, and preheat over medium-high heat. Add the chicken to the skillet, and cook for 2 to 3 minutes on each side, or until nicely browned. Remove the skillet from the heat, and set aside.

3. Place the tomatoes and tomato paste in a large bowl, and stir to mix well. Add the zucchini, mushrooms, and onion, and stir to mix well. Spread the vegetable mixture over and around the chicken in the skillet.

**4.** Cover the skillet with aluminum foil, and bake at 350°F for about 35 minutes, or until the vegetables are tender and the chicken is no longer pink inside. Serve hot with brown rice or pasta, if desired.

## NUTRITIONAL FACTS
### (Per Serving)

| | | | |
|---|---|---|---|
| Cal: 220 | Carbs: 13 g | Chol: 82 mg | Fat: 2 g |
| Fiber: 3.4 g | Protein: 35 g | Sodium: 484 mg | |

# Baked Chicken Paprika

## Yield: 4 servings

4 bone-in skinless chicken breast halves (about 8 ounces each)

1/4 teaspoon salt

1/4 teaspoon ground black pepper

1/2 teaspoon garlic powder

1 medium-large Spanish onion, sliced and separated into rings

1 tablespoon ground paprika

1/4 cup plus 2 tablespoons tomato juice

SAUCE

2 teaspoons cornstarch

2 teaspoons chicken broth

1/2 cup nonfat sour cream

**1.** Rinse the chicken, and pat it dry with paper towels. Place the salt, pepper, and garlic powder in a small bowl, and stir to mix well. Rub both sides of the chicken with the spice mixture.

**2.** Coat a large nonstick oven-proof skillet with nonstick cooking spray, and preheat over medium-high heat. Place the chicken in the skillet, and cook for about 2 minutes on each side, or until nicely browned. Transfer the chicken to a plate, and set aside.

**3.** Arrange half of the onion rings over the bottom of the skillet, and sprinkle with 1 teaspoon of the paprika. Pour the tomato juice over the onions, and lay the chicken over the onions and tomato juice. Sprinkle 1 teaspoon of the remaining paprika over the chicken, top with the remaining onion rings, and sprinkle with the remaining paprika.

**4.** Cover the pan tightly with aluminum foil, and bake at 350°F for 40 minutes. Remove the foil, and bake for 20 additional minutes, or until the chicken is tender and no longer pink inside. Transfer the chicken and onions to a serving platter, and cover to keep warm.

**5.** Measure the pan juices; there should be 1 cup. Adjust the amount if necessary by adding chicken broth, and return the juices to the skillet.

**6.** Place the cornstarch and chicken broth in a small bowl, and stir to mix well. Add the mixture to the skillet. Stir the sour cream, and add it to the skillet mixture, whisking until smooth.

**7.** Place the skillet over medium heat, and cook, stirring constantly, for about 2 minutes, or until the mixture is thickened and bubbly. Transfer the sauce to a warmed gravy boat or pitcher, and serve hot with the chicken. Serve with noodles or brown rice if desired.

## NUTRITIONAL FACTS
### (Per Serving)

| | | | |
|---|---|---|---|
| Cal: 216 | Carbs: 12 g | Chol: 82 mg | Fat: 2.1 g |
| Fiber: 1.4 g | Protein: 35 g | Sodium: 316 mg | |

# Cajun Red Beans and Rice

### Yield: 5 servings

1 1/2 cups sliced smoked sausage or kielbasa, at least 97% lean (about 8 ounces)

1/3 cup chopped onion

1/3 cup chopped green bell pepper

1/3 cup chopped celery

3/4 teaspoon dried thyme

1 1/4 cups water or unsalted chicken broth

1 can (8 ounces) unsalted tomato sauce

1 1/2 cups quick-cooking brown rice

1 can (15 ounces) red kidney beans, drained

1. Coat a large nonstick skillet with nonstick cooking spray, and preheat over medium heat. Add the sausage, onion, bell pepper, celery, and thyme, and stir to mix. Cover and cook, stirring occasionally, for about 4 minutes, or until the vegetables begin to soften.

2. While the sausage and vegetables are cooking, place the water or broth and the tomato sauce in a medium-sized bowl, and stir to mix well.

3. Add the rice, beans, and tomato sauce mixture to the skillet, and stir to mix well. Increase the heat to medium-high, and allow the mixture to come to a boil. Reduce the heat to low, cover, and simmer without stirring for 10 minutes, or until the liquid is absorbed and the rice is tender. Remove the skillet from the heat, and let sit for 5 minutes before serving.

### NUTRITIONAL FACTS
(Per 1 1/2-cup serving)

Cal: 365    Carbs: 66 g    Chol: 22 mg    Fat: 3.1 g
Fiber: 12 g    Protein: 20.1 g    Sodium: 485 mg

# Down-Home Chicken and Dumplings

### Yield: 6 servings

1/2 cup skim or 1% low-fat milk

1/4 cup plus 2 tablespoons unbleached flour

3 cups chicken broth

1/4 teaspoon poultry seasoning

1/8 teaspoon ground white pepper

1 medium carrot, peeled, halved lengthwise, and sliced

1 stalk celery, thinly sliced (include the leaves)

1/2 cup chopped onion

2 cups diced cooked chicken breast (about 10 ounces)

1 cup frozen (thawed) green peas

DUMPLINGS

1 1/2 cups unbleached flour

2 teaspoons baking powder

1 teaspoon sugar

3/4 cup nonfat or low-fat buttermilk

1. Place the milk and flour in a jar with a tight-fitting lid, and shake until smooth. Set aside.

2. Place the broth, poultry seasoning, pepper, carrot, celery, and onion in a 4-quart pot or a large, deep nonstick skillet (at least 3-quart capacity), and bring to a boil over high heat. Reduce the heat to low, cover, and simmer for 5 minutes, or until the vegetables are almost tender.

3. Add the chicken and peas to the pot, and increase the heat to return the mixture to a boil. Reduce the heat to medium, shake the flour-milk mixture, and slowly pour it into the pot while stirring constantly. Cook and

stir for a minute or 2, or until the mixture is thickened and bubbly. Reduce the heat to low.

4. To make the dumplings, place the flour, baking powder, and sugar in a medium-sized bowl, and stir to mix well. Add the buttermilk, and stir just until moistened. Add a little more buttermilk if needed to make a thick batter.

5. Drop heaping teaspoonfuls of the batter onto the simmering stew. Cover and simmer over low heat for 10 to 12 minutes, or until the dumplings are fluffy and cooked through. Serve hot.

## NUTRITIONAL FACTS
### (Per 1 1/2-Cup Serving)

| Cal: 241 | Carbs: 36 g | Chol: 34 mg | Fat: 1.2 g |
|---|---|---|---|
| Fiber: 2.7 g | Protein: 20 g | Sodium: 591 mg | |

# Glazed Turkey Tenderloins

*For variety, substitute pork tenderloin for the turkey tenderloins.*

### Yield: 4 servings

2 turkey breast tenderloins (about 8 ounces each)

1/4 teaspoon garlic powder

1/4 teaspoon salt

1/4 teaspoon coarsely ground black pepper

1 teaspoon dried fines herbes* or dried rosemary

GLAZE

1/4 cup orange marmalade

1/4 cup chicken broth

1 tablespoon balsamic vinegar

1 1/2 teaspoons Dijon mustard

* A blend of thyme, oregano, sage, rosemary, marjoram, and basil, fines herbes can be found in the dried spice section of most grocery stores.

1. To make the glaze, place all of the glaze ingredients in a small bowl, and stir to mix well. Set aside.

2. Rinse the turkey, and pat it dry with paper towels. Cut each tenderloin crosswise into 4 slices to make 8 medallions. Using a meat mallet, pound each medallion to 1/4-inch thickness.

3. Place the garlic powder, salt, pepper, and fines herbes or rosemary in a small bowl, and stir to mix well. Rub some of the herb mixture over both sides of each medallion.

4. Coat a large nonstick skillet with nonstick cooking spray, and preheat over medium-high heat. Place the medallions in the skillet, and cook for about 2 minutes on each side, or until nicely browned and no longer pink inside. (Note that you will need to cook the medallions in 2 batches.) Transfer the medallions to a plate, and cover to keep warm.

5. Reduce the heat under the skillet to medium. Stir the glaze mixture, and pour it into the skillet. Cook, stirring constantly, for about 1 minute, or until the glaze is reduced by about a third and is thickened and bubbly.

6. Return the medallions to the skillet, and turn them in the glaze to coat well. Serve hot, accompanied by brown rice or whole wheat couscous, if desired.

## NUTRITIONAL FACTS
### (Per Serving)

| Cal: 181 | Carbs: 14 g | Chol: 70 mg | Fat: 1 g |
|---|---|---|---|
| Fiber: 0.1 g | Protein: 28 g | Sodium: 296 mg | |

# Szechuan Stir-Fry

## Yield: 4 servings

12 ounces boneless skinless chicken breast, shrimp, scallops, pork tenderloin, or beef top sirloin

3 cups broccoli florets

1 cup sliced fresh mushrooms

1 small yellow onion, cut into thin wedges

1 medium red bell pepper, cut into thin strips

1 can (8 ounces) sliced water chestnuts, bamboo shoots, or baby corn, drained

SAUCE

1 cup unsalted chicken broth*

3 tablespoons reduced-sodium soy sauce

2 tablespoons dry sherry

2 tablespoons dark brown sugar

1 tablespoon plus 1 teaspoon Szechuan seasoning**

2 teaspoons sesame oil

1 tablespoon plus 1 teaspoon cornstarch

\* If you are using beef, substitute beef broth for the chicken broth.

\*\* A mixture of ginger, garlic, pepper, and Asian seasonings, Szechuan seasoning can be found in the spice section of most grocery stores. Or combine 1 teaspoon ground ginger, 3/4 teaspoon dry mustard, 3/4 teaspoon lemon pepper, 1/2 teaspoon garlic powder, and 1/2 teaspoon crushed red pepper.

**1.** Rinse the chicken, seafood, or meat, and pat it dry with paper towels. If you are using chicken, pork, or beef, slice the meat across the grain into thin strips. (It is easiest to do this if the meat is partially frozen.) If you are using shrimp or scallops, leave them whole. Place in a shallow nonmetal container, and set aside.

**2.** Place all of the sauce ingredients except for the cornstarch in a small bowl, and stir to mix well. Pour 1/4 cup of the sauce over the chicken, seafood, pork, or beef. Toss to mix well, and set aside to marinate at room temperature for 20 minutes. Stir the cornstarch into the remaining sauce, and set aside.

**3.** Coat a large nonstick skillet or wok with nonstick cooking spray, and preheat over medium-high heat. Add the chicken, seafood, pork, or beef, along with the sauce it is marinating in, and stir-fry for about 4 minutes, or until all of the liquid has evaporated and the meat is thoroughly cooked and nicely browned. Transfer the meat to a medium-sized bowl, and cover to keep warm.

**4.** Respray the skillet with cooking spray, and add the broccoli, mushrooms, onion, and red pepper to the skillet. Stir-fry for about 3 minutes, or until the vegetables are crisp-tender. Cover the skillet periodically if it begins to dry out. (The steam from the cooking vegetables will moisten the skillet.) Add a few teaspoons of water only if needed.

**5.** Add the cooked meat or seafood and the water chestnuts, bamboo shoots, or corn to the skillet, and toss to mix well. Stir the sauce, and pour it over the meat and vegetables. Cook and stir for a minute or 2, or until the sauce thickens. Serve hot over brown rice or noodles, if desired.

## NUTRITIONAL FACTS
(Per 1 1/2-Cup Serving)

Cal: 223   Carbs: 22.6 g   Chol: 49 mg   Fat: 3.7 g
Fiber: 4.4 g   Protein: 24 g   Sodium: 461 mg

# Salsa and Spice Chili

## Yield: 8 servings

1 pound ground beef or turkey, at least 95% lean

1 can (14$\frac{1}{2}$ ounces) unsalted tomatoes

1 can (8 ounces) unsalted tomato sauce

1 cup bottled salsa, mild or medium

2 cans (15 ounces each) red kidney beans, drained

1 cup chopped onion

2 tablespoons chili powder

1 teaspoon dried oregano

$\frac{1}{2}$ teaspoon ground cumin

$\frac{1}{2}$ teaspoon ground cinnamon

TOPPINGS

$\frac{1}{2}$ cup shredded nonfat or reduced-fat Cheddar cheese

$\frac{1}{2}$ cup nonfat sour cream

$\frac{1}{2}$ cup chopped scallions

**1.** Coat a 3-quart pot with nonstick cooking spray, and preheat over medium heat. Add the ground beef or turkey, and cook, stirring to crumble, until the meat is no longer pink.

**2.** Add the tomatoes, tomato sauce, salsa, beans, onion, chili powder, oregano, cumin, and cinnamon to the pot, and stir to mix. Increase the heat to medium-high, and bring the mixture to a boil. Reduce the heat to low, cover, and simmer, stirring occasionally, for 25 to 30 minutes, or until the onions are soft and the flavors are well blended.

**3.** Serve hot, topping each serving with some of the cheese, sour cream, and scallions.

### NUTRITIONAL FACTS
(Per 1-Cup Serving Plus Toppings)

Cal: 259     Carbs: 32 g     Chol: 36 mg     Fat: 3 g
Fiber: 11 g   Protein: 25 g   Sodium: 260 mg

# Chili Macaroni Skillet

## Yield: 6 servings

1 pound 95% lean ground beef

1 can (14$\frac{1}{2}$ ounces) unsalted tomatoes, crushed

1 can (8 ounces) unsalted tomato sauce

1 can (15 ounces) kidney beans, drained

$\frac{1}{2}$ cup chopped onion

8 ounces ziti pasta (about 2$\frac{2}{3}$ cups)

2 cups water

1 tablespoon chili powder

2 teaspoons instant beef bouillon granules

$\frac{1}{2}$ teaspoon dried oregano

$\frac{1}{2}$ teaspoon ground cumin

**1.** Coat a large, deep nonstick skillet with nonstick cooking spray, and preheat over medium heat. Add the ground beef, and cook, stirring to crumble, until the meat is no longer pink.

**2.** Add all of the remaining ingredients to the skillet, and stir to mix well. Increase the heat to medium-high, and allow the mixture to come to a boil. Reduce the heat to low, cover, and simmer, stirring occasionally, for about 12 minutes, or until the ziti is tender and most of the liquid has been absorbed. Serve hot.

### NUTRITIONAL FACTS
(Per 1$\frac{1}{2}$-Cup Serving)

Cal: 360     Carbs: 51 g     Chol: 46 mg     Fat: 3.9 g
Fiber: 9.5 g   Protein: 29 g   Sodium: 464 mg

# Garden Meat Loaf

*"Lean" meat loaf pans are great for low-fat cooking. These pans have a perforated inner liner that allows the fat to drain into the bottom of the pan instead of being reabsorbed into the meat.*

### Yield: 8 servings

1 pound 95% lean ground beef

1 cup frozen (thawed) meatless burger-style recipe crumbles or Tofu Crumbles

$\frac{1}{2}$ cup finely chopped onion

$\frac{1}{2}$ cup finely chopped green bell pepper

$\frac{1}{2}$ cup finely shredded carrots

$\frac{3}{4}$ cup quick-cooking oats

$\frac{1}{4}$ cup plus 2 tablespoons fat-free egg substitute

$1\frac{1}{2}$ teaspoons dried thyme

$1\frac{1}{2}$ teaspoons dried sage

$1\frac{1}{2}$ teaspoons crushed fresh garlic

$\frac{1}{2}$ teaspoon ground black pepper

$\frac{1}{2}$ cup canned vegetable juice, like V-8 vegetable juice

$\frac{1}{2}$ cup ketchup

**1.** Place all of the ingredients except for the ketchup in a large bowl, and mix well. Coat a 9-x-5-inch meat loaf pan with nonstick cooking spray, and press the mixture into the pan to form a loaf.

**2.** Bake uncovered at 350°F for 45 minutes. Spread the ketchup over the top of the loaf, and bake for 30 additional minutes, or until the meat is no longer pink inside or an instant-read thermometer inserted in the center of the loaf reads 160°F.

**3.** Remove the loaf from the oven, and let sit for 10 minutes before slicing and serving.

### NUTRITIONAL FACTS
#### (Per Serving)

| | | | |
|---|---|---|---|
| Cal: 151 | Carbs: 13 g | Chol: 30 mg | Fat: 3.1 g |
| Fiber: 2.4 g | Protein: 17.2 g | Sodium: 287 mg | |

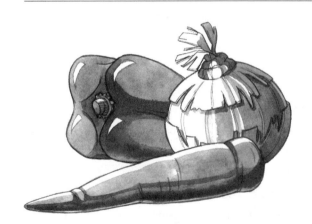

## Sneaking in Soy

*Looking for a way to get more nutritious soy into your diet? Try substituting Tofu Crumbles, texturized vegetable protein (TVP), or frozen meatless recipe crumbles for part or all of the meat in any of the ground-beef recipes in this chapter. In addition to reducing both the fat content and the cholesterol content of your dish, this simple strategy will add health-promoting isoflavones and other nutrients. Just follow the guidelines for substitution presented on page 55, and replace up to half the ground meat in most recipes with little or no detectable difference in flavor or texture.*

# Roasted Eggplant Lasagna

## Yield: 8 servings

2 large eggplants (1 pound each)

1 tablespoon plus 1 teaspoon balsamic vinegar

Ground black pepper

Nonstick olive oil cooking spray

2 tablespoons grated nonfat or regular Parmesan cheese

1 cup shredded nonfat or reduced-fat mozzarella cheese

### CHEESE FILLING

3 cups nonfat ricotta cheese

$\frac{1}{3}$ cup grated nonfat or regular Parmesan cheese

$\frac{1}{4}$ cup fat-free egg substitute

$\frac{1}{4}$ cup finely chopped fresh parsley

### SAUCE

12 ounces 95% lean ground beef

1 cup chopped onion

2 teaspoons crushed fresh garlic

1 can (14$\frac{1}{2}$ ounces) unsalted tomatoes, crushed

$\frac{1}{2}$ cup tomato paste

$\frac{1}{2}$ cup dry red wine or beef broth

2 teaspoons dried oregano

2 teaspoons instant beef bouillon granules

1. Trim the ends off the eggplants, and slice them into $\frac{1}{2}$-inch rounds. Brush both sides of the eggplant slices lightly with the balsamic vinegar, and sprinkle lightly with the pepper.

2. Coat a large nonstick baking sheet with the olive oil cooking spray, and arrange the slices in a single layer on the sheet. Spray the tops lightly with the cooking spray, and bake at 450°F for 10 minutes. Turn and bake for 5 additional minutes, or until nicely browned and tender. Remove from the oven and set aside.

3. To make the cheese filling, place all of the filling ingredients in a medium-sized bowl, and stir to mix well. Set aside.

4. To make the sauce, spray a large nonstick skillet with nonstick cooking spray, and preheat over medium heat. Add the beef, and cook, stirring to crumble, until the meat is no longer pink.

5. Add all of the remaining sauce ingredients to the skillet, and stir to mix. Increase the heat to high, and allow the mixture to come to a boil. Reduce the heat to low, cover, and simmer, stirring occasionally, for about 15 minutes, or until the onions are tender. Remove the skillet from the heat, and set aside.

6. To assemble the lasagna, coat a 9-x-13-inch pan with nonstick cooking spray. Arrange half of the eggplant slices over the bottom of the pan in a single layer. Top with half of the cheese filling and half of the sauce. Repeat the eggplant, cheese, and sauce layers. Sprinkle with the 2 tablespoons of Parmesan.

7. Bake uncovered at 350°F for about 35 minutes, or until bubbly around the edges. Top with the mozzarella, and bake for 10 additional minutes, or until the cheese is melted. Remove the dish from the oven, and let sit for 5 minutes before cutting into squares and serving.

## NUTRITIONAL FACTS
### (Per Serving)

| | | | |
|---|---|---|---|
| Cal: 256 | Carbs: 24 g | Chol: 40 mg | Fat: 2 g |
| Fiber: 4.4 g | Protein: 34 g | Sodium: 541 mg | |

## Presto Paella

### Yield: 5 servings

2 cups reduced-sodium chicken broth

1/2 teaspoon loosely packed saffron threads

8 ounces cleaned raw shrimp or scallops

1 1/4 cups sliced smoked sausage or kielbasa, at least 97% lean (about 6 ounces)

1/2 cup chopped green bell pepper

1/2 cup chopped onion

1 teaspoon crushed fresh garlic

1/2 teaspoon dried thyme

1/2 teaspoon dried oregano

2 cups quick-cooking brown rice

1 cup frozen (thawed) green peas

1. Place the broth and saffron in a blender, and process until the saffron is finely ground and the broth turns bright yellow. Set aside.

2. Rinse the seafood, and pat it dry with paper towels. Set aside.

3. Coat a large nonstick skillet with nonstick cooking spray, and preheat over medium-high heat. Add the sausage, green pepper, onion, garlic, thyme, and oregano. Stir-fry for about 4 minutes, or just until the sausage nicely browned and the vegetables begin to soften. Cover the skillet periodically if it begins to dry out. (The steam from the cooking vegetables will moisten the skillet.)

4. Add the rice, tomatoes, shrimp or scallops, and broth mixture to the skillet. Stir to mix well, and bring the mixture to a boil. Reduce the heat to low, cover, and simmer without stirring for about 7 minutes.

5. Add the peas to the skillet, and stir to mix. Cover and cook for 3 additional minutes, or until the liquid is absorbed and the rice is tender. Remove the skillet from the heat, and let sit covered for 5 minutes before serving.

### NUTRITIONAL FACTS
(Per 1 1/3-Cup Serving)

Cal: 274    Carbs: 44 g    Chol: 79 mg    Fat: 2.7 g
Fiber: 4.1 g    Protein: 20 g    Sodium: 575 mg

## Shrimp Fried Rice

*For variety, substitute diced skinless chicken breast or pork tenderloin for the shrimp.*

### Yield: 4 servings

1–2 teaspoons sesame oil

1 cup diced cleaned raw shrimp (about 6 ounces)

1/2 cup thinly sliced scallions

1/2 cup thinly sliced celery

1 teaspoon dark brown sugar

3 1/2 cups cooked brown rice

3/4 cup frozen (thawed) green peas

3 tablespoons reduced-sodium soy sauce

1/2 cup fat-free egg substitute

1. Coat a large nonstick skillet with nonstick cooking spray. Add the sesame oil, and preheat over medium-high heat. Add the shrimp, and stir-fry for about 3 minutes, or until the shrimp turn opaque and are thoroughly cooked.

2. Add the scallions, celery, and brown sugar to the skillet, and stir-fry for about 2 minutes, or until the vegetables are crisp-tender. Cover the skillet periodically if it begins to dry out. (The steam from the cooking vegetables will moisten the skillet.) Add a few teaspoons of water or broth to the skillet only if necessary.

3. Add the rice, peas, and soy sauce to the skillet, and stir-fry for about 1 minute, or just until the mixture is heated through. Add a few teaspoons of water or broth if the skillet becomes too dry.

4. Make a well in the center of the skillet mixture, and respray the center of the skillet lightly. Add the egg substitute. Reduce the heat to medium, and let the eggs cook without stirring for a couple of minutes, or just until set. Gently stir the cooked eggs into the rice mixture, and serve immediately.

### NUTRITIONAL FACTS
(Per 1½-Cup Serving)

| Cal: 288 | Carbs: 48 g | Chol: 60 mg | Fat: 3 g |
|---|---|---|---|
| Fiber: 5.3 g | Protein: 17 g | Sodium: 422 mg | |

# Dilled Salmon Burgers

### Yield: 4 servings

Nonstick cooking spray
4 multigrain burger buns
4 slices tomato
4 leaves lettuce

BURGERS
1½ slices whole wheat or multigrain bread
2 cans (6½ ounces each) water-packed boneless skinless pink salmon

2 egg whites, or ¼ cup fat-free egg substitute
2 tablespoons finely chopped fresh parsley
2 tablespoons finely chopped onion
¼ teaspoon dried dill
¼ teaspoon coarsely ground black pepper

DRESSING
3 tablespoons nonfat or reduced-fat mayonnaise
2 tablespoons nonfat sour cream
¼ teaspoon dried dill

1. To make the dressing, place all of the dressing ingredients in a small bowl, and stir to mix well. Set aside.

2. To make the burgers, tear the bread into pieces, place in a blender or food processor, and process into fine crumbs. Measure the crumbs; there should be ¾ cup. Adjust the amount if necessary.

3. Place the bread crumbs and all of the remaining burger ingredients in a medium-sized bowl, and stir to mix well. Shape the mixture into 4 (4-inch) patties.

4. Coat a large nonstick skillet with nonstick cooking spray, and preheat over medium heat. Cook the burgers for about 3 minutes, or until the bottoms are nicely browned. Spray the tops of the burgers lightly with the cooking spray, turn, and cook for 3 additional minutes, or until the burgers are nicely browned on the second side.

5. To serve, place each salmon burger on the bottom half of a bun. Top with some of the dressing, 1 slice of tomato, 1 lettuce leaf, and the remaining bun half. Serve hot.

### NUTRITIONAL FACTS
(Per Serving)

| Cal: 321 | Carbs: 35 g | Chol: 65 mg | Fat: 5.3 g |
|---|---|---|---|
| Fiber: 4.4 g | Protein: 33 g | Sodium: 527 mg | |

# *Fast and Flavorful Spice Rubs*

*Bursting with flavor, spice rubs can transform bland and boring meat, seafood, and poultry into delicious culinary creations—without adding a lot of fat or salt to your meal.*

*To apply the rub, rinse the food and pat it dry with paper towels. Then, using your fingers, rub the outside surface of the meat with the seasoning blend. If you have time, allow the food to stand at room temperature for fifteen to thirty minutes before cooking. This will enable the seasonings to permeate the food. (Refrigerate if you are going to let the food stand for more than 1 hour.) Spray the food lightly with nonstick cooking spray, and grill, broil, or roast, as desired. Then enjoy great flavor without added fat!*

*The following recipes will remain flavorful for several months, so make a double or triple batch of your favorite rubs, and store the mixtures in airtight containers so that you'll always have a supply on hand. Note that each of the following recipes will make enough rub to season 2 pounds of meat, poultry, or seafood.*

## Cajun Spice Rub

### Yield: about 5 tablespoons

1 $1/2$ tablespoons ground paprika
1 tablespoon light brown sugar
1 $1/2$ teaspoons garlic powder
1 teaspoon onion powder
1 teaspoon dried thyme
1 teaspoon dried oregano
$3/4$ teaspoon ground black pepper
$3/4$ teaspoon cayenne pepper
$1/2$ teaspoon salt

1. Place all of the ingredients in a small bowl, and stir to mix well.
2. Apply the rub according to the directions given above, and grill, broil, or roast the meat as desired.

### NUTRITIONAL FACTS
(Per $2^1/_2$-Teaspoon Serving)

| Cal: 16 | Carbs: 3.6 g | Chol: 0 mg | Fat: 0.2 g |
|---|---|---|---|
| Fiber: 0.6 g | Protein: 0.4 g | Sodium: 79 mg | |

## Lemon-Herb Rub

### Yield: about 5 tablespoons

2 tablespoons dried crushed oregano or thyme
1 tablespoon dried grated lemon rind
1 tablespoon light brown sugar
$3/4$ teaspoon coarsely ground black pepper
$3/4$ teaspoon garlic powder
$1/2$ teaspoon salt

1. Place all of the ingredients in a small bowl, and stir to mix well.
2. Apply the rub according to the directions given above, and grill, broil, or roast the meat as desired.

### NUTRITIONAL FACTS
(Per $2^1/_2$-Teaspoon Serving)

| Cal: 12 | Carbs: 2.9 g | Chol: 0 mg | Fat: 0.1 g |
|---|---|---|---|
| Fiber: 0.6 g | Protein: 0.2 g | Sodium: 156 mg | |

## Spicy Tex-Mex Rub

### Yield: about 5 tablespoons

1 tablespoon chili powder
1 tablespoon ground paprika
1 tablespoon light brown sugar
2 teaspoons lemon pepper
1 teaspoon ground cumin
$1/2$ teaspoon garlic powder
$1/4$ teaspoon salt

1. Place all of the ingredients in a small bowl, and stir to mix well.
2. Apply the rub according to the directions given above, and grill, broil, or roast the meat as desired.

### NUTRITIONAL FACTS
(Per $2^1/_2$-Teaspoon Serving)

| Cal: 15 | Carbs: 3.1 g | Chol: 0 mg | Fat: 0.2 g |
|---|---|---|---|
| Fiber: 0.5 g | Protein: 0.2 g | Sodium: 47 mg | |

# Savory Stuffed Fish

## Yield: 4 servings

4 long, thin fish fillets (4 ounces each), such as flounder, sole, or orange roughy
Nonstick butter-flavored cooking spray
Ground paprika

STUFFING
3 slices whole wheat or multigrain bread
1/4 cup finely chopped onion
1/4 cup finely chopped celery
3/4 teaspoon lemon pepper
1/4 teaspoon dried thyme
1/4 cup chicken broth, divided
3/4 cup finely chopped cooked crab meat, or 1 can (6 ounces) crab meat, drained

1. Rinse the fish, and pat it dry with paper towels. Set aside.

2. To make the stuffing, tear the bread into pieces, place in a blender or food processor, and process into coarse crumbs. Measure the crumbs; there should be 1 1/2 cups. Adjust the amount if necessary, and set aside.

3. Coat a large nonstick skillet with nonstick cooking spray, and preheat over medium heat. Add the onion, celery, lemon pepper, thyme, and 1 tablespoon of the broth, and stir to mix. Cover and cook, stirring occasionally, for about 3 minutes, or until the vegetables are tender. Add a little more, broth to the skillet if it becomes too dry.

4. Remove the skillet from the heat, and toss the bread crumbs and crab meat into the vegetable mixture. Gently toss in the remaining broth, 1 tablespoon at a time, until the

mixture is moist but not wet, and holds together nicely. Add a little more broth or water if needed.

5. Arrange the fish fillets on a flat surface, and spread a quarter of the stuffing over the bottom half of each fillet, gently pressing the stuffing onto the fish so that it holds together. Fold the tops over to enclose the filling, and secure each fillet with a wooden toothpick.

6. Coat a 9-inch nonstick square pan with nonstick cooking spray, and arrange the fillets in the pan. Spray the top of each fillet lightly with the cooking spray, and sprinkle with the paprika. Bake uncovered at 400°F for 20 minutes, or until the fish flakes easily with a fork. Serve hot.

## NUTRITIONAL FACTS
(Per Serving)

Cal: 184    Carbs: 11 g    Chol: 71 mg    Fat: 2.6 g
Fiber: 1.9 g    Protein: 28 g    Sodium: 306 mg

# Grilled Lemon-Herb Fish

*For variety, substitute Cajun Spice Rub (page 163) for the Lemon-Herb Rub.*

## Yield: 4 servings

6 firm-fleshed fish steaks (5 ounces each), such as tuna, salmon, mahi-mahi, grouper, or amberjack
1 recipe Lemon-Herb rub (page 163)
Nonstick olive oil or butter-flavored cooking spray

1. Rinse the fish, and pat it dry with paper towels. Coat both sides of each fish steak with some of the rub, and set aside for 15 to 30 minutes.

2. Spray the steaks lightly with the cooking spray, and cook, covered, over medium coals or broil 6 inches under a preheated broiler for 5 minutes on each side, or until the meat is easily flaked with a fork. Serve hot.

## NUTRITIONAL FACTS
### (Per Serving)

Cal: 170    Carb: 3.6 g    Chol: 63 mg    Fat: 1.7 g
Fiber: 0.7 g    Protein: 33 g    Sodium: 247 mg

# Tempting Tuna Skillet

### Yield: 5 servings

$^1/_2$ cup plus 2 tablespoons chopped fresh mushrooms

$^1/_4$ cup plus 2 tablespoons finely chopped onion

$^1/_4$ teaspoon dried thyme

8 ounces seashell pasta (about 3 cups)

2$^1/_2$ cups reduced-sodium chicken broth

1$^1/_4$ cups skim or 1% low-fat milk, divided

1 tablespoon plus 1$^1/_2$ teaspoons cornstarch

$^1/_8$ teaspoon ground white pepper

3 tablespoons instant nonfat dry milk powder

$^3/_4$ cup frozen (thawed) green peas

3 ounces nonfat or reduced-fat process Cheddar cheese or reduced-fat Cheddar cheese, shredded or diced (about $^3/_4$ cup)

1 can (12 ounces) water-packed albacore tuna, drained

1. Spray a large deep nonstick skillet with nonstick cooking spray, and preheat over medium heat. Add the mushrooms, onion, and thyme, and stir to mix. Cover and cook, stirring occasionally, for about 3 minutes, or until the vegetables are tender. Add a little water or broth if the skillet becomes too dry.

2. Add the pasta and the broth to the skillet, stir to mix, and increase the heat slightly to bring the mixture to a boil. Reduce the heat to medium-low, cover, and simmer, stirring occasionally, for about 9 minutes, or until the pasta is almost al dente and most of the liquid has been absorbed.

3. While the pasta is cooking, place 2 tablespoons of the milk and all of the cornstarch and pepper in a small bowl. Stir to dissolve the cornstarch, and set aside.

4. Add the remaining 1$^1/_8$ cups of milk the milk powder, and the peas to the skillet, and stir to mix. Increase the heat to medium, and bring the mixture to a boil, stirring frequently. Stir the cornstarch mixture, and add it to the skillet. Cook and stir for a minute or 2, or until the sauce is slightly thickened and bubbly.

5. Reduce the heat to medium-low. Add the cheese to the skillet, and continue to cook, stirring frequently, for a minute or 2, or until the cheese melts.

6. Stir the tuna into the skillet mixture, and cook for another minute, or until the tuna is heated through. Add a little more milk if the mixture seems too dry. Serve hot.

## NUTRITIONAL FACTS
### (Per 1$^1/_3$-Cup Serving)

Cal: 351    Carbs: 44 g    Chol: 31 mg    Fat: 2.6 g
Fiber: 2.7 g    Protein: 35 g    Sodium: 498 mg

## *Fish Is the Dish*

*Fish has long been associated with a reduced risk of heart disease. And a 1997 study added to the evidence, further supporting the health benefits of fish. In this study, researchers discovered that men who eat on average at least 35 grams (about 1¼ ounces) of fish per day are about 40 percent less likely to die of heart disease than are men who eat no fish at all.*

*How does fish protect against heart disease?*

*The omega-3 fatty acids in fish help prevent deadly blood clots from forming, reduce blood pressure, reduce blood triglycerides, and prevent abnormal heart rhythms that can lead to heart attack. And when you eat fish instead of fatty meats like prime rib and pork chops, you trim saturated fat from your diet—which adds to the benefits. So to maximize your health, be sure to include fish in your diet several times a week.*

# Crispy Oven-Fried Fish

### Yield: 4 servings

1 pound cod, grouper, orange roughy, or other white fish fillets, cut into 4 equal pieces

¼ cup plus 2 tablespoons fat-free egg substitute

½ cup corn flake crumbs or dried bread crumbs

1 teaspoon ground paprika

1–2 teaspoons lemon pepper

Nonstick cooking spray

TANGY TARTAR SAUCE

¼ cup nonfat or reduced-fat mayonnaise

2–3 teaspoons sweet pickle relish

2 teaspoons finely chopped onion

¼ teaspoon dry mustard

1. To make the tartar sauce, place all of the sauce ingredients in a small bowl, and stir to mix well. Cover and chill while you prepare the fish.

2. Rinse the fish, and pat it dry with paper towels. Set aside.

3. Place the egg substitute in a shallow bowl. Place the corn flake or bread crumbs, paprika, and lemon pepper in another shallow bowl, and stir to mix well.

4. Dip the fish pieces first in the egg substitute and then in the crumb mixture, turning to coat both sides well.

5. Coat a medium-sized baking sheet with nonstick cooking spray, and arrange the fish pieces on the sheet in a single layer. Spray the tops lightly with the cooking spray, and bake at 450°F for about 15 minutes, or until the outside is crisp and golden and the fish flakes easily with a fork. Serve hot, accompanied by the tartar sauce.

### NUTRITIONAL FACTS
#### (Per Serving)

| Cal: 159 | Carbs: 13 g | Chol: 48 mg | Fat: 0.7 g |
|---|---|---|---|
| Fiber: 0.4 g | Protein: 23 g | Sodium: 357 mg | |

# Mediterranean Foil-Baked Fish

### Yield: 4 servings

4 firm-fleshed fish fillets or steaks (5 ounces each), such as orange roughy, grouper, tuna, mahi-mahi, or salmon

2 teaspoons lemon pepper

12 thin slices tomato

12 thin slices onion

$1/4$ cup sliced black olives

2 tablespoons fresh dill, or 2 teaspoons dried

1. Rinse the fish, and pat it dry with paper towels.

2. Coat four 12-x-12-inch pieces of aluminum foil with nonstick olive oil cooking spray, and center a fish fillet on the lower half of each piece. Sprinkle $1/2$ teaspoon of the lemon pepper over each fillet. Top each fillet with 3 of the tomato slices, 3 of the onion slices, and a tablespoon of olives. Sprinkle a quarter of the dill over the top.

3. Fold the upper half of the foil over the fish to meet the bottom half. Seal the edges together by making a tight $1/2$-inch fold; then fold again to double-seal. Allow space for heat circulation and expansion. Use this technique to seal the remaining sides.

4. Arrange the pouches on a baking sheet, and bake at 450°F for about 18 minutes, or until the fish is opaque and the thickest part is easily flaked with a fork. Open each packet by carefully cutting an "X" in the top of the foil (steam will escape), and serve hot.

### NUTRITIONAL FACTS
(Per Serving)

Cal: 171    Carbs: 13 g    Chol: 28 mg    Fat: 3.1 g
Fiber: 2.8 g    Protein: 23 g    Sodium: 295 mg

# 11.

# Meatless Main Dishes

What's one of the best ways to get the fat and cholesterol out of your diet, and at the same time boost your intake of fiber and other health-promoting nutrients? Eat more meatless meals! The vegetables, soy products, legumes, and grains featured in vegetarian cuisine are naturally free of cholesterol, low in saturated fat, and rich in fiber. And, as vegetarians have long known, these foods are also powerful preventive medicines against cancer, heart disease, high blood pressure, obesity, and many other health problems.

There is one small catch, though. Vegetarian meals that are made with whole-milk cheeses, full-fat sour cream, and other high-fat dairy products are no more healthful than meat-based meals. If this is difficult to believe, consider this: Just one ounce of full-fat cheese, such as Cheddar, contains more than twice as much fat as a three-ounce serving of top beef round. The solution? Simply replace full-fat milk, cheese, sour cream, and other dairy products with their low- or no-fat counterparts. By doing this—as well as making a few other simple recipe adjustments—you can enjoy healthy versions of many of your meatless favorites, including crusty pizzas and cheese-topped burritos. And by adding ultra-lean meat alternatives to your pantry, you can even make luscious burgers, spicy sloppy Joes, and tempting tacos—all with just a fraction of the fat that's usually found in these dishes.

Can you get all the protein you need without eating meat? Most definitely. Properly planned vegetarian meals that feature beans, tofu, grains, nonfat or low-fat dairy products, and egg whites or fat-free egg substitutes provide all the protein you need to support your immune system and help maintain muscles—without providing the protein overload that can contribute to health problems like osteoporosis.

So if you're trying to eliminate meat from your diet—or if you simply want a change from the usual lunch and dinner fare—you've come to the right place. In the following pages, a variety of taste-tempting recipes will prove to you once and for all that dishes made without meat can be not only healthful and low in fat, but also absolutely delicious.

# Spicy Lentils and Rice

## Yield: 4 servings

$^3/_4$ cup brown lentils, cleaned (page 102)

$1^3/_4$ cups plus 2 tablespoons vegetable or chicken broth, divided

$1^1/_2$ cups coarsely chopped fresh mushrooms

1 medium yellow onion, chopped

2 teaspoons curry paste

$1^1/_2$ teaspoons crushed fresh garlic

$^1/_2$ teaspoon ground cumin

$^1/_2$ teaspoon ground ginger

$2^1/_2$ cups cooked brown rice

$^3/_4$ cup frozen (thawed) green peas

1. Place the lentils and $1^1/_2$ cups of the broth in a $1^1/_2$-quart pot, and bring to a boil over high heat. Reduce the heat to low, cover, and simmer for about 20 minutes, or until the lentils are tender and the liquid is absorbed. Set aside.

2. Coat a large nonstick skillet with nonstick cooking spray, and preheat over medium heat. Add the mushrooms, onions, curry paste, garlic, cumin, ginger, and 2 tablespoons of the broth. Cover and cook, stirring occasionally, for about 4 minutes, or until the onions and mushrooms are tender.

3. Add the rice, peas, lentils, and remaining $^1/_4$ cup of broth to the skillet, and stir to mix. Cook over medium heat, stirring frequently, for about 3 minutes, or until well mixed and heated through. Serve hot.

## NUTRITIONAL FACTS
### (Per $1^1/_3$-Cup Serving)

| | | | |
|---|---|---|---|
| Cal: 313 | Carbs: 56 g | Chol: 0 mg | Fat: 2.9 g |
| Fiber: 9.4 g | Protein: 15.6 g | Sodium: 322 mg | |

# Curried Vegetable Stew

## Yield: 8 cups

1 can (19 ounces) chickpeas, rinsed and drained, or 2 cups cooked chickpeas, divided

$1^1/_2$ cups vegetable or chicken broth, divided

2 cups $^1/_2$-inch cubes white potatoes or butternut squash

2 cups small cauliflower florets

1 cup sliced fresh mushrooms

1 can ($14^1/_2$ ounces) unsalted stewed tomatoes, crushed

2–3 teaspoons curry paste

1 cup frozen (thawed) green peas

1. Place $^1/_2$ cup of the chickpeas and $^1/_2$ cup of the broth in a blender, and process until smooth. Set aside.

2. Place the remaining chickpeas, the remaining broth, and the potatoes or squash, cauliflower, mushrooms, tomatoes with their juice, and curry paste in a 3-quart pot, and bring to a boil over high heat. Reduce the heat to medium-low, cover, and cook, stirring occasionally, for 20 minutes, or until the potatoes or squash and the cauliflower are tender.

3. Add the peas and the chickpea-broth mixture to the pot, and stir to mix. Cover and simmer for 5 to 10 additional minutes, or until the mixture is heated through and the flavors are well blended. Serve hot over whole wheat couscous, brown rice, or pasta, if desired.

## NUTRITIONAL FACTS
### (Per 1-Cup Serving)

| | | | |
|---|---|---|---|
| Cal: 138 | Carbs: 24 g | Chol: 0 mg | Fat: 2 g |
| Fiber: 4.3 g | Protein: 7 g | Sodium: 304 mg | |

# Vegetable-Brown Rice Curry

Yield: 5 servings

1 1/2 cups small cauliflower florets

1 cup finely chopped peeled tomatoes (about 1 1/2 medium)

3/4 cup chopped onion

1/2 cup finely chopped carrot

2–3 teaspoons curry paste

2 teaspoons crushed fresh garlic

1/2 teaspoon ground ginger

1/4 teaspoon salt

2 tablespoons vegetable or chicken broth

4 cups cooked brown rice

1 can (15 ounces) red kidney beans, rinsed and drained, or 1 recipe Crispy Tofu Cubes (page 180)

3/4 cup frozen (thawed) green peas

1. Place the cauliflower, tomatoes, onion, carrot, curry paste, garlic, ginger, salt, and broth in a large nonstick skillet. Cover and cook over medium heat, stirring occasionally, for 5 to 7 minutes, or until the vegetables are tender. Add a little more broth if the skillet becomes too dry.

2. Add the rice, beans or tofu, and peas to the skillet. Cook and stir over medium heat until the mixture is heated through, and serve hot.

## NUTRITIONAL FACTS
### (Per 1 2/3-Cup Serving)

| Cal: 318 | Carbs: 61 g | Chol: 0 mg | Fat: 3g |
|---|---|---|---|
| Fiber: 12.4 g | Protein: 12 g | Sodium: 382 mg | |

# Roasted Ratatouille

Yield: 4 servings

1 1/3 cups brown rice

3 1/3 cups water

1 pound fresh plum tomatoes, quartered lengthwise (about 6 medium)

2 cups 3/4-inch cubes peeled eggplant (about 1 small)

1 medium-large zucchini, halved lengthwise and sliced 1/2-inch thick

1 medium green bell pepper, cut into 1/2-inch-thick strips

1 medium yellow onion, cut into 1/2-inch-thick wedges

2 teaspoons crushed fresh garlic

3/4 teaspoon dried thyme

1/2 teaspoon salt

1/8 teaspoon ground black pepper

1 tablespoon balsamic vinegar

1 tablespoon extra virgin olive oil

1/2 cup crumbled nonfat or reduced-fat feta cheese

1. Place the rice and water in a 2 1/2-quart nonstick pot, and bring to a boil over high heat. Stir, reduce the heat to low, and cover. Allow to simmer for 45 to 50 minutes, or until the water is absorbed and the rice is tender. Do not stir during cooking.

2. While the rice is cooking, place the vegetables, garlic, thyme, salt, pepper, vinegar, and the olive oil in a large bowl, and toss to mix well.

3. Coat a 9-x-13-inch nonstick roasting pan with nonstick olive oil cooking spray, and spread the mixture evenly in the pan. Cover the pan with aluminum foil.

4. Bake at 450°F for 15 minutes. Then remove the foil and bake for 15 additional minutes. Turn the vegetables, and bake for 15 minutes more, or until the tomatoes are soft and the vegetables are nicely browned.

5. Place 1 cup of rice on each of 4 serving plates, and top with 1 cup of the vegetable mixture. Serve hot, topping each serving with 2 tablespoons of the feta cheese.

## NUTRITIONAL FACTS
### (Per Serving)

| Cal: 352 | Carbs: 59 g | Chol: 1 mg | Fat: 5.7 g |
|---|---|---|---|
| Fiber: 7 g | Protein: 10.8 g | Sodium: 548 mg | |

# Roasted Vegetable Sandwiches

### Yield: 4 servings

2 medium-large zucchini, each diagonally cut into 8 ($^3/_8$-inch) slices

2 Portabella mushrooms, each cut into 8 ($^1/_2$-inch) slices

2 medium red bell peppers, each cut into 6 (1$^1/_2$-inch) strips

1 medium-large Spanish or red onion, cut into 8 ($^3/_8$-inch) slices

Nonstick olive oil cooking spray

1 teaspoon dried fines herbs* or dried Italian seasoning

$^1/_4$ teaspoon salt

4 whole wheat submarine-sandwich rolls (6 inches each)

4 ounces nonfat or reduced-fat mozzarella or provolone cheese, thinly sliced

$^1/_4$ cup crumbled nonfat or reduced-fat feta cheese

2 tablespoons plus 2 teaspoons bottled fat-free balsamic vinaigrette or Italian salad dressing

\* A blend of thyme, oregano, sage, rosemary, marjoram, and basil, fines herbes can be found in the dried spice section of most grocery stores.

1. Coat a large baking sheet with olive oil cooking spray, and arrange the vegetables in a single layer on the sheet. Spray the vegetables lightly with the cooking spray, and sprinkle with the herbs and salt.

2. Bake uncovered at 450°F degrees for 12 minutes. Turn the vegetables, and bake for 8 additional minutes, or until tender and nicely browned. Remove the vegetables from the oven, and set aside.

3. Split the rolls in half, and place the halves on a large baking sheet, cut sides up. Place under a preheated broiler, and broil for a minute or 2, or until lightly toasted. Place the bottom half of each roll on an individual serving plate, and set aside. Lay 1 ounce of the mozzarella or provolone cheese on the inside of the top half of each roll, and return the rolls to the broiler for about 1 minute, or until the cheese is melted.

4. Layer 4 zucchini slices, 4 mushroom slices, 3 red pepper strips, and 2 onion slices on the bottom half of each roll. Sprinkle with 1 tablespoon of the feta cheese and 2 teaspoons of the dressing. Place the top half of the roll, cheese side down, over the vegetables, and serve hot.

## NUTRITIONAL FACTS
### (Per Serving)

| Cal: 310 | Carbs: 49 g | Chol: 0 mg | Fat: 2.9 g |
|---|---|---|---|
| Fiber: 6.1 g | Protein: 22 g | Sodium: 696 mg | |

# Portabella Mushroom Sandwiches

## Yield: 4 servings

Nonstick olive oil cooking spray

20 slices (each $3/4$-inch thick) Portabella mushroom (about 4 medium-large)

$1/8$ teaspoon salt

$1/8$ teaspoon coarsely ground black pepper

$1/2$ teaspoon dried fines herbes* or dried Italian seasoning

4 sourdough rolls, onion rolls, or multigrain burger buns (2 ounces each)

4 ounces nonfat or reduced-fat mozzarella or provolone cheese, sliced

### TOPPINGS

$1/4$ cup nonfat or low-fat mayonnaise

4 teaspoons Dijon mustard

4 slices red onion

4 slices tomato

12 tender fresh spinach or arugula leaves

\* A blend of thyme, oregano, sage, rosemary, marjoram, and basil, fines herbes can be found in the dried spice section of most grocery stores.

1. Coat a large baking sheet with the cooking spray, and arrange the mushrooms in a single layer on the sheet. Spray the tops of the mushrooms lightly with the cooking spray, and sprinkle with the salt, pepper, and herbs.

2. Bake uncovered at 450°F for 10 minutes. Turn the slices, and bake for 5 additional minutes, or until nicely browned. Remove the sheet from the oven, and set aside.

3. While the mushrooms are cooking, place the mayonnaise and mustard in a small bowl, and stir to mix well. Set aside.

4. Cut the rolls in half, and place the halves on a large baking sheet, cut sides up. Place under a preheated broiler, and broil for a minute or 2, or until lightly toasted. Spread each of the cut sides with some of the mayonnaise mixture. Set the roll tops aside, leaving the bottoms on the baking sheet.

5. Place first a quarter of the mushroom slices, and then a quarter of the cheese over the bottom half of each roll. Return to the broiler for about 1 minute, or until the cheese is melted.

6. Top the melted cheese on each roll with 1 slice of onion, 1 slice of tomato, 3 spinach or arugula leaves, and a roll half. Serve hot.

### NUTRITIONAL FACTS
(Per Serving)

| | | | |
|---|---|---|---|
| Cal: 264 | Carbs: 44 g | Chol: 3 mg | Fat: 2.7 g |
| Fiber: 3.7 g | Protein: 16.6 g | Sodium: 834 mg | |

# Black Bean Burritos

## Yield: 4 servings

$1^1/2$ cups cooked black beans, or 1 can (15 ounces) black beans, drained

1 teaspoon chili powder

4 flour tortillas (8-inch rounds)

1 cup frozen (thawed) whole kernel corn

$1/2$ cup bottled salsa

$1/2$ cup shredded nonfat or reduced-fat Cheddar cheese

### TOPPINGS

1 cup shredded lettuce

$1/2$ cup chopped tomatoes

$1/2$ cup nonfat sour cream

$1/4$ cup sliced scallions

1. Place the beans and chili powder in a 1-quart pot, and mash lightly with a fork or a potato masher, leaving the beans slightly chunky. Cover and cook over medium heat, stirring occasionally, for about 2 minutes, or until heated through. Set aside.

2. Warm the tortillas according to package directions. Lay a warm tortilla on a flat surface, and spoon a quarter of the beans along the right side of the tortilla, stopping $1^{1}/_{2}$ inches from the bottom. Top the beans with a quarter of the corn.

3. Fold the bottom edge of the tortilla up about 1 inch. (This fold will prevent the filling from falling out.) Then, beginning at the right edge, roll the tortilla up jelly-roll style. Repeat with the remaining ingredients to make 4 burritos. (See the figure on page 176.)

4. Coat a 9-x-13-inch pan with nonstick cooking spray, and arrange the burritos, seam side down, in a single layer in the pan. Spread the salsa over the tops of the burritos, and sprinkle with the cheese. Cover the pan with aluminum foil.

5. Bake at 350°F for 20 minutes, or until the burritos are heated through and the cheese is melted. Top each burrito with $^{1}/_{4}$ cup of lettuce, 2 tablespoons of tomatoes, 2 tablespoons of sour cream, and a tablespoon of the scallions, and serve hot.

### NUTRITIONAL FACTS
(Per Buritto)

| | | | |
|---|---|---|---|
| Cal: 286 | Carbs: 50 g | Chol: 1 mg | Fat: 2.5 g |
| Fiber: 8.1 g | Protein: 15 g | Sodium: 467 mg | |

# Unfried Falafel Pockets

### Yield: 6 servings

Nonstick olive oil cooking spray

3 whole wheat or oat bran pita pockets (6-inch rounds), cut in half

18 thin slices cucumber

6 slices tomato

$1^{1}/_{2}$ cups alfalfa sprouts or shredded romaine lettuce

FALAFEL MIXTURE

1 can (19 ounces) chickpeas, rinsed and drained, or 2 cups cooked chickpeas

1 cup diced cooked sweet potato (about 1 medium)

4 scallions, chopped

$^{1}/_{4}$ cup plus 2 tablespoons chopped fresh parsley

2 teaspoons crushed fresh garlic

1 teaspoon ground cumin

1 teaspoon ground coriander

$^{1}/_{2}$ teaspoon coarsely ground black pepper

$^{1}/_{3}$ cup toasted wheat germ

DRESSING

$^{1}/_{4}$ cup plain nonfat yogurt

2–3 tablespoons toasted sesame tahini (sesame seed paste)

2 tablespoons seasoned rice vinegar

$^{1}/_{2}$ teaspoon crushed fresh garlic

$^{1}/_{4}$ teaspoon ground ginger

1. To make the dressing, place all of the dressing ingredients in a blender or mini-food processor, and blend until smooth. Set aside.

2. To make the falafel, place all of the falafel mixture ingredients except for the wheat germ in a food processor, and process until

puréed, but still slightly chunky. Add a few teaspoons of plain yogurt or water if the mixture seems too dry to shape into patties.

3. Coat a large baking sheet with nonstick cooking spray, and set aside.

4. Place the wheat germ in a shallow dish. Shape the falafel mixture into 12 (2-inch) patties and, 1 at a time, lay the patties in the dish containing the wheat germ, turning to coat both sides. Arrange the patties in a single layer on the prepared baking sheet.

5. Spray the tops of the patties lightly with the cooking spray, and bake at 400°F for 10 minutes. Turn the patties, and bake for 10 additional minutes, or until the patties are nicely browned.

6. To heat the pita pockets, place them on a microwave-safe plate. Cover with a damp paper towel, and microwave on high power for about 45 seconds, or until warm.

7. To assemble the sandwiches, place 2 patties in each pita half. Add 3 slices of cucumber, 1 slice of tomato, and $1/4$ cup of sprouts or lettuce. Drizzle with the dressing, and serve immediately.

## NUTRITIONAL FACTS
(Per Serving)

| | | | |
|---|---|---|---|
| Cal: 253 | Carbs: 44 g | Chol: 0 mg | Fat: 5 g |
| Fiber: 8.9 g | Protein: 12 g | Sodium: 331 mg | |

# Spicy Rice Casserole

Yield: 6 servings

$3/4$ cup chopped onion
$3/4$ cup chopped green bell pepper
1 teaspoon crushed fresh garlic

4 cups cooked brown rice
1 can (15 ounces) red kidney beans, pinto beans, or black beans, drained
1 cup plus 2 tablespoons frozen (thawed) whole kernel corn
1 can ($14^1/2$ ounces) Mexican-style stewed tomatoes, drained and chopped
2 teaspoons chili powder
1 cup shredded nonfat or reduced-fat Cheddar cheese

1. Coat a large nonstick skillet with nonstick cooking spray, and preheat over medium heat. Add the onion, green pepper, and garlic, and stir to mix. Cover the skillet and cook, stirring occasionally, for about 3 minutes, or until the vegetables begin to soften. Add a few teaspoons of water if the skillet seems too dry.

2. Remove the skillet from the heat. Add the rice, beans, corn, tomatoes, and chili powder, and stir to mix well. Add the cheese, and stir to mix well.

3. Coat a $2^1/2$-quart casserole dish with nonstick cooking spray, and spread the mixture evenly in the dish. Cover with aluminum foil, and bake at 350°F for 45 minutes, or until the mixture is heated through and the cheese is melted. Remove the dish from the oven, and let sit for 5 minutes before serving.

## NUTRITIONAL FACTS
(Per $1^1/3$-Cup Serving)

| | | | |
|---|---|---|---|
| Cal: 318 | Carbs: 60 g | Chol: 2 mg | Fat: 1.6 g |
| Fiber: 10.7 g | Protein: 16.5 g | Sodium: 348 mg | |

# Vegetarian Roll-Ups

## Yield: 4 servings

4 flour tortillas (8- to 10-inch rounds)

1 1/3 cups Spicy Garbanzo Spread (page 94)
  or Healthy Hummus (page 92)

1 cup alfalfa sprouts or shredded lettuce

1/2 cup diced tomatoes

1/4 cup sliced black olives

**1.** Warm the tortillas according to package directions. Lay a warm tortilla on a flat surface, and spoon 1/3 cup of the Spicy Garbanzo Dip or Healthy Hummus along the right side of the tortilla, stopping 1 1/2 inches from the bottom. Top the filling with 1/4 cup of sprouts or lettuce, 2 tablespoons of chopped tomatoes, and 1 tablespoon of olives.

**2.** Fold the bottom edge of the tortilla up about 1 inch. (This fold will prevent the filling from falling out.) Then, beginning at the right edge, roll the tortilla up jelly-roll style.

**3.** Repeat with the remaining ingredients to make 4 roll-ups, and serve.

### NUTRITIONAL FACTS
#### (Per Roll-Up)

| | | | |
|---|---|---|---|
| Cal: 244 | Carbs: 43 g | Chol: 0 mg | Fat: 3.7 g |
| Fiber: 8 g | Protein: 9.5 g | Sodium: 398 mg | |

# Making Vegetarian Roll-Ups

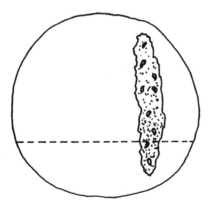

**a.** Arrange the filling along the right side of the tortilla.

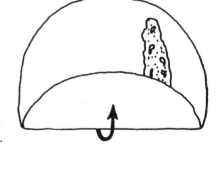

**b.** Fold up the bottom edge of the tortilla.

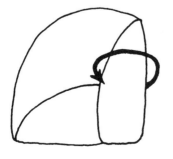

**c.** Fold the right side over the filling.

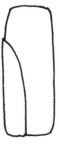

**d.** Continue folding to form a roll.

# Veggie Primo Pizza

## Yield: 8 slices

### CRUST

1¼ cups plus 2 tablespoons bread flour or unbleached flour

⅓ cup quick-cooking oats

1½ teaspoons Rapid Rise yeast

1 teaspoon sugar

¼ teaspoon salt

½ cup plus 2 tablespoons skim milk or low-fat soymilk

### TOPPINGS

¾ cup Chunky Garden Marinara Sauce (page 143) or bottled fat-free marinara sauce

2 tablespoons grated nonfat or regular Parmesan cheese

¾ cup frozen (thawed) ground meatless crumbles

1 cup shredded nonfat or reduced-fat mozzarella cheese

⅓ cup sliced fresh mushrooms

5 thin rings red bell pepper

3 thin slices onion, separated into rings

¼ cup sliced black olives

1. To make the crust, place ¾ cup of the flour and all of the oats, yeast, sugar, and salt in a large bowl, and stir to mix well. Place the milk in a small saucepan, and heat until very warm (125°F to 130°F). Add the milk to the flour mixture, and stir for 1 minute. Stir in enough of the remaining flour, 2 tablespoons at a time, to form a soft dough.

2. Sprinkle 2 tablespoons of the remaining flour over a flat surface, and turn the dough onto the surface. Knead the dough for 5 minutes, gradually adding enough of the remaining flour to form a smooth, satiny ball. (Be careful not to make the dough too stiff, or it will be hard to roll out.)

3. Coat a large bowl with nonstick cooking spray, and place the ball of dough in the bowl. Cover the bowl with a clean kitchen towel, and let rise in a warm place for about 35 minutes, or until doubled in size.

4. When the dough has risen, punch it down, shape it into a ball, and turn it onto a lightly floured surface. Using a rolling pin, roll the dough into a 14-inch circle. (For a thick crust, roll the dough into a 12-inch circle.) Coat a 14-inch (or 12-inch) pizza pan with nonstick cooking spray. Place the dough on the pan, forming a slight rim around the edges. Set the crust aside for 5 to 10 minutes.

5. Spread the sauce over the crust to within ½ inch of the edges. Sprinkle first the Parmesan and then the meatless crumbles over the sauce. Top with the mozzarella. Then arrange the mushrooms, red pepper rings, onion rings, and olives over the top.

6. Bake at 425°F for about 12 minutes, or until the cheese is melted and the crust is lightly browned. Slice and serve immediately.

## NUTRITIONAL FACTS
### (Per Slice)

| | | | |
|---|---|---|---|
| Cal: 127 | Carbs: 19 g | Chol: 2 mg | Fat: 1.1 g |
| Fiber: 2 g | Protein: 10 g | Sodium: 254 mg | |

# Greek Pizza

## Yield: 8 slices

CRUST

1¼ cups plus 2 tablespoons bread flour or unbleached flour

⅓ cup quick-cooking oats

1½ teaspoons Rapid Rise yeast

1 teaspoon sugar

¼ teaspoon salt

½ cup plus 2 tablespoons skim milk or low-fat soymilk

TOPPINGS

1 cup finely chopped tomatoes (about 3 medium)

¾ cup shredded nonfat or reduced-fat mozzarella cheese

½ cup crumbled nonfat or reduced-fat feta cheese

1 tablespoon finely chopped fresh oregano, or 1 teaspoon dried

3–4 slices red onion, separated into rings

¼ cup sliced black olives

1. To make the crust, place ¾ cup of the flour and all of the oats, yeast, sugar, and salt in a large bowl, and stir to mix well. Place the milk in a small saucepan, and heat until very warm (125°F to 130°F). Add the milk to the flour mixture, and stir for 1 minute. Stir in enough of the remaining flour, 2 tablespoons at a time, to form a soft dough.

2. Sprinkle 2 tablespoons of the remaining flour over a flat surface, and turn the dough onto the surface. Knead the dough for 5 minutes, gradually adding enough of the remaining flour to form a smooth, satiny ball. (Be careful not to make the dough too stiff, or it will be hard to roll out.)

3. Coat a large bowl with nonstick cooking spray, and place the ball of dough in the bowl. Cover the bowl with a clean kitchen towel, and let rise in a warm place for about 35 minutes, or until doubled in size.

4. When the dough has risen, punch it down, shape it into a ball, and turn it onto a lightly floured surface. Using a rolling pin, roll the dough into a 14-inch circle. (For a thick crust, roll the dough into a 12-inch circle.) Coat a 14-inch (or 12-inch) pizza pan with nonstick cooking spray. Place the dough on the pan, forming a slight rim around the edges. Set the crust aside for 5 to 10 minutes.

5. Spread the tomatoes over the crust to within ½ inch of the edges. Sprinkle first the mozzarella and then the feta over the tomatoes. Sprinkle with the oregano; then spread with the onions. Top with the olives.

6. Bake at 425°F for about 12 minutes, or until the cheese is melted and the crust is lightly browned. Slice and serve immediately.

## NUTRITIONAL FACTS
### (Per Slice)

| | | | |
|---|---|---|---|
| Cal: 126 | Carbs: 19 g | Chol: 2 mg | Fat: 1.1 g |
| Fiber: 1.7 g | Protein: 9.7 g | Sodium: 333 mg | |

## Time-Saving Tip

To make the dough for Greek Pizza or Veggie Primo Pizza (page 177) in a bread machine, place all of the dough ingredients except for 2 tablespoons of the flour in the machine's bread pan. (Do not heat the milk.) Turn the machine to the "rise," "dough," "manual," or equivalent setting so that the machine will mix, knead, and let the dough rise once. Check the dough about 5 minutes after the machine has started. If the dough seems too sticky, add more of the flour, a tablespoon at a time. When the dough is ready, proceed to shape, top, and bake it as directed in the recipe.

# Tofu Soft Tacos

*Like Skinny Sloppy Joes (page 185), this dish can be made with 8 ounces of browned 95% lean ground beef or ground turkey and only half the amount of meat alternative, if you prefer.*

### Yield: 8 servings

1 package (10 ounces) Tofu Crumbles, 2 cups frozen (unthawed) ground meatless crumbles, or 1 cup texturized vegetable protein (TVP) hydrated with $7/8$ cup water or broth (page 55)

1 cup bottled chunky salsa

1 tablespoon chili powder

$1/2$ teaspoon ground cumin

8 flour tortillas (6-inch rounds)

TOPPINGS

$1/2$ cup shredded nonfat or reduced-fat Cheddar cheese

$1/2$ cup nonfat sour cream

$1/2$ cup diced tomatoes

1 cup shredded lettuce

**1.** To make the filling, place the Tofu Crumbles, ground meatless crumbles, or TVP in a large nonstick skillet. Add the salsa, chili powder, and cumin, and bring to a boil over medium-high heat. Reduce the heat to low, cover, and simmer, stirring occasionally, for 10 minutes, or until the flavors are well blended. (Add a little water or broth during cooking if the skillet seems too dry.) Simmer uncovered for a few minutes if the sauce seems too thin.

**2.** Heat the tortillas according to package directions. Lay a warm tortilla on a flat surface, and cover the bottom half with $1/4$ cup of the filling. Top the filling with 1 tablespoon of cheese, 1 tablespoon of sour cream, 1 tablespoon of tomatoes, and 2 tablespoons of lettuce. Fold the top half over to cover the bottom half.

**3.** Repeat with the remaining ingredients to make 8 tacos, and serve hot.

### NUTRITIONAL FACTS
### (Per Taco)

Cal: 139    Carbs: 21 g    Chol: 21 mg    Fat: 3.6 g
Fiber: 3.9 g    Protein: 8 g    Sodium: 376 mg

# Tofu Chop Suey

### Yield: 5 servings

1 pound reduced-fat firm or extra-firm tofu, frozen, thawed, and squeezed dry (page 182)

Nonstick cooking spray

2 teaspoons crushed fresh garlic

1 medium yellow onion, cut into thin wedges

1 cup diagonally sliced carrots

1 cup diagonally sliced celery

1 small green bell pepper, cut into thin strips

$1^1/2$ cups sliced fresh mushrooms

2 cups fresh mung bean sprouts

SAUCE

1 cup vegetable or chicken broth

$1/4$ cup reduced-sodium soy sauce

3 tablespoons dry sherry

2 tablespoons dark brown sugar

2–3 teaspoons sesame oil

1 teaspoon ground ginger

1 tablespoon plus 1 teaspoon cornstarch

1. Cut the tofu into $1/2$-inch cubes, and arrange in a shallow nonmetal container.

2. To make the sauce, place all of the sauce ingredients except for the cornstarch in a small bowl, and stir to mix well. Pour $1/4$ cup of the sauce mixture over the tofu, tossing to mix, and set aside for 10 minutes. (The tofu will soak up the sauce.) Add the cornstarch to the remaining sauce, stir to dissolve the cornstarch, and set aside.

3. Coat a large baking sheet with nonstick cooking spray. Arrange the tofu cubes in a single layer over the baking sheet, and spray the tops lightly with the nonstick cooking spray.

4. Bake at 375°F for 10 minutes. Turn the cubes, and bake for 10 additional minutes, or until nicely browned and crisp. Set aside.

5. Coat a large deep nonstick skillet or a nonstick wok with nonstick cooking spray, and preheat over medium-high heat. Add the garlic, onion, carrots, celery, green pepper, and mushrooms, and stir-fry for about 4 minutes, or until crisp-tender. Cover the skillet or wok periodically if it begins to dry out. (The steam from the cooking vegetables will moisten the skillet.). Add a few teaspoons of water or broth to the skillet or wok only if necessary.

6. Add the bean sprouts to the skillet or wok. Stir-fry for another minute or 2, or just until the sprouts start to wilt.

7. Stir the sauce, and add it to the skillet. Stir-fry the mixture for another minute or 2, or until the sauce thickens. Add the tofu cubes, and toss to mix well. Serve hot over brown rice, if desired.

## NUTRITIONAL FACTS
(Per 1$2/3$-Cup Serving)

| | | | |
|---|---|---|---|
| Cal: 162 | Carbs: 17 g | Chol: 0 mg | Fat: 5.5 g |
| Fiber: 3 g | Protein: 11.6 g | Sodium: 532 mg | |

# Crispy Tofu Cubes

*Tofu prepared this way has a pleasant crispy-chewy texture, much like that of deep-fried tofu. Use Crispy Tofu Cubes instead of meat in stir-fries, stews, and casseroles. You can use either fresh or previously frozen and thawed tofu for this recipe.*

## Yield: 5 servings

1 pound reduced-fat firm or extra-firm tofu

Nonstick cooking spray

MARINADE

$3/4$ cup vegetable, chicken, or beef broth

2 tablespoons reduced-sodium soy sauce

1 teaspoon ground ginger, or 1 tablespoon freshly grated ginger root

1 teaspoon crushed fresh garlic

1 teaspoon sesame oil (optional)

1. Cut the tofu into $1/2$-inch cubes, and arrange in a single layer in a shallow nonmetal container.

2. To make the marinade, place all of the marinade ingredients in a small bowl, and stir to mix well. Pour the marinade over the tofu cubes, and set aside at room temperature for 30 minutes, or cover and refrigerate for several hours or overnight.

3. Coat a large baking sheet with nonstick cooking spray. Remove the tofu cubes from the marinade, and discard the marinade.

Arrange the tofu cubes in a single layer over the baking sheet, and spray the tops with the nonstick cooking spray.

4. Bake at 375°F for 10 minutes. Turn the cubes, and bake for 20 additional minutes, or until golden brown and crisp on the outside, and chewy on the inside. (The longer the cubes bake, the crisper and chewier they will become.) If you are using frozen thawed tofu for this recipe, bake for only about 20 minutes, turning after 10 minutes, as the frozen tofu is more porous and will cook faster.

5. Add the tofu cubes to stir-fries, stews, casseroles, and other dishes.

## NUTRITIONAL FACTS
### (Per Serving)

Cal: 73     Carbs: 2.5 g     Chol: 0 mg     Fat: 4 g
  Fiber: 0 g   Protein: 8.3 g   Sodium: 156 mg

# Teriyaki Tofu

### Yield: 5 servings

1 pound reduced-fat firm or extra-firm tofu, frozen, thawed, and squeezed dry (page 182)

Nonstick cooking spray

MARINADE

1 cup unsweetened pineapple juice

3 tablespoons reduced-sodium soy sauce

1 tablespoon plus 1 teaspoon dark brown sugar

2 teaspoons crushed fresh garlic

1 teaspoon ground ginger, or 1 tablespoon freshly grated ginger root

1 tablespoon plus 1 teaspoon peanut butter, or 2 teaspoons sesame oil (optional)

1. To make the marinade, place all of the marinade ingredients in a blender, and process for about 30 seconds, or until well mixed.

2. Cut the block of tofu crosswise into 10 slices. Arrange the tofu slices in a shallow nonmetal container, and pour the marinade over the tofu, lifting the tofu slices to allow the marinade to flow beneath them. Cover and refrigerate for at least 2 hours.

3. When ready to cook the tofu, coat a large baking sheet with nonstick cooking spray. Remove the tofu from the marinade, reserving the marinade, and arrange the tofu in a single layer on the sheet. Spray the tops lightly with the nonstick cooking spray.

4. Bake at 375°F for 15 minutes. Turn the slices, and cook for 10 to 15 additional minutes, or until nicely browned on both sides. (The longer the slices bake, the firmer and crisper they will become.)

5. A few minutes before the tofu is done, place the remaining marinade in a nonstick 1-quart pot, and bring to a boil over medium heat. Cook uncovered, stirring frequently, for several minutes, or until the marinade is reduced by almost half.

6. Arrange the baked tofu on a serving platter. Pour the marinade over the tofu, and serve hot.

## NUTRITIONAL FACTS
### (Per Serving)

Cal: 144     Carbs: 16 g     Chol: 0 mg     Fat: 4 g
  Fiber: 0 g   Protein: 11.2 g   Sodium: 393 mg

# *Tofu Tips*

*Made from soybeans in a process similar to cheese-making, tofu has been a staple throughout Asia for thousands of years. Many Americans also appreciate this protein-rich food. And over the past few years, thanks to research demonstrating the numerous health benefits of soy foods, tofu has gained increasing popularity in this country. Let's look at the various types of tofu available, and then learn some tofu tips that will help you make the most of this versatile food.*

## *Types of Tofu*

*These days, you can easily find fresh tofu in the produce section of most grocery stores, as well as in the shelf-stable packaging found on grocery store shelves. Several types of tofu are available, including extra-firm, firm, soft, and silken. What's the difference between these various forms? Primarily, the amount of water they contain. The firmer the tofu, the lower its water content and the higher its protein and fat contents. For instance, extra-firm tofu contains about 11 grams of protein and 5 grams of fat per 3-ounce serving, while silken tofu has about 5 grams of protein and 2 grams of fat in the same size serving. Fortunately, low-fat and reduced-fat brands of all types of tofu are now available, with only 1 to 4 grams of fat per serving. Following is a general description of the tofus you are likely to find in local grocery and specialty stores, as well as suggestions for including tofu in your dishes.*

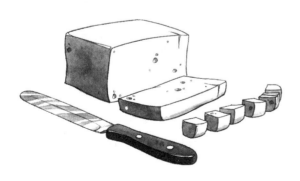

*Extra-Firm Tofu. This tofu has a dense, spongy texture, making it an excellent meat substitute in stir-fries, casseroles, soups, and other dishes. Extra-firm tofu can also be sliced and baked, broiled, or grilled; crumbled and used as a ground meat substitute in chili, tacos, and other dishes; or crumbled, mixed with bread crumbs and seasonings, and made into burgers.*

*Firm Tofu. Although not as dense as extra-firm tofu, firm tofu can be diced and used in stir-fries, casseroles, and soups; sliced and baked or grilled; or crumbled and used as a ground meat substitute. Firm tofu can also be crumbled and used to replace all or part of the eggs in egg salad, or processed in a blender and used as a base for quiches and cheesecakes. You can even mash or blend firm tofu until smooth, and use it as a substitute for cottage or ricotta cheese in dishes such as lasagna.*

*Soft Tofu. Higher in water than firm and extra-firm tofu, soft tofu has the consistency of sour cream or yogurt when blended, making it a perfect base for dips, spreads, and dressings. Soft tofu can also be crumbled and used to replace part or all of the eggs in scrambled eggs.*

*Silken Tofu. This tofu has a finer, smoother texture than other forms of tofu, making it especially well suited for use in cheesecakes, puddings, sauces, and other dishes in which a creamy smooth texture is desirable. Like regular tofu, silken tofu is available in extra-firm, firm, and soft textures. Use blended silken extra-firm or firm tofu as a base for cheesecakes, quiches, puddings, cream pies, dips, and dressings. Blended silken soft tofu can replace yogurt and sour cream in dips and spreads, or can be used as a base for cream soups or shakes. Unlike regular tofu, silken tofu should not be frozen.*

*As you can see, each type of tofu is best suited for certain culinary needs. Experiment with different forms and brands to find the ones that give you the results you desire.*

## Keeping Tofu Fresh

*Tofu is highly perishable and must be handled properly to avoid spoilage. When purchasing fresh tofu, be sure to check the expiration date on the package and to use the tofu before that date. Once the package has been opened, use the tofu as soon as possible. Place any unused tofu in a sealed container, cover with water, and store it in the refrigerator for several days, changing the water daily. Unopened tofu packaged in shelf-stable containers can be stored in your pantry until the expiration date on the package. Fresh tofu has a bland, slightly sweet smell. If your tofu smells sour, it is past its prime, and should be discarded.*

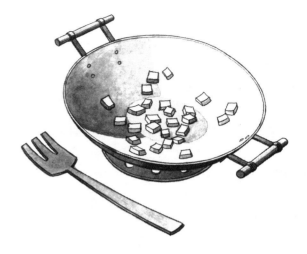

## Freezing Tofu

*Not wild about the texture of tofu? Try freezing it. Freezing causes tofu to take on a meaty, chewy texture that is perfect in stir-fries, stews, and chilis, and is also wonderful when grilled or baked. Freezing also improves tofu's ability to soak up marinades and sauces.*

*To freeze tofu, place the unopened container in the freezer for at least twenty-four hours, and for as long as several months. Keep in mind that when frozen, tofu takes on a yellowish color, but that this color will disappear when the product is thawed.*

*To thaw frozen tofu, place it in the refrigerator for approximately twenty-four hours, or thaw at room temperature by immersing it in cool water. When it is thawed, press the tofu between your palms to squeeze out any excess liquid. The tofu is now ready to marinate or cook. Freeze only nonsilken firm and extra-firm tofu. Silken tofu is not suitable for freezing.*

## Pressing Tofu

*Like freezing, pressing changes the texture of tofu. Denser, smoother, and firmer than tofu taken straight from the package, pressed tofu stands up well in stir-fries and stews, and when grilled and baked.*

*To press tofu, remove it from its package and drain off any water. Slice the tofu block in half hori-* zontally to form two slabs, each about one-inch thick, and place the slabs side by side on a large dinner plate. Then place another plate on top of the tofu, and top with a couple of two-pound cans (or several one-pound cans) from your pantry. Place just enough weight on the plate to cause the sides of the tofu to bulge slightly, but not so much that the tofu splits.*

*Allow the tofu to sit this way for thirty minutes. Then drain off any liquid that has accumulated on the plate. For an even firmer texture, press the tofu for another thirty minutes, or for as long as several hours. If you are going to press the tofu for longer than an hour, be sure to place it in the refrigerator.*

## Baking Tofu

*When using tofu in a stir-fry or casserole, you can greatly enhance its texture and its flavor by cutting it into cubes and baking it before you add it to your dish. As the tofu bakes, some of its water evaporates and it takes on a pleasant crisp-chewy texture, as well as a golden color reminiscent of deep-fried tofu. The recipe for Crispy Tofu Cubes on page 180 will show you how to bake tofu with delicious results. Even people who claim that they don't like tofu give it rave reviews when it is prepared this way.*

# Vegetarian Fried Rice

## Yield: 5 servings

1½ teaspoons crushed fresh garlic
1½ cups sliced fresh mushrooms
1 cup thinly sliced celery
½ cup plus 2 tablespoons sliced scallions
1¼ cups frozen (thawed) green peas
1 recipe Crispy Tofu Cubes (page 180)
4 cups cooked brown rice
¼ cup reduced-sodium soy sauce

1. Coat a large nonstick skillet with nonstick cooking spray, and preheat over medium-high heat. Add the garlic, mushrooms, celery, and scallions, and stir-fry for about 3 minutes, or until the vegetables are crisp-tender. Cover the skillet periodically if it begins to dry out. (The steam released from the cooking vegetables will moisten the skillet.) Add a few teaspoons of broth or water to the skillet only if necessary.

2. Add the peas and tofu to the skillet mixture, and toss to mix well. Add the rice and soy sauce, and cook, tossing gently, for another minute or 2, or until the mixture is thoroughly heated and the flavors are well blended. Add a little broth or water if the mixture seems too dry. Serve hot.

### NUTRITIONAL FACTS
(Per 1½-Cup Serving)

| | | | |
|---|---|---|---|
| Cal: 281 | Carbs: 47 g | Chol: 0 mg | Fat: 4.6 g |
| Fiber: 5.4 g | Protein: 15 g | Sodium: 473 mg | |

# Savory Stuffed Peppers

## Yield: 4 servings

4 large green bell peppers

FILLING
½ cup plus 1 tablespoon dried brown lentils, cleaned (page 102)
1 cup plus 2 tablespoons unsalted vegetable, chicken, or beef broth
¾ cup chopped fresh mushrooms
¼ cup plus 2 tablespoons chopped onion
¼ cup chopped celery
2 teaspoons crushed fresh garlic
1 teaspoon dried thyme
2½ cups cooked brown rice
⅓ cup grated nonfat or regular Parmesan cheese
¼ cup chopped soy nuts or walnuts

SAUCE
½ teaspoon dried thyme
¼ teaspoon salt
1 can (1 pound) unsalted tomato sauce

1. To make the filling, place the lentils and broth in a 1-quart pot, and bring to a boil over high heat. Reduce the heat to low, cover, and simmer for 20 minutes, or until the lentils are tender and the broth has been absorbed. Remove the pot from the heat.

2. Coat a large nonstick skillet with nonstick cooking spray, and preheat over medium heat. Add the mushrooms, onion, celery, garlic, and thyme, and stir to mix. Cover and cook, stirring occasionally, for about 3 minutes, or until the mushrooms begin to brown and release their juices. Add a few teaspoons of water or broth if the skillet seems too dry.

3. Remove the skillet from the heat, and stir in first the rice and lentils, and then the Parmesan cheese. Stir in the nuts, and set aside.

4. Cut the tops off the peppers, and remove the seeds and membranes. Divide the filling among the peppers, and replace the pepper tops.

5. To make the sauce, stir the thyme and salt into the tomato sauce. Arrange the peppers upright in an 8-x-8-inch casserole dish, and pour the sauce around the peppers. Cover the pan with aluminum foil, and bake at 350°F for about 1 hour, or until the peppers are tender. Serve hot.

## NUTRITIONAL FACTS
### (Per Serving)

| Cal: 340 | Carbs: 64 g | Chol: 6 mg | Fat: 3.2 g |
|---|---|---|---|
| Fiber: 13.6 g | Protein: 17.6 g | Sodium: 429 mg | |

# Skinny Sloppy Joes

*If you have never used a ground meat alternative, you might want to start out by substituting 8 ounces of browned 95% lean ground beef or ground turkey for half of the meat alternative in this recipe the first time you make it. You can then gradually increase the proportion of meatless crumbles, Tofu Crumbles, or TVP each time you make this dish until you have an entirely vegetarian version.*

### Yield: 6 servings

1 cup chopped onion

3/4 cup chopped green bell pepper

2 cups frozen (unthawed) ground meatless crumbles, 1 package (10 ounces) Tofu Crumbles, or 1 cup texturized vegetable protein (TVP) hydrated with 7/8 cup water or broth (page 55)

1 can (1 pound) unsalted tomato sauce

1 tablespoon spicy brown mustard

1 tablespoon Worcestershire sauce

1/4 cup tomato paste

2 tablespoons dark brown sugar

2 teaspoons chili powder

1/2 teaspoon dried oregano

1/4 teaspoon salt

1/4 teaspoon ground black pepper

6 whole wheat or multigrain hamburger buns

1. Coat a large nonstick skillet with nonstick cooking spray, and preheat over medium heat. Add the onion and green pepper, cover, and cook, stirring frequently, for about 4 minutes, or until the vegetables start to soften.

2. Add all of the remaining ingredients except for the buns to the skillet, and bring to a boil over medium-high heat. (If you used Tofu Crumbles or TVP instead of ground meatless crumbles, you may want to increase the salt to 1/2 teaspoon.)

3. Reduce the heat to low, cover, and simmer, stirring occasionally, for about 15 minutes, or until the onions and peppers are soft and the flavors are well blended. Allow the mixture to simmer uncovered for a few minutes if the sauce seems too thin.

4. Spoon 1/2 cup of the mixture onto the bottom half of each bun, top with the remaining half, and serve hot.

## NUTRITIONAL FACTS
### (Per Serving)

| Cal: 230 | Carbs: 39 g | Chol: 0 mg | Fat: 3 g |
|---|---|---|---|
| Fiber: 6.3 g | Protein: 14 g | Sodium: 393 mg | |

# 12.

# Smart Side Dishes

Mom was right when she told you to eat your vegetables. The most nutrient-rich of all foods, veggies are loaded with vitamins, minerals, phytochemicals, and fiber—all powerful preventive medicines in the fight against cancer, heart disease, and many other disorders. As for fat and cholesterol, vegetables contain neither. And they're low in calories, too. A half cup of nonstarchy vegetables like asparagus, broccoli, cauliflower, green beans, or summer squash provides only about 25 calories. Even starchy vegetables like potatoes and corn have only about 80 calories per half cup. Compare this with the other foods on your plate—a three-ounce portion of roast chicken can have anywhere from 140 to 250 calories, for instance—and it's clear that veggies are a calorie counter's best friend.

Because of the many health benefits of vegetables, health professionals recommend that your diet contain at least three to five servings per day. This isn't as much as it may seem, as a serving is only half a cup of cooked vegetables, or one cup of raw leafy vegetables. In other words, if your dinner includes a two-cup side salad, a cup of broccoli, and a medium-sized sweet potato, you will enjoy the equivalent of five servings in just one meal!

Of course, when vegetables have been fried in oil or blanketed in buttery sauces, nutritionally, they are not much better than a bowl of chips. But once you learn the secrets of light and healthy cooking, you will find that there are many ways to make vegetables tasty and appealing without excessive amounts of butter or other high-fat ingredients. The recipes in this chapter use herbs, spices, nonfat dairy products, and a variety of other ingredients to give side dishes flavor with little or no fat—and without an unhealthy dose of sodium. As an added bonus, these recipes often replace boiling with stir-frying and other cooking techniques that minimize nutrient loss while keeping veggies bright in color and bursting with garden-fresh flavor. The result? Your vegetable dishes will be not just tasty, but also rich in the nutrients that make them such an important part of your diet. Mom would be proud!

# Spicy Green Beans and Potatoes

### Yield: 5 servings

8 ounces fresh green beans

1 cup vegetable or chicken broth

2 cups ½-inch cubes peeled white or sweet potato (about 2 medium)

1 cup finely chopped peeled tomato

¼ cup finely chopped onion

2 teaspoons curry paste

1. Rinse the beans with cool water. Trim the ends, and snap the beans into 1½-inch pieces. Measure the beans; there should be 2 cups. Adjust the amount if necessary.

2. Place the beans and broth in a large non-stick skillet, and bring to a boil over high heat. Reduce the heat to medium-low, cover, and cook for 6 minutes.

3. Add the potatoes to the skillet, and increase the heat to return the mixture to a boil. Reduce the heat to medium-low, cover, and cook for 6 additional minutes, or until the vegetables are tender. If necessary, add a little more broth during cooking, but only enough to keep the skillet moist.

4. Using a slotted spoon, transfer the green beans and potatoes to a large bowl. Cover to keep warm, and set aside.

5. Add the tomato, onion, and curry paste to the liquid remaining in the skillet, and bring to a boil over medium-high heat. Reduce the heat to medium-low, cover, and cook, stirring occasionally, for about 5 minutes, or until the tomatoes are very soft and the liquid is thick.

6. Return the green beans and potatoes to the skillet, and toss to mix well. Cover and cook for about 2 minutes, or until the flavors are well blended. Serve hot.

## NUTRITIONAL FACTS
### (Per ¾-Cup Serving)

| | | | |
|---|---|---|---|
| Cal: 100 | Carbs: 20 g | Chol: 0 mg | Fat: 1.4 g |
| Fiber: 4 g | Protein: 2.9 g | Sodium: 150 mg | |

# Greek Cottage Fries

*For variety, substitute peeled sweet potatoes for the baking potatoes.*

### Yield: 4 servings

1½ pounds unpeeled baking potatoes (about 4 medium)

2–3 teaspoons extra virgin olive oil

1 teaspoon crushed fresh garlic

¾ teaspoon dried rosemary, finely crumbled

¼ teaspoon salt

1. Scrub the potatoes well, and cut lengthwise into strips that are ⅜-inch thick and ¾-inch wide. Place the strips in a large bowl.

2. Drizzle the olive oil over the potatoes. Add the garlic, rosemary, and salt, and toss to mix well.

3. Coat a large nonstick baking sheet with nonstick olive oil cooking spray. Arrange the potatoes in a single layer on the sheet, being sure that the strips don't touch one another.

4. Bake at 400°F for 20 minutes. Turn the potatoes, and bake for 10 additional minutes, or until nicely browned and tender. Serve hot.

## NUTRITIONAL FACTS
### (Per Serving)

| | | | |
|---|---|---|---|
| Cal: 167 | Carbs: 34 g | Chol: 0 mg | Fat: 2.4 g |
| Fiber: 3.1 g | Protein: 3.2 g | Sodium: 152 mg | |

# Spiced Spinach and Potatoes

## Yield: 6 servings

$1/3$ cup finely chopped onion

2 teaspoons crushed fresh garlic

1 teaspoon whole cumin seeds

$1/2$ teaspoon ground ginger

$1/4$ teaspoon coarsely ground black pepper

1 pound white or sweet potatoes, peeled and cut into $3/4$-inch chunks (about $3 1/2$ cups)

2 cups chicken or vegetable broth

5 cups (moderately packed) coarsely chopped fresh spinach (about 1 pound)

1. Coat a large nonstick skillet with nonstick cooking spray, and preheat over medium-high heat. Add the onion, garlic, cumin seeds, ginger, and pepper, and stir to mix. Cover and cook, stirring frequently, for about 2 minutes, or until the onions begin to soften and the mixture is fragrant. Add a little broth or water to the skillet if it becomes too dry.

2. Add the potatoes and broth to the skillet, and allow the mixture to come to a boil. Reduce the heat to medium-low, cover, and cook, stirring occasionally, for 10 to 15 minutes, or until the potatoes are tender.

3. Remove the lid from the skillet, increase the heat to medium-high, and cook uncovered for several minutes, or until all but about $1/2$ cup of the cooking liquid has evaporated.

4. Add the spinach to the skillet, and stir-fry for about 2 minutes, or just until the spinach has wilted. Serve hot.

## NUTRITIONAL FACTS
(Per $3/4$-Cup Serving)

Cal: 71    Carbs: 16 g    Chol: 0 mg    Fat: 0.2 g
Fiber: 2.6 g    Protein: 2.7 g    Sodium: 229 mg

# Southwestern Roasted Sweet Potatoes

## Yield: 6 servings

$1 3/4$ pounds unpeeled sweet potatoes (about 3 medium-large)

3–4 teaspoons chili powder

$1/4$ teaspoon salt

1 tablespoon extra virgin olive oil

1. Peel the potatoes, and cut into $1/4$-inch-thick slices. Measure the potatoes; there should be 5 cups. Adjust the amount if necessary.

2. Place the potatoes in a large bowl. Sprinkle with the chili powder and salt, and drizzle with the olive oil. Toss well to coat.

3. Coat a nonstick 9-x-13-inch pan with non-stick cooking spray, and spread the potatoes evenly in the pan. Cover the pan with aluminum foil, and bake at 400°F for 15 minutes. Remove the foil, and bake for 10 additional minutes. Turn the potatoes, and bake for 10 minutes more, or until tender. Serve hot.

## NUTRITIONAL FACTS
(Per $2/3$-Cup Serving)

Cal: 106    Carbs: 20 g    Chol: 0 mg    Fat: 2.5 g
Fiber: 2.8 g    Protein: 1.6 g    Sodium: 109 mg

# Garlic Mashed Potatoes

## Yield: 6 servings

2 pounds Yukon Gold or russet potatoes (about 6 medium)

5–6 cloves garlic, peeled

1/2 cup plain nonfat yogurt or nonfat sour cream

1/4 teaspoon salt

Pinch ground white pepper

1. Peel the potatoes, and cut them into chunks. Place the potatoes and the garlic in a 3-quart pot, add water just to cover, and bring to a boil over high heat. Reduce the heat to medium, cover, and cook for about 12 minutes, or until soft.

2. Drain the potatoes and garlic, reserving 1/2 cup of the cooking liquid. Return the vegetables to the pot, and stir in the yogurt or sour cream, salt, pepper, and 1/4 cup of the reserved cooking liquid.

3. Beat the potatoes with an electric mixer or mash with a potato masher until smooth. If the potatoes are too stiff, add enough of the reserved cooking liquid to achieve the desired consistency. Serve hot.

## NUTRITIONAL FACTS
### (Per 3/4-Cup Serving)

| Cal: 130 | Carbs: 29 g | Chol: 0 mg | Fat: 0.2 g |
|---|---|---|---|
| | Fiber: 2 g | Protein: 3.6 g | Sodium: 111 mg |

# Sweet Potato-Apple Casserole

## Yield: 8 servings

1 3/4 pounds unpeeled sweet potatoes (about 3 medium-large)

4 medium apples

1/4 cup plus 2 tablespoons dark raisins

3 tablespoons orange juice

2 tablespoons honey

2 tablespoons light brown sugar

1 1/2 teaspoons cornstarch

1 teaspoon dried grated orange rind

1. Peel the potatoes, halve lengthwise, and cut into 1/8-inch-thick slices. Measure the potatoes; there should be 5 cups. Adjust the amount if necessary.

2. Peel the apples, and cut into 1/4-inch-thick slices. Measure the apples; there should be 3 cups. Adjust the amount if necessary.

3. Coat a 2-quart casserole dish with nonstick butter-flavored cooking spray, and spread half of the potatoes over the bottom of the dish. Top with half of the apples and half of the raisins. Repeat the layers.

4. Place all of the remaining ingredients in a small bowl, and stir until the cornstarch is dissolved. Pour the juice mixture over the casserole. Cover the dish with aluminum foil, and, using a sharp knife, cut four 1-inch slits in the foil to allow steam to escape.

5. Bake at 350°F for 1 hour, or until all of the layers are tender. Serve hot.

## NUTRITIONAL FACTS
### (Per 2/3-Cup Serving)

| Cal: 131 | Carbs: 33 g | Chol: 0 mg | Fat: 0.2 g |
|---|---|---|---|
| | Fiber: 2.7 g | Protein: 1.3 g | Sodium: 8 mg |

# Spiced Sweet Potato Soufflé

### Yield: 8 servings

2 pounds unpeeled sweet potatoes (about 4 medium)

$\frac{1}{2}$ cup apple or orange juice

3 tablespoons maple syrup or honey

$\frac{1}{2}$ teaspoon ground cinnamon

$\frac{1}{2}$ teaspoon ground nutmeg

$\frac{1}{4}$ cup plus 2 tablespoons golden raisins or chopped dates

3 egg whites, brought to room temperature

$\frac{1}{2}$ teaspoon cream of tartar

TOPPING

$\frac{1}{4}$ cup light brown sugar

$\frac{1}{4}$ cup honey crunch wheat germ or finely chopped pecans

3 tablespoons shredded sweetened coconut

1. To cook the sweet potatoes in a conventional oven, bake them at 400°F for about 45 minutes, or until tender. To cook in a microwave oven, prick each potato in several places with a fork, and microwave on high power for about 15 minutes, or until tender. Set aside to cool.

2. To make the topping, place all of the topping ingredients in a small bowl, and stir to mix well. Set aside.

3. When the potatoes have cooled, peel them and cut into chunks. Place the potatoes, fruit juice, maple syrup or honey, cinnamon, and nutmeg in a large bowl, and, using an electric mixer or a potato masher, beat or mash the potatoes until smooth. Stir in the raisins or dates, and set the mixture aside.

4. Place the egg whites in a large glass bowl, and sprinkle the cream of tartar over the top. Using an electric mixer, beat for several minutes, or until stiff peaks form when the beaters are lifted. Gently fold the egg whites into the potato mixture.

5. Coat a 2-quart casserole dish with nonstick cooking spray, and spread the sweet potato mixture evenly in the dish. Sprinkle the topping over the potatoes.

6. Bake at 350°F for about 45 minutes, or until the topping is golden brown and a sharp knife inserted near the center of the casserole comes out clean. Cover the casserole loosely with aluminum foil during the last few minutes of cooking if the top starts to brown too quickly. Serve hot.

## NUTRITIONAL FACTS
### (Per $\frac{2}{3}$-Cup Serving)

| | | | |
|---|---|---|---|
| Cal: 168 | Carbs: 37 g | Chol: 0 mg | Fat: 1.2 g |
| Fiber: 2.6 g | Protein: 3.5 g | Sodium: 35 mg | |

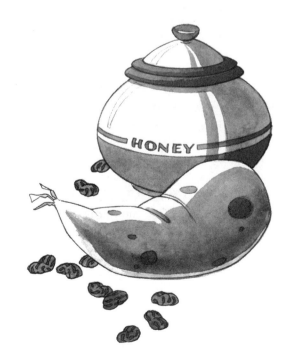

# Braised Cabbage With Bacon and Onions

### Yield: 4 servings

1/2 medium-large head cabbage (about 1 pound)

3 strips extra-lean turkey bacon, diced

1/2 medium onion, thinly sliced

1/4 cup chicken or vegetable broth

1/8 teaspoon ground black pepper

1. Cut the cabbage in half lengthwise, and trim away the core. Then cut each piece into 1/2-inch slices. Set aside.

2. Coat a large nonstick skillet with nonstick cooking spray, and preheat over medium heat. Add the bacon, and cook, stirring frequently, for about 3 minutes, or until nicely browned.

3. Add the cabbage, onion, broth, and pepper to the skillet. Cover and cook over medium heat, stirring occasionally, for about 5 minutes, or until the cabbage begins to wilt. Add a few more tablespoons of broth if the skillet seems too dry, but only enough to keep the cabbage from scorching.

4. Reduce the heat to medium-low, cover, and cook for 10 additional minutes, or until the cabbage is wilted and tender. Serve hot.

### NUTRITIONAL FACTS
(Per 3/4-Cup Serving)

| | | | |
|---|---|---|---|
| Cal: 44 | Carbs: 6 g | Chol: 11 mg | Fat: 0.7 g |
| Fiber: 3.2 g | Protein: 3.9 g | Sodium: 153 mg | |

# Asparagus With Honey Mustard Sauce

### Yield: 5 servings

1 1/2 pounds fresh asparagus spears

SAUCE

1/4 cup plus 2 tablespoons nonfat or reduced-fat mayonnaise

1 tablespoon plus 1 teaspoon Dijon mustard

1 tablespoon plus 1 teaspoon lemon juice

1 tablespoon plus 1 teaspoon honey

1. Rinse the asparagus under cool running water, and snap off the tough stem ends. Arrange the asparagus spears in a microwave or conventional steamer. Cover and cook at high power or over medium-high heat for about 4 minutes, or just until the spears are crisp-tender. Transfer to a serving dish.

2. While the asparagus are cooking, place all of the sauce ingredients in a 1-quart saucepan, and stir to mix well. Cook over medium-low heat, stirring constantly, just until the sauce is heated through. Alternatively, place the sauce in a microwave-safe bowl, and microwave uncovered at high power for 1 to 2 minutes, or just until heated through. Add a few teaspoons of water if the sauce seems too thick.

3. Drizzle the sauce over the asparagus, and serve hot.

### NUTRITIONAL FACTS
(Per Serving)

| | | | |
|---|---|---|---|
| Cal: 61 | Carbs: 12 g | Chol: 0 mg | Fat: 0.6 g |
| Fiber: 2.5 g | Protein: 2.9 g | Sodium: 221 mg | |

# Stuffed Acorn Squash

Yield: 4 servings

2 medium acorn squash (1 pound each)

FILLING

$1/2$ cup quick-cooking brown rice

1 can (8 ounces) crushed pineapple in juice, undrained

$1/4$ cup finely chopped onion

$1/4$ cup finely chopped celery

$1/4$ cup golden raisins

$1/4$ cup vegetable or chicken broth

1 teaspoon curry paste

1. Cut each squash in half crosswise, and scoop out the seeds. If necessary, trim a small piece off the bottom of each half to allow it to sit upright. Set aside.

2. To make the filling, place all of the filling ingredients in a 1-quart pot, and stir to mix well. Bring to a boil over medium-high heat. Reduce the heat to low, cover, and simmer without stirring for about 10 minutes, or until the rice is tender and the liquid has been absorbed. Spoon a quarter of the mixture into the cavity of each squash half.

3. Coat a 9-x-13-inch pan with nonstick cooking spray, and arrange the filled squash halves in the pan. Cover the pan with aluminum foil, and bake at 350°F for 50 to 60 minutes, or until tender. Serve hot.

## NUTRITIONAL FACTS
### (Per Serving)

Cal: 201    Carbs: 44 g    Chol: 0 mg    Fat: 1.3 g
Fiber: 7.5 g   Protein: 3.3 g   Sodium: 92 mg

# Dilled Zucchini and Carrots

Yield: 5 servings

2 medium-large zucchini, unpeeled

3 medium-large carrots

2–3 teaspoons extra virgin olive oil

1 teaspoon crushed fresh garlic

$1^1/2$ teaspoons finely chopped fresh dill, or $1/2$ teaspoon dried

$1/4$ teaspoon salt

1. Diagonally cut the zucchini into $1/4$-inch-thick slices. Measure the zucchini; there should be 3 cups. Adjust the amount if necessary.

2. Peel the carrots, and diagonally cut into $1/8$-inch-thick slices. Measure the carrots; there should be 3 cups. Adjust the amount if necessary.

3. Coat a large, deep nonstick skillet with the olive oil, and preheat over medium-high heat. Add all of the remaining ingredients, and cook, stirring frequently, for about 4 minutes, or until the vegetables are crisp-tender. Cover the skillet periodically if it begins to dry out. (The steam released from the cooking vegetables will moisten the skillet.) Serve hot.

## NUTRITIONAL FACTS
### (Per $3/4$-Cup Serving)

Cal: 61    Carbs: 10 g    Chol: 0 mg    Fat: 2 g
Fiber: 3.3 g   Protein: 1.7 g   Sodium: 146 mg

# Glazed Rosemary Carrots

## Yield: 5 servings

1 pound carrots (about 7 medium)
$1/2$ cup plus 2 tablespoons apple juice
$1/2$ teaspoon dried rosemary, finely crumbled
$1/8$ teaspoon salt
1 tablespoon light brown sugar or honey
1 tablespoon plus 1 teaspoon reduced-fat margarine or light butter

1. Peel the carrots, and cut them into matchstick-sized pieces. Measure the carrots; there should be 4 cups. Adjust the amount if necessary.

2. Place the carrots, apple juice, rosemary, and salt in a large nonstick skillet, and stir to mix well. Bring the mixture to a boil over high heat. Reduce the heat to medium-low, cover, and cook, stirring occasionally, for about 6 minutes, or until the carrots are tender. Add a little more juice if the skillet becomes too dry.

3. Remove the cover from the skillet, and stir in the brown sugar or honey and the margarine or butter. Increase the heat to medium-high, and cook for a few additional minutes, or until most of the liquid has evaporated. Serve hot.

## NUTRITIONAL FACTS
### (Per $2/3$-Cup Serving)

| | | | |
|---|---|---|---|
| Cal: 75 | Carbs: 15 g | Chol: 0 mg | Fat: 1.7 g |
| Fiber: 2.6 g | Protein: 0.9 g | Sodium: 109 mg | |

# Italian Oven-Fried Eggplant

## Yield: 4 servings

1 large eggplant (about 1 pound)
$1/4$ cup fat-free egg substitute
$1/3$ cup Italian-style seasoned dried bread crumbs
3 tablespoons grated Parmesan cheese*
1 tablespoon plus 1 teaspoon unbleached flour
Nonstick olive oil cooking spray

* In this recipe, use regular Parmesan cheese, not a fat-free product.

1. Trim a couple of inches off each end of the eggplant, and discard. Slice the eggplant crosswise into eight rounds, each $1/2$-inch thick. Set aside.

2. Coat a large baking sheet with nonstick olive oil cooking spray, and set aside.

3. Place the egg substitute in a shallow bowl. Place the bread crumbs, Parmesan cheese, and flour in another shallow bowl, and stir to mix well. Dip the eggplant slices first in the egg substitute, and then in the crumb mixture, turning to coat both sides well. Arrange the slices in a single layer on the prepared sheet, and spray the tops lightly with the cooking spray.

4. Bake at 400°F for 10 minutes. Turn the slices and bake for 10 additional minutes, or until golden brown and tender. Serve hot.

## NUTRITIONAL FACTS
### (Per Serving)

| | | | |
|---|---|---|---|
| Cal: 87 | Carbs: 13 g | Chol: 3 mg | Fat: 1.7 g |
| Fiber: 2.5 g | Protein: 5.4 g | Sodium: 229 mg | |

# Glorious Green Bean Casserole

## Yield: 6 servings

$1/2$ cup evaporated skim milk

3 tablespoons unbleached flour

$1/8$ teaspoon ground white pepper

1 pound frozen (unthawed) French-cut or regular-cut green beans

$1/2$ cup chicken or vegetable broth

1 can (4 ounces) sliced mushrooms, drained

3 tablespoons toasted sliced almonds

1 medium-small yellow onion, very thinly sliced and separated into rings

TOPPING

2 tablespoons grated Parmesan cheese*

2 tablespoons Italian-style seasoned dried bread crumbs

Nonstick butter-flavored cooking spray

\* In this recipe, use regular Parmesan cheese, not a fat-free brand.

1. To make the topping, place the Parmesan cheese and bread crumbs in a small dish, and stir to mix well. Set aside.

2. Place the evaporated milk, flour, and pepper in a jar with a tight-fitting lid, and shake until smooth. Set aside.

3. Place the green beans and broth in a $2^1/2$-quart pot, and bring to a boil over high heat. Reduce the heat to medium, cover, and cook for about 1 minute, or just until the beans are completely thawed and heated through.

4. Shake the milk mixture, and, stirring constantly, add it to the pot. Continue to cook and stir for a minute or 2, or until the mixture is thickened and bubbly. Remove the pot from the heat, and stir in the mushrooms and almonds.

5. Coat a shallow 1-quart casserole dish or a 9-inch deep dish pie pan with nonstick cooking spray, and spread the green bean mixture evenly in the dish. Spread the onion rings over the top, and sprinkle with the topping. Spray lightly with the cooking spray.

6. Bake at 350°F for 30 minutes, or until bubbly and nicely browned. Remove the dish from the oven, and let sit for 5 minutes before serving.

## NUTRITIONAL FACTS
### (Per $1/2$-Cup Serving)

| | | | |
|---|---|---|---|
| Cal: 92 | Carbs: 12 g | Chol: 2 mg | Fat: 2.6 g |
| Fiber: 3 g | Protein: 5.2 g | Sodium: 244 mg | |

## Crazy for Cruciferous Vegetables

*Cruciferous vegetables such as broccoli; Brussels sprouts; cabbage; cauliflower; rutabagas; and turnip, mustard, and collard greens are among the superstars of vegetables. Why? These veggies are unique because of their high contents of specific cancer-fighting phytochemicals. For instance, the isothiocyanates in cruciferous vegetables stimulate enzymes that detoxify carcinogens. And indole-3-carbinol stimulates enzymes that make estrogen less effective, which may reduce the risk of breast and endometrial cancers. Don't forget that these foods also provide a wealth of fiber, vitamins, and minerals—nutrients that offer additional protection against cancer and many other diseases.*

*So make cruciferous veggies a regular part of your diet. Whether cooked into a savory side dish, tossed into a fresh salad, or added to a stir-fry or casserole, these vegetables provide a delicious way to enhance your health and improve longevity.*

# Celery Crunch Casserole

## Yield: 8 servings

$3/4$ cup evaporated skim milk

3 tablespoons plus 1 teaspoon unbleached flour

3 cups thinly sliced celery (about 6 medium stalks)

1 tablespoon water

1 cup chicken broth

1 can (8 ounces) sliced water chestnuts, drained

1 can (4 ounces) sliced mushrooms, drained

2 tablespoons toasted sliced almonds (optional)

TOPPING

2 tablespoons grated Parmesan cheese*

2 tablespoons plain dried bread crumbs

Nonstick butter-flavored cooking spray

\* In this recipe, use regular Parmesan cheese, not a fat-free product.

**1.** To make the topping, place the Parmesan cheese and bread crumbs in a small dish, and stir to mix well. Set aside.

**2.** Place the evaporated milk and flour in a jar with a tight-fitting lid, and shake until smooth. Set aside.

**3.** Place the celery and water in a large nonstick skillet. Cover and cook over medium heat, stirring frequently, for about 3 minutes, or until the celery is crisp-tender. (Add a little more water if the skillet becomes too dry.) Carefully drain off any excess liquid.

**4.** Add the broth to the skillet, and allow the mixture to come to a boil. Shake the milk mixture, and, stirring constantly, add it to the celery mixture. Reduce the heat to medium, and continue to cook and stir for another minute or 2, or until the mixture is thickened and bubbly.

**5.** Remove the skillet from the heat, and stir in the water chestnuts, mushrooms, and if desired, the almonds. Set aside.

**6.** Coat a shallow $1\frac{1}{2}$-quart casserole dish or gratin dish with nonstick cooking spray, and spread the vegetable mixture evenly in the dish. Sprinkle the topping over the vegetables, and spray the top lightly with the cooking spray.

**7.** Bake at 350°F for about 23 minutes, or until the mixture is bubbly around the edges and the top is nicely browned. Remove the dish from the oven, and let sit for 5 minutes before serving.

## NUTRITIONAL FACTS
### (Per $\frac{1}{2}$-Cup Serving)

| | | | |
|---|---|---|---|
| Cal: 67 | Carbs: 12 g | Chol: 2 mg | Fat: 0.8 g |
| Fiber: 2.5 g | Protein: 3.7 g | Sodium: 235 mg | |

# Summer Squash Casserole

## Yield: 6 servings

$1\frac{1}{2}$ pounds fresh yellow squash (8–10 medium)

$1/2$ cup chopped onion

2 tablespoons water

$1/8$ teaspoon ground black pepper

1 tablespoon unbleached flour

$3/4$ cup nonfat or low-fat cottage cheese

$3/4$ cup fat-free egg substitute

$3/4$ cup shredded nonfat or reduced-fat Cheddar cheese

2 tablespoons Italian-style seasoned dried bread crumbs

Nonstick butter-flavored cooking spray

1. Cut each squash in half lengthwise. Then cut into slices slightly less than $1/4$-inch thick. Measure the squash; there should be 5 cups. Adjust the amount if necessary.

2. Place the squash, onion, water, and pepper in a large nonstick skillet, and stir to mix. Cover and cook over medium heat for about 4 minutes, or until the squash starts to soften. Reduce the heat to medium-low, and cook, stirring occasionally, for 7 additional minutes, or until the squash is tender. Add a little water during cooking if needed, but only enough to prevent sticking and burning.

3. If any excess water remains in the skillet cook uncovered until the liquid evaporates. Remove the skillet from the heat, and set aside for about 10 minutes to cool slightly.

4. Stir the flour into the cottage cheese. Then add the cottage cheese to the squash, stirring to mix well. Stir in first the egg substitute and then the cheese.

5. Coat an 8-inch square (2-quart) baking dish with nonstick cooking spray, and spread the mixture evenly in the pan. Sprinkle the bread crumbs over the top, and spray the top lightly with the cooking spray.

6. Bake at 375°F for about 45 minutes, or until the mixture is bubbly around the edges, the top is lightly browned, and a sharp knife inserted in the center of the casserole comes out clean. Remove the dish from the oven, and let sit for 10 minutes before serving.

## NUTRITIONAL FACTS
### (Per $3/4$-Cup Serving)

| | | | |
|---|---|---|---|
| Cal: 96 | Carbs: 10 g | Chol: 4 mg | Fat: 0.4 g |
| Fiber: 2.4 g | Protein: 13.4 g | Sodium: 321 mg | |

# Garden Rice

*For variety, substitute whole wheat couscous or bulgur wheat for the rice.*

## Yield: 4 servings

$2/3$ cup chopped fresh broccoli

$2/3$ cup fresh or frozen (unthawed) whole kernel corn

$1/3$ cup chopped red bell pepper

$1/3$ cup chopped fresh mushrooms

3 tablespoons sliced scallions

2 cups cooked brown rice

2 tablespoons vegetable broth, chicken broth, or nonfat or reduced-fat margarine

$1/4$ teaspoon salt

1. Coat a large nonstick skillet with nonstick butter-flavored cooking spray, and preheat over medium-high heat. Add the broccoli, corn, red pepper, mushrooms, and scallions. Cover and cook, stirring frequently, for about 3 minutes, or until the vegetables are crisp-tender. Add a little water if the skillet becomes too dry.

2. Add the rice, broth or margarine, and salt to the skillet, and cook uncovered for another minute or 2, or until the mixture is heated through. Add a little more broth or margarine if the mixture seems too dry. Serve hot.

## NUTRITIONAL FACTS
### (Per $7/8$-Cup Serving)

| | | | |
|---|---|---|---|
| Cal: 139 | Carbs: 30 g | Chol: 0 mg | Fat: 1 g |
| Fiber: 3.2 g | Protein: 4 g | Sodium: 144 mg | |

# Country Corn Pudding

## Yield: 7 servings

2 cups skim or 1% low-fat milk

$1/2$ cup quick-cooking yellow corn grits*

$1/4$ cup finely chopped onion

1 tablespoon sugar

$1/8$ teaspoon ground white pepper

1 can (8 ounces) creamed corn

1 can (8 ounces) whole kernel corn, drained

$1/4$ cup plus 2 tablespoons evaporated skim milk

$3/4$ cup fat-free egg substitute

$1/2$ teaspoon baking powder

* Look for grits that cook in 3 to 5 minutes.

1. Place the milk, grits, onion, sugar, and pepper in a $2^1/_2$-quart nonstick pot, and stir to mix. Cook over medium heat, stirring frequently, until the mixture begins to boil. Reduce the heat to low, cover, and simmer, stirring frequently, for about 5 minutes, or until thick and bubbly.

2. Remove the pot from the heat, and stir in first the creamed and whole kernel corn, then the evaporated milk, and, finally, the egg substitute. Sprinkle the baking powder over the top, and stir to mix well.

3. Coat a 2-quart casserole dish with nonstick cooking spray, and pour the pudding mixture into the dish. Place the dish in a large roasting pan, and add hot tap water to the pan until it reaches halfway up the sides of the dish.

4. Bake uncovered at 350°F for 50 minutes, or until a sharp knife inserted in the center of the dish comes out clean. Remove the dish from the oven, and let sit for 10 minutes before serving.

---

## *Beyond Beta-Carotene*

*Beta-carotene has received much attention in recent years. Why? Researchers have discovered that because this nutrient is a powerful antioxidant, diets high in beta-carotene-rich vegetables and fruits offer impressive protection against heart disease and cancer.*

*But before you run out to your health foods store for a bottle of beta-carotene capsules, you should be aware that several large studies have shown that beta-carotene supplements do not seem to provide the protection supplied by nutrient-rich foods. In fact, in some cases, people who took supplements of this nutrient actually had an increased rate of heart disease or cancer.*

*How can this be? Beta-carotene is just one of many different carotenoids that occur in foods. Scientists are beginning to discover that some of these other carotenoids—like the lycopene found in tomatoes and the lutein found in green leafy vegetables—may offer as much or more protection against cancer and heart disease than beta-carotene does. Furthermore, large doses of beta-carotene may suppress the absorption and utilization of these other carotenoids, actually contributing to poor health. It has become clear that carotenoids work best as a team—which is the way they occur naturally in vegetables and fruits.*

*What amount of carotenoids do you need each day? There is no set recommendation yet, but researchers agree that if you eat five to nine servings of vegetables and fruits each day, you will receive all of the carotenoids you need for good health. Deep orange vegetables and fruits like sweet potatoes, winter squash, pumpkin, carrots, cantaloupe, and apricots; leafy green vegetables like spinach, greens, and kale; and tomatoes are some of the best sources of these valuable nutrients.*

## NUTRITIONAL FACTS
(Per ⅔-Cup Serving)

Cal: 136     Carbs: 25 g     Chol: 2 mg     Fat: 0.6 g
Fiber: 1.3 g   Protein: 8 g   Sodium: 259 mg

# Savory Baked Tomatoes

*For variety, substitute sweet onions for the tomatoes.*

### Yield: 4 servings

2 large tomatoes, halved crosswise

3 tablespoons grated Parmesan cheese*

½ teaspoon dried Italian seasoning or dried basil

* In this recipe, use regular Parmesan cheese, not a fat-free product.

1. Coat an 8-inch square baking dish with nonstick cooking spray, and arrange the tomatoes, cut side up, in the pan.

2. Place the Parmesan cheese and Italian seasoning or basil in a small bowl, and stir to mix well. Sprinkle some of the mixture over the top of each tomato half.

3. Bake uncovered at 350°F for 30 to 35 minutes, or until the tomatoes are tender and the topping is lightly browned. Serve hot.

### NUTRITIONAL FACTS
(Per Serving)

Cal: 45     Carbs: 6 g     Chol: 3 mg     Fat: 1.7 g
Fiber: 1.8 g   Protein: 2.9 g   Sodium: 97 mg

# Spinach-Noodle Casserole

### Yield: 8 servings

*For variety, substitute frozen chopped broccoli for the spinach.*

4 ounces no-yolk noodles (about 2⅔ cups)

1 package (10 ounces) frozen chopped spinach, thawed and squeezed dry

1 cup nonfat or low-fat cottage cheese

1 cup shredded nonfat or reduced-fat mozzarella cheese

½ cup evaporated skim milk

½ cup fat-free egg substitute

TOPPING

3 tablespoons grated Parmesan cheese*

1 tablespoon plus 1½ teaspoons Italian-style seasoned dried bread crumbs

Nonstick butter-flavored cooking spray

* In this recipe, use regular Parmesan cheese, not a fat-free product.

1. Cook the noodles al dente according to package directions. Drain well, and return to the pot.

2. Add the spinach, cottage cheese, mozzarella, milk, and egg substitute to the noodles, and toss to mix well. Set aside.

3. To make the topping, place the Parmesan cheese and bread crumbs in a small dish, and stir to mix well. Set aside.

4. Coat an 8-inch square (2-quart) baking dish with nonstick cooking spray. Spread the spinach mixture evenly in the dish, and sprinkle with the topping. Spray the top lightly with the cooking spray.

5. Cover the dish with aluminum foil, and bake at 350°F for 35 minutes. Remove the foil and bake for 10 additional minutes, or until the mixture is bubbly around the edges and the top is lightly browned.

6. Remove the dish from the oven, and let sit for 10 minutes before cutting into squares and serving.

## NUTRITIONAL FACTS
### (Per ¾-Cup Serving)

| | | | |
|---|---|---|---|
| Cal: 138 | Carbs: 16 g | Chol: 6 mg | Fat: 1.1 g |
| Fiber: 1.2 g | Protein: 15 g | Sodium: 335 mg | |

---

## *The Preventive Powers of Onions*

*Like garlic, onions are members of the allium family, and they provide many of the health benefits offered by garlic. Studies have shown that people who eat half an onion daily have about half the risk of getting stomach cancer as people who eat no onions at all. In addition, onions can help protect against cardiovascular disease both by lowering blood cholesterol levels and by preventing blood clots from forming.*

*Although all onions are healthful, pungent, strong-flavored varieties provide more protection than do milder onions. Why? The phytochemicals known as organosulfides, which are responsible for the onion's preventive powers, are the same compounds that give onions their pungent flavor and smell. And, as is true of garlic, the less the onion is cooked, the more protection it appears to offer.*

---

# Herb-Roasted Onions

## Yield: 6 servings

2 pounds Spanish or sweet onions (about 4 large)

1 tablespoon balsamic vinegar

1½ teaspoons dried thyme or rosemary, or 1½ tablespoons chopped fresh

¼ teaspoon salt

¼ teaspoon ground black pepper

1 tablespoon extra virgin olive oil (optional)

Nonstick olive oil cooking spray

1. Peel the onions, trim the ends off, and slice into ¾-inch-thick wedges. Measure the onions; there should be about 6 cups. Adjust the amount if necessary.

2. Place the onions in a large bowl, and add the vinegar, thyme or rosemary, salt, pepper, and, if desired, the olive oil. Toss to mix well.

3. Coat a 9-x-13-inch pan with the cooking spray, and spread the onions over the bottom of the pan. If you did not use the olive oil, spray the tops of the onions with the cooking spray.

4. Bake at 450°F for 20 minutes. Stir well, and bake for 15 additional minutes, or until tender and nicely browned. Serve hot.

## NUTRITIONAL FACTS
### (Per ¾-Cup Serving)

| | | | |
|---|---|---|---|
| Cal: 52 | Carbs: 12 g | Chol: 0 mg | Fat: 0.2 g |
| Fiber: 2.2 g | Protein: 1.6 g | Sodium: 93 mg | |

# 13.

# Deceptively Decadent Desserts

Dessert is one of the simplest yet greatest pleasures of life. But, as everyone knows, most desserts are loaded with fat, sugar, and calories, leaving them little place in a healthy diet. Take your typical chocolate fudge cake, for instance. With two cups of sugar, almost a half pound of chocolate, a stick of butter, and a cup of oil, even a moderate portion of this delight contains over 500 calories and almost 30 grams of fat! And desserts like cheesecake, mousses, streusel-topped pies, and buttery pastries are no better.

Does this mean you must give up dessert to live a healthy low-fat lifestyle? Definitely not. After all, what good is living longer if you are deprived of the foods you love? As you will see, with just a little thought, you can still have your dessert and eat it too. The recipes in this chapter combine wholesome ingredients with creative cooking techniques to bring you the best of both worlds—great taste *and* good nutrition in a variety of treats that are sure to delight family and friends.

Each and every recipe in this chapter is designed to keep fat and calories to a minimum, to use only moderate amounts of sugar, and to provide a respectable amount of nutrition. For instance, many of the fruit desserts in this chapter provide a full serving of fruit. Delightfully sweet cobbler and fruit-pie toppings include nutrient-rich ingredients like whole grain flours, oats, wheat germ, and nuts. Rich and creamy custards, puddings, cheesecake, and frozen desserts feature nonfat and low-fat dairy products that add calcium and protein—but not unwanted fat—to your diet. And cakes are made super-moist and meltingly tender with puréed fruits, juices, and nonfat buttermilk—not unhealthy amounts of shortening or oil.

So get ready to enjoy sweet satisfaction without an excess of calories, fat, or sugar. From Cherry-Berry Cobbler to Black Forest Fudge Cake, you will find a galaxy of deceptively decadent desserts that are right for any occasion. Skip dessert? There's no need—not once you know the secrets of cooking for long life.

# Blueberry Bread Pudding

### Yield: 8 servings

5 cups $\frac{1}{2}$-inch cubes firm multigrain, oatmeal, or oat bran bread

$1\frac{3}{4}$ cups skim milk or low-fat vanilla soymilk

$\frac{1}{2}$ cup nonfat sour cream

$\frac{3}{4}$ cup fat-free egg substitute

$\frac{1}{2}$ cup plus 1 tablespoon sugar, divided

$1\frac{1}{2}$ teaspoons vanilla extract

$\frac{3}{4}$ cup fresh or frozen (unthawed) blueberries

**1.** Place the bread cubes in a large bowl, and set aside.

**2.** Place the milk, sour cream, egg substitute, $\frac{1}{2}$ cup of the sugar, and vanilla extract in a large bowl, and whisk until smooth. Pour the milk mixture over the bread cubes, and set aside for 10 minutes. Stir in the blueberries.

**3.** Coat a 2-quart casserole dish with nonstick cooking spray, and pour the bread mixture into the dish. Sprinkle the remaining tablespoon of sugar over the top.

**4.** Bake uncovered at 350°F for 55 minutes to 1 hour, or until a sharp knife inserted in the center of the dish comes out clean. Allow to cool at room temperature for 45 minutes before serving. Serve warm or at room temperature, refrigerating any leftovers.

### NUTRITIONAL FACTS
(Per $\frac{3}{4}$-Cup Serving)

| | | | |
|---|---|---|---|
| Cal: 164 | Carbs: 32 g | Chol: 1 mg | Fat: 0.6 g |
| Fiber: 1.6 g | Protein: 7.2 g | Sodium: 179 mg | |

# Deep, Dark, Delicious Chocolate Pudding

### Yield: 5 servings

2 packages (12.3 ounces each) light silken extra-firm tofu

$\frac{3}{4}$ cup plus 2 tablespoons dark brown sugar

$\frac{1}{3}$ cup plus 1 tablespoon Dutch processed cocoa powder

2 teaspoons vanilla extract

2 tablespoons coffee liqueur

**1.** Place all of the ingredients in a food processor, and, scraping down the sides as needed, process for about 3 minutes, or until the mixture is smooth and creamy.

**2.** Divide the pudding among five 8-ounce serving dishes or wine glasses, cover with plastic wrap, and chill for at least 2 hours before serving.

### NUTRITIONAL FACTS
(Per $\frac{2}{3}$-Cup Serving)

| | | | |
|---|---|---|---|
| Cal: 214 | Carbs: 35 g | Chol: 0 mg | Fat: 1.5 g |
| Fiber: 1.9 g | Protein: 11.2 g | Sodium: 125 mg | |

### Variation

To make Deep, Dark, Delicious Chocolate Mousse, gently fold 2 cups of fat-free or light whipped topping into the pudding. Divide the mixture among seven 8-ounce serving dishes or wine glasses, cover with plastic wrap, and chill for at least 2 hours before serving.

### NUTRITIONAL FACTS
(Per $\frac{3}{4}$-Cup Serving)

| | | | |
|---|---|---|---|
| Cal: 190 | Carbs: 31.5 g | Chol: 0 mg | Fat: 1.8 g |
| Fiber: 1.4 g | Protein: 8 g | Sodium: 102 mg | |

# Apple Streusel Pie

### Yield: 8 servings

FILLING

1/3 cup light brown sugar

1 tablespoon plus 2 teaspoons cornstarch

1/2 teaspoon ground cinnamon

1/4 teaspoon ground nutmeg

1/4 cup plus 1 tablespoon apple juice

6 cups sliced peeled Golden delicious or Rome apples (about 8 medium)

1/4 cup dark raisins or dried cranberries (optional)

CRUST

1/2 cup plus 2 tablespoons quick-cooking oats

1/2 cup plus 1 tablespoon unbleached flour

1/8 teaspoon salt

2–3 tablespoons walnut or canola oil

2 tablespoons skim or 1% low-fat milk

TOPPING

1/3 cup honey crunch wheat germ or toasted finely chopped pecans or walnuts

1/3 cup light brown sugar

1/4 cup whole wheat pastry flour

1/2 teaspoon ground cinnamon

1 tablespoon chilled tub-style nonfat margarine, or 1 tablespoon plus 1 1/2 teaspoons tub-style reduced-fat margine

1. To make the crust, place the oats, flour, and salt in a medium-sized bowl, and stir to mix. Add the oil and milk, and stir until the mixture is moist and crumbly, and holds together when pinched. Add a little more milk if needed.

2. Coat a 9-inch deep dish pie pan with nonstick cooking spray. Pinch off pieces of dough, and press them in a thin layer against the sides of the pan. Then fill in the bottom with the remaining dough. Set aside.

3. To make the filling, place the brown sugar, cornstarch, cinnamon, and nutmeg in a 4-quart pot, and stir to mix well. Add the apple juice, and stir to mix well. Place the pot over medium heat, and cook, stirring constantly, until the mixture comes to a boil. Add the apples, and if desired, the raisins or cranberries, and cook, stirring constantly for another minute or 2, or until the fruit is coated with a thick glaze.

4. Spread the filling evenly in the crust. Spray the underside of a square of aluminum foil with nonstick cooking spray, and cover the pie loosely with the foil. Bake at 400°F for about 25 minutes, or until the apples begin to soften and release their juices.

5. While the pie is baking, prepare the topping by placing the wheat germ or nuts, brown sugar, flour, and cinnamon in a small bowl. Stir to mix well. Add the margarine, and stir until the mixture is moist and crumbly. Add a little more margarine if the mixture seems too dry.

6. Remove the pie from the oven, and sprinkle the topping over the pie. Reduce the oven temperature to 375°F, and bake uncovered for 25 to 30 additional minutes, or until the topping is nicely browned and the filling is bubbly around the edges. Cover loosely with aluminum foil during the last few minutes of baking if the topping starts to brown too quickly.

7. Allow the pie to cool at room temperature for at least 1 hour before cutting into wedges and serving. Serve warm or at room temperature.

## NUTRITIONAL FACTS
### (Per Serving)

| | | | |
|---|---|---|---|
| Cal: 240 | Carbs: 48 g | Chol: 0 mg | Fat: 4.5 g |
| Fiber: 3.4 g | Protein: 3.9 g | Sodium: 58 mg | |

# Honey-Vanilla Custard

## Yield: 6 servings

1 1/2 cups skim or 1% low-fat milk
1 can (12 ounces) evaporated skim milk
1 cup fat-free egg substitute
1/4 cup plus 1 tablespoon sugar
1/4 cup honey
1 tablespoon vanilla extract
Ground nutmeg (garnish)

1. Place all of the ingredients except for the nutmeg in a blender or food processor, and process for at least 30 seconds to mix well.

2. Coat a 1 1/2-quart casserole dish with non-stick cooking spray. Pour the custard mixture into the dish, and sprinkle with the nutmeg. Place the dish in a pan filled with 1 inch of hot water.

3. Bake uncovered at 350°F for about 1 hour, or until a sharp knife inserted midway between the center of the custard and the rim of the dish comes out clean. Allow the custard to cool to room temperature. Then cover and chill for at least 2 hours before serving.

## NUTRITIONAL FACTS
### (Per 3/4-Cup Serving)

| | | | |
|---|---|---|---|
| Cal: 167 | Carbs: 31 g | Chol: 3 mg | Fat: 0.2 g |
| Fiber: 0 g | Protein: 10.4 g | Sodium: 164 mg | |

# Autumn Fruit Crisp

## Yield: 8 servings

5 cups sliced peeled pears (about 5 medium)
1/3 cup dark raisins, dried cranberries, or dried pitted cherries
3 tablespoons sugar
2 teaspoons cornstarch

TOPPING
1/4 cup plus 2 tablespoons quick-cooking oats
1/4 cup plus 2 tablespoons whole wheat pastry flour
1/3 cup light brown sugar
1/2 teaspoon ground cinnamon
1/4 teaspoon ground nutmeg
2 tablespoons maple syrup
1/4 cup toasted chopped pecans or walnuts
2 tablespoons honey crunch wheat germ

1. To make the filling, place the pears and the raisins, cranberries, or cherries in a large bowl, and toss to mix well. Set aside.

2. Place the sugar and cornstarch in a small bowl, and stir to mix well. Sprinkle the mixture over the fruit, and toss to mix. Coat a 9-inch deep dish pie pan with nonstick cooking spray, and spread the mixture evenly in the pan. Set aside.

3. To make the topping, place the oats, flour, brown sugar, cinnamon, and nutmeg in a small bowl, and stir to mix well. Add the maple syrup, and stir until the mixture is moist and crumbly. Add a little more maple syrup if the mixture seems too dry. Stir in the nuts and wheat germ, and sprinkle the topping over the filling.

4. Bake uncovered at 375°F for 35 to 40 minutes, or until the filling is bubbly and the topping is golden brown. Cover loosely with aluminum foil during the last few minutes of baking if the topping starts to brown too quickly. Allow to cool at room temperature for at least 15 minutes before serving. Serve warm or at room temperature.

## NUTRITIONAL FACTS
### (Per Serving)

Cal: 200    Carbs: 41 g    Chol: 0 mg    Fat: 3.4 g
Fiber: 4 g    Protein: 2.6 g    Sodium: 4 mg

### Variation

To make Autumn Fruit Crisp with apples, substitute 5 cups of sliced peeled Rome or golden Delicious apples plus 3 tablespoons of apple juice for the pears.

# Cherry-Berry Cobbler

### Yield: 8 servings

3 cups fresh or frozen (partially thawed) pitted sweet cherries

2$\frac{1}{2}$ cups fresh or frozen (partially thawed) blueberries, blackberries, or raspberries

$\frac{1}{3}$ cup sugar

1 tablespoon plus 1 teaspoon cornstarch

2 tablespoons orange juice

BISCUIT TOPPING

$\frac{3}{4}$ cup unbleached flour

$\frac{1}{3}$ cup quick-cooking oats or oat bran

$\frac{1}{4}$ cup plus 1$\frac{1}{2}$ teaspoons sugar, divided

1$\frac{1}{2}$ teaspoons baking powder

$\frac{3}{4}$ cup plus 1 tablespoon nonfat or low-fat vanilla yogurt

1. To make the filling, place the cherries and berries in a large bowl, and toss to mix well. Set aside.

2. Place the sugar and cornstarch in a small bowl, and stir to mix well. Sprinkle the mixture over the fruit, and toss to mix well. (If the fruit is tart, you may need to add another couple of tablespoons of sugar.) Add the juice, and toss to mix well.

3. Coat a 2-quart casserole dish with nonstick cooking spray, and spread the cherry mixture evenly in the dish. Cover the dish with aluminum foil, and bake at 375°F for 30 to 40 minutes, or until hot and bubbly.

4. To make the biscuit topping, place the flour, oats or oat bran, $\frac{1}{4}$ cup of sugar, and all of the baking powder in a medium-sized bowl, and stir to mix well. Add just enough of the yogurt to make a moderately thick batter, stirring just until the dry ingredients are moistened.

5. Drop heaping tablespoonfuls of the batter onto the hot cherry filling to make 8 biscuits. Sprinkle the remaining 1$\frac{1}{2}$ teaspoons of sugar over the tops of the biscuits.

6. Bake uncovered at 375°F for about 18 minutes, or until the biscuits are lightly browned. Allow to cool at room temperature for at least 10 minutes before serving warm.

## NUTRITIONAL FACTS
### (Per Serving)

Cal: 205    Carbs: 46 g    Chol: 1 mg    Fat: 0.5 g
Fiber: 3.3 g    Protein: 3.7 g    Sodium: 110 mg

# Cherry-Peach Crumble

Yield: 8 servings

4 cups sliced peeled peaches (about 6 medium)

1 1/2 cups fresh or frozen (partially thawed) pitted sweet cherries

1/4 cup sugar

1 tablespoon plus 1/2 teaspoon cornstarch

TOPPING

1/4 cup plus 2 tablespoons quick-cooking oats

1/4 cup plus 2 tablespoons whole wheat pastry flour

1/3 cup light brown sugar

1/2 teaspoon ground cinnamon

2 tablespoons frozen white grape juice concentrate, thawed

1/4 cup toasted chopped almonds or pecans

2 tablespoons honey crunch wheat germ

1. To make the filling, place the peaches and cherries in a large bowl, and toss to mix well. Set aside.

2. Place the sugar and cornstarch in a small bowl, and stir to mix well. Sprinkle the mixture over the fruit, and toss to mix. Coat a 9-inch deep dish pie pan with nonstick cooking spray, and spread the mixture evenly in the pan. Set aside.

3. To make the topping, place the oats, flour, brown sugar, and cinnamon in a small bowl, and stir to mix well. Add the juice concentrate, and stir until the mixture is moist and crumbly. Stir in the nuts and wheat germ, and sprinkle the topping over the filling.

4. Bake uncovered at 375°F for 35 to 40 minutes, or until the filling is bubbly and the topping is golden brown. Cover loosely with aluminum foil during the last few minutes of baking if the topping starts to brown too

quickly. Allow to cool at room temperature for at least 15 minutes before serving. Serve warm or at room temperature.

## NUTRITIONAL FACTS
(Per Serving)

Cal: 184    Carbs: 38 g    Chol: 0 mg    Fat: 2.6 g
Fiber: 3.8 g    Protein: 3.4 g    Sodium: 3 mg

# Triple Berry Sundaes

Yield: 4 servings

3/4 cup sliced strawberries

1/2 cup raspberries

1/2 cup blueberries

1 tablespoon plus 1 1/2 teaspoons sugar

1 tablespoon orange or amaretto liqueur

3 cups nonfat or low-fat vanilla ice cream

1/4 cup toasted sliced almonds (optional)

1. Place the berries in a small bowl. Sprinkle the sugar over the berries, and toss to mix. Allow to sit at room temperature for 10 minutes.

2. Add the liqueur to the berry mixture, and toss to mix well. Cover and chill for 1 to 3 hours.

3. To assemble the sundaes, place 3/4 cup of ice cream in each of four 10-ounce balloon wine glasses. Top the ice cream in each glass with a quarter of the berry mixture, and sprinkle with a tablespoon of almonds, if desired. Serve immediately.

## NUTRITIONAL FACTS
(Per Serving)

Cal: 193    Carbs: 41 g    Chol: 3 mg    Fat: 0.3 g
Fiber: 1.6 g    Protein: 5 g    Sodium: 84 mg

# Applesauce Spice Cake

### Yield: 18 servings

1 stick (¹/₂ cup) reduced-fat margarine or light butter, softened to room temperature

1¹/₂ cups light brown sugar

¹/₄ cup plus 2 tablespoons fat-free egg substitute

2 teaspoons vanilla extract

1¹/₄ cups unbleached flour

1¹/₄ cups oat flour

2 teaspoons baking powder

1 teaspoon baking soda

1 teaspoon ground cinnamon

¹/₂ teaspoon ground nutmeg

1 cup unsweetened applesauce

¹/₂ cup apple butter

¹/₂ cup dark raisins or chopped dates

¹/₂ cup chopped walnuts or toasted pecans (optional)

GLAZE

1¹/₂ cups powdered sugar

¹/₄ cup apple butter

1. Place the margarine or butter in a large bowl. Using an electric mixer, beat in the brown sugar ¹/₂ cup at a time. Add the egg substitute and vanilla extract, and beat to mix well. Set aside.

2. Place the flours, baking powder, baking soda, cinnamon, and nutmeg in a medium-sized bowl, and stir to mix well. Add the flour mixture, the applesauce, and the apple butter to the margarine mixture, and stir with a wooden spoon just until well mixed. Stir in the raisins or dates and, if desired, the nuts.

3. Coat a 9-x-13-inch pan with nonstick cooking spray, and spread the batter evenly in the pan. Bake at 325°F for about 35 minutes, or just until the top springs back when lightly touched, and a wooden toothpick inserted in the center of the cake comes out clean. Be careful not to overbake. Remove the cake from the oven, and set aside.

4. To make the glaze, place the powdered sugar and apple butter in a medium-sized bowl, and stir to mix well. Spread the glaze over the hot cake. Allow the cake to cool to room temperature before serving.

## NUTRITIONAL FACTS
### (Per Serving)

| | | | |
|---|---|---|---|
| Cal: 225 | Carbs: 48 g | Chol: 0 mg | Fat: 2.9 g |
| Fiber: 1.6 g | Protein: 2.5 g | Sodium: 172 mg | |

## *An Apple a Day . . .*

*An apple a day just might keep the doctor away. This old adage has received support from a study that investigated the effects of a class of phytochemicals known as flavonoids. Researchers found that people who eat generous amounts of flavonoid-rich vegetables and fruits are about 20 percent less likely to develop cancer of any type than are people who eat few flavonoid-rich foods. Of the foods studied, apples stood out as being especially protective against lung cancer. In fact, people who consume the most apples appear to be 58 percent less likely to develop lung cancer than people who eat the fewest apples. What is it about apples that might offer cancer protection? These fruits are rich in a flavonoid known as quercetin, which is a potent antioxidant and cancer fighter.*

# Apple Tunnel Cake

## Yield: 18 servings

2 cups unbleached flour

1 cup whole wheat pastry flour

1½ cups sugar

1 teaspoon baking soda

1 teaspoon baking powder

¼ teaspoon salt

1 cup plus 2 tablespoons nonfat or low-fat buttermilk

¼ cup plus 2 tablespoons fat-free egg substitute

¼ cup plus 2 tablespoons walnut or canola oil

2 teaspoons vanilla extract

### FILLING

¾ cup unsweetened apple juice, divided

1 tablespoon plus 1 teaspoon cornstarch

¼ cup sugar

½ teaspoon ground cinnamon

3 cups finely chopped peeled golden Delicious or Rome apples (about 5 medium)

⅓ cup dark raisins, chopped dried apricots, dried pitted cherries, or dried cranberries

### GLAZE

½ cup powdered sugar

⅛ teaspoon ground cinnamon

2 teaspoons skim milk

½ teaspoon vanilla extract

1 tablespoon chopped walnuts (optional)

1. To make the filling, place 2 tablespoons of the apple juice and all of the cornstarch in a small bowl, and stir to dissolve the cornstarch. Set aside.

2. Place the sugar and cinnamon in a 2-quart pot, and stir to mix well. Add the remaining apple juice, and stir to mix well. Add the apples and the dried fruit, and stir to mix well.

3. Bring the apple mixture to a boil over medium-high heat. Reduce the heat to medium-low, cover, and simmer, stirring occasionally, for 5 minutes, or until the apples are tender. Stir the cornstarch mixture, and add it to the apples. Cook and stir for another minute, or until the mixture is thick and bubbly. Allow to cool to room temperature.

4. To make the batter, place the flours, sugar, baking soda, baking powder, and salt in a large bowl, and stir to mix well. Add the buttermilk, egg substitute, oil, and vanilla extract, and stir just until the dry ingredients are moistened.

5. Coat a 12-cup bundt pan with nonstick cooking spray, and spread three-fourths of the batter evenly in the pan. Spoon the filling in a ring over the center of the batter. Then top with the remaining batter.

6. Bake at 350°F for about 45 minutes, or until the top is golden brown, and a wooden toothpick inserted near the sides of the cake comes out clean. Allow the cake to cool in the pan for 1 hour. Then invert onto a serving platter, and cool to room temperature.

7. To make the glaze, place the powdered sugar and cinnamon in a small bowl, and stir to mix well. Add the milk and vanilla extract, and stir until smooth. Add a little more milk if the mixture seems too thick.

8. Drizzle the glaze over the cake, and sprinkle with the walnuts, if desired. Allow the cake to sit for at least 15 minutes before slicing and serving.

## NUTRITIONAL FACTS
### (Per Serving)

| | | | |
|---|---|---|---|
| Cal: 229 | Carbs: 44 g | Chol: 0 mg | Fat: 4.8 g |
| Fiber: 1.6 g | Protein: 3.5 g | Sodium: 158 mg | |

# Phyllo Apple Dumplings

## Yield: 6 servings

3 tablespoons sugar

$1/4$ teaspoon ground cinnamon

6 medium golden Delicious or Rome apples

3 tablespoons dark raisins, dried cranberries, or chopped dried apricots

3 tablespoons toasted chopped almonds, pecans, or walnuts

5 tablespoons honey, divided

6 sheets (about 12 x 18 inches) phyllo pastry (about 5 ounces)

Nonstick butter-flavored cooking spray

1. Place the sugar and cinnamon in a small bowl, and stir to mix well. Set aside.

2. Starting at the stem end, core the apples without cutting through the opposite end. Then peel the apples, and set aside.

3. Place the dried fruit and nuts in a small bowl, and toss to mix well. Stuff 1 tablespoon of the mixture into the cavity of each apple, and drizzle 1 teaspoon of honey over the fruit-nut mixture. Set aside.

4. Spread the phyllo dough out on a clean, dry surface, with the short end facing you. Cover the dough with plastic wrap to prevent it from drying out as you work. (Remove the sheets as you need them, being sure to re-cover the remaining dough.)

5. Remove 1 sheet of the phyllo dough, and lay it on a clean dry surface. Spray the sheet lightly with the cooking spray, and sprinkle with 1 teaspoon of the cinnamon mixture. Fold the bottom up to form a double layer

of phyllo measuring approximately 12 x 9 inches.

6. Stand an apple upright in the center of the folded phyllo sheet. Bring 1 corner of the sheet up and over the top of the apple and down the other side. Repeat with the other 3 corners to completely cover the apple. Use your hands to press the phyllo dough over the apple to make it conform to the shape of the apple. Repeat this procedure with the remaining ingredients to make 6 phyllo-wrapped apples.

7. Coat a large baking sheet with nonstick cooking spray, and stand the wrapped apples upright on the sheet. Spray the tops and sides of the apples lightly with the cooking spray, and sprinkle with the remaining sugar mixture.

8. Bake at 350°F for 35 minutes, or the phyllo is nicely browned and the apples are tender when pierced with a sharp knife. Cover the apples loosely with aluminum foil during the last 10 minutes of baking if they begin to brown too quickly.

9. Remove the apples from the oven, and allow to cool for 10 minutes. To serve, cut each apple in half lengthwise and drizzle with $1^{1}/_{2}$ teaspoons of the remaining honey. Serve warm.

## NUTRITIONAL FACTS
### (Per Serving)

| | | | |
|---|---|---|---|
| Cal: 224 | Carbs: 47 g | Chol: 1 mg | Fat: 3.9 g |
| Fiber: 2.7 g | Protein: 2.5 g | Sodium: 94 mg | |

# Maple Jumbles

## Yield: 40 cookies

1 cup plus 2 tablespoons whole wheat pastry flour

$3/4$ cup light brown sugar

$1/4$ teaspoon ground cinnamon

1 teaspoon baking soda

$1/4$ cup maple syrup

$1/4$ cup water

1 teaspoon vanilla extract

2 cups bran flake and raisin cereal

$1/2$ cup chopped dried apricots

$3/4$ cup toasted chopped pecans, almonds, or walnuts

1. Place the flour, brown sugar, and cinnamon in a large bowl, and stir to mix well. Use the back of a spoon to press out any lumps in the brown sugar.

2. Add the baking soda to the flour mixture, and stir to mix well. Add the maple syrup, water, and vanilla extract, and stir to mix well. Finally, add the cereal, apricots, and nuts, and stir to mix well.

3. Coat a baking sheet with nonstick cooking spray. Drop rounded teaspoonfuls of dough onto the sheet, placing them $1^1/2$ inches apart. Slightly flatten each cookie with a tip of a spoon. (Note that the dough will be slightly crumbly, so that you may have to press it together slightly to make it hold its shape.)

4. Bake at 275°F for about 17 minutes, or until lightly browned. Cool the cookies on the pan for 2 minutes. Then transfer the cookies to wire racks, and cool completely. Serve immediately, or transfer to an airtight con-

tainer and arrange in single layers separated by sheets of waxed paper. If the cookies become too chewy during storage, place an apple wedge or a $1^1/2$-inch piece of bread in with each layer, and let the cookies sit for several hours or overnight. The moisture from the apple or bread will seep into the cookies and soften them up.

## NUTRITIONAL FACTS
### (Per Cookie)

| | | | |
|---|---|---|---|
| Cal: 59 | Carbs: 11 g | Chol: 0 mg | Fat: 1.6 g |
| Fiber: 1.2 g | Protein: 1.0 g | Sodium: 51 mg | |

# Glazed Mocha Brownies

## Yield: 12 brownies

1 tablespoon hot tap water

1 teaspoon instant coffee granules

$2/3$ cup oat flour

$1/4$ cup Dutch processed cocoa powder

2 tablespoons instant nonfat dry milk powder

1 pinch baking soda

$1/8$ teaspoon salt

$3/4$ cup light brown sugar

$1/4$ cup plus 2 tablespoons fat-free egg substitute

$1/4$ cup chocolate syrup

$1^1/2$ teaspoons vanilla extract

$1/3$ cup toasted chopped pecans or almonds (optional)

GLAZE

$1/2$ cup powdered sugar

$1/2$ teaspoon vanilla extract

$1/4$ teaspoon instant coffee granules

2 teaspoons skim or 1% low-fat milk

1. To make the batter, place hot water and coffee granules in a small bowl, and stir to mix well. Set aside.

2. Place the flour, cocoa powder, milk powder, baking soda, and salt in a medium-sized bowl, and stir to mix well. Add the brown sugar, and stir to mix well. Use the back of a wooden spoon to press out any lumps in the brown sugar. Add the egg substitute, chocolate syrup, vanilla extract, and coffee mixture, and stir to mix well. Set the batter aside for 15 minutes.

3. If desired, stir the nuts into the batter. Coat the *bottom only* of an 8-x-8-inch pan with nonstick cooking spray, and spread the mixture in the pan. Bake at 325°F for about 22 minutes, or just until the edges are firm and the center is almost set. Be careful not to overbake. Cool to room temperature.

4. To make the glaze, place the powdered sugar in a small bowl. Place the vanilla extract in another small bowl, add the coffee granules, and stir to dissolve the granules. Add the vanilla mixture and milk to the sugar, and stir to mix well, adding a little more milk if the glaze seems too thick. Microwave on high power for about 30 seconds, or until hot and runny.

5. Drizzle the hot glaze back and forth over the cooled brownies. Allow the brownies to sit for at least 15 minutes before cutting into squares and serving. For easier cutting, rinse the knife off periodically.

## NUTRITIONAL FACTS
### (Per Brownie)

| | | | |
|---|---|---|---|
| Cal: 115 | Carbs: 25 g | Chol: 0 mg | Fat: 0.6 g |
| Fiber: 1.3 g | Protein: 2.2 g | Sodium: 56 mg | |

# Black Forest Fudge Cake

### Yield: 18 servings

1¼ cups unbleached flour

¾ cup oat flour

½ cup Dutch processed cocoa powder

1½ cups sugar

1½ teaspoons baking soda

½ teaspoon salt

2½ cups frozen (thawed) pitted sweet cherries (12 ounces)

½ cup coffee, cooled to room temperature

¼ cup vegetable oil

2 teaspoons vanilla extract

FROSTING

1 package (4-serving size) instant white chocolate pudding mix

1 cup nonfat or low-fat vanilla yogurt

2 cups nonfat or light whipped topping

3 tablespoons toasted sliced almonds (optional)

1. Place the flours, cocoa, sugar, baking soda, and salt in a large bowl, and stir with a wire whisk to mix well. Set aside.

2. Place the cherries, including the juice that has accumulated during thawing, and the coffee in a blender, and process until smooth. Add the cherry mixture, oil, and vanilla extract to the flour mixture, and whisk until well mixed.

3. Coat a 9-x-13-inch pan with nonstick cooking spray, and spread the batter evenly in the pan. Bake at 325°F for about 30 minutes, or just until the top springs back when lightly touched and a wooden toothpick inserted in the center of the cake comes out

clean or coated with a few fudgy crumbs. Allow the cake to cool to room temperature.

4. To make the frosting, place the pudding mix and yogurt in a medium-sized bowl, and whisk for about 1 minute, or until well mixed and thickened. Gently fold the whipped topping into the pudding mixture, and immediately spread the frosting over the cake. Sprinkle with the almonds, if desired.

5. Cover the cake, and refrigerate for at least 2 hours before cutting into squares and serving.

### NUTRITIONAL FACTS
#### (Per Serving)

| Cal: 195 | Carbs: 39 g | Chol: 0 mg | Fat: 3.8 g |
|---|---|---|---|
| Fiber: 1.8 g | Protein: 2.7 g | Sodium: 257 mg | |

## Spiked Strawberries

*For variety, substitute sliced fresh peaches for the strawberries, and amaretto liqueur for the orange liqueur.*

### Yield: 4 servings

4 cups strawberry halves

3 tablespoons sugar

3 tablespoons orange liqueur, such as curaçao, Grand Marnier, or Triple Sec

1/2 cup nonfat or light whipped topping (optional)

1. Place the berries in a medium-sized bowl. Sprinkle the sugar over the berries, and toss to mix. (If the berries are tart, you may need to add another tablespoon of sugar.)

2. Add the liqueur to the berry mixture, and toss to mix well. Cover and chill for 4 to 6 hours, stirring occasionally.

3. When ready to serve, divide the mixture among four 10-ounce balloon wine glasses. Top each serving with 2 tablespoons of the whipped topping, if desired, and serve immediately.

### NUTRITIONAL FACTS
#### (Per Serving)

| Cal: 132 | Carbs: 26 g | Chol: 0 mg | Fat: 0.6 g |
|---|---|---|---|
| Fiber: 2.5 g | Protein: 1 g | Sodium: 3 mg | |

## Old-Fashioned Strawberry Shortcake

*For variety, substitute diced peaches for the strawberries, and amaretto for the raspberry or orange liqueur. Or substitute fresh raspberries or blueberries for part of the strawberries.*

### Yield: 6 servings

BISCUITS

1 cup unbleached flour

1/4 cup oat bran

1/3 cup sugar

2 teaspoons baking powder

2–3 tablespoons chilled reduced-fat margarine or light butter, cut into pieces

1/2 cup plus 1 tablespoon nonfat or low-fat buttermilk

BERRY MIXTURE

4 cups sliced strawberries

1/3 cup sugar

2 tablespoons Chambord raspberry liqueur or orange liqueur (optional)

TOPPING

1 cup nonfat or light whipped topping

1/3 cup nonfat or low-fat vanilla yogurt

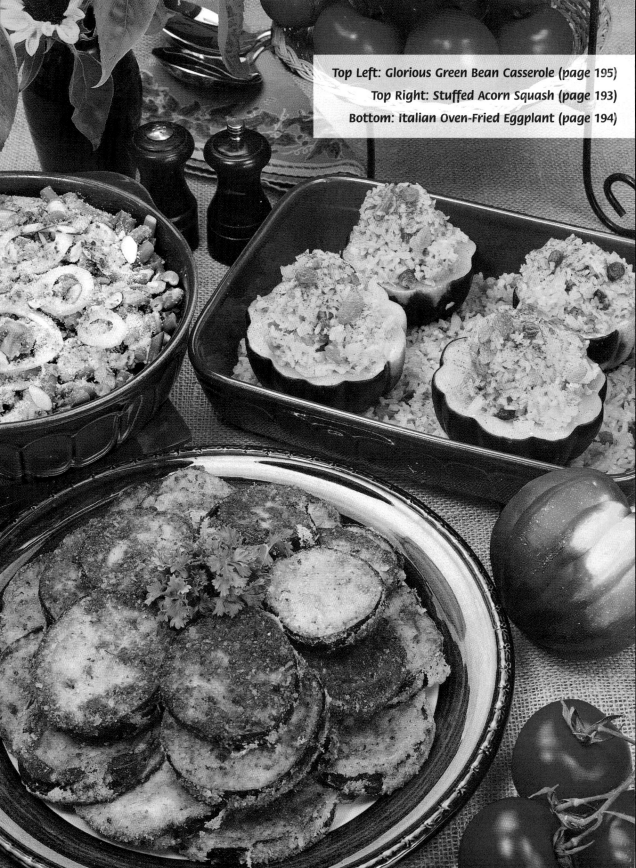

Top Left: Glorious Green Bean Casserole (page 195)
Top Right: Stuffed Acorn Squash (page 193)
Bottom: Italian Oven-Fried Eggplant (page 194)

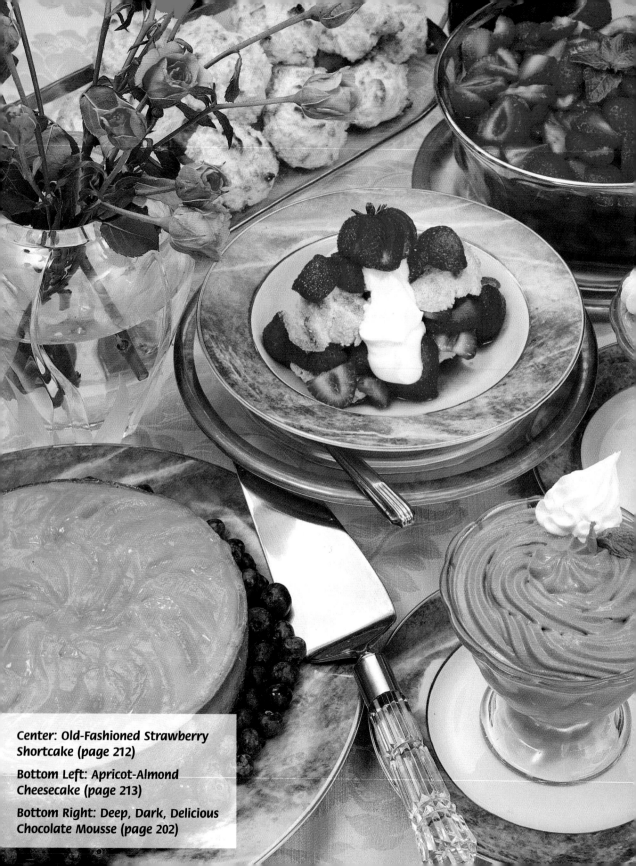

**Center:** Old-Fashioned Strawberry Shortcake (page 212)

**Bottom Left:** Apricot-Almond Cheesecake (page 213)

**Bottom Right:** Deep, Dark, Delicious Chocolate Mousse (page 202)

1. To make the berry mixture, place 1 cup of the strawberries in a medium-sized bowl. Add the sugar, and mash with a fork. Add the remaining berries and, if desired, the liqueur, and stir to mix well. Cover and chill for 2 to 5 hours to allow the juices to develop.

2. To make the topping, place the whipped topping in a small bowl, and gently fold in the yogurt. Cover and chill until ready to serve.

3. To make the biscuits, place the flour, oat bran, sugar, and baking powder in a medium-sized bowl, and stir to mix well. Using a pastry cutter or 2 knives, cut in the margarine or butter just until the mixture resembles coarse crumbs. Add the buttermilk, and stir just until moistened. Add a little more buttermilk if needed to make a moderately thick batter.

4. Coat a medium-sized baking sheet with nonstick cooking spray, and drop heaping tablespoons of the batter onto the sheet to make 6 biscuits. Bake at 400°F for about 15 minutes, or until the biscuits are lightly browned. Be careful not to overbake. Remove the biscuits from the oven, and let sit for 5 minutes.

5. To assemble the desserts, use a serrated knife to split each biscuit open, and place each biscuit bottom on an individual dessert plate. Top the biscuit half with ¼ cup of the berry mixture, the top half of the biscuit, and 2 more tablespoons of the berry mixture. Crown with a dollop of the topping. Repeat with the remaining ingredients to make 6 desserts, and serve immediately.

### NUTRITIONAL FACTS
(Per Serving)

Cal: 252    Carbs: 53 g    Chol: 2 mg    Fat: 3 g
Fiber: 3.6 g    Protein: 4.9 g    Sodium: 227 mg

# Apricot-Almond Cheesecake

*For variety, substitute a 20-ounce can of light (reduced-sugar) apple or cherry pie filling for the apricot topping.*

## Yield: 12 servings

CRUST

24 reduced-fat vanilla wafers

2 tablespoons sugar

1 tablespoon tub-style nonfat margarine

¼ cup plus 2 tablespoons toasted sliced almonds

FILLING

2 blocks (8 ounces each) nonfat cream cheese, softened to room temperature

2 teaspoons vanilla extract

2 tablespoons plus 1 teaspoon cornstarch

1 can (14 ounces) fat-free sweetened condensed milk

½ cup plus 2 tablespoons fat-free egg substitute

1 cup vanilla yogurt cheese (page 47)

TOPPING

1 can (15 ounces) apricot halves packed in juice or light syrup, undrained

2 tablespoons sugar

1 tablespoon cornstarch

1. To make the crust, break the vanilla wafers into pieces, place in a food processor, and process into fine crumbs. Measure the crumbs; there should be ¾ cup. Adjust the amount if necessary.

2. Return the crumbs to the food processor, add the sugar, and process for a few seconds to mix well. Add the margarine, and process for about 20 seconds, or until moist and crumbly. Add the almonds, and process for a few seconds more, or until the almonds are finely chopped.

3. Coat a 9-inch springform pan with nonstick cooking spray, and use the back of a spoon to press the crumb mixture against the bottom and 1 inch up the sides of the pan, forming an even layer of crust. Then use your fingers to finish pressing the crust firmly against the bottom and sides of the pan.

4. Bake the crust at 350°F for about 8 minutes, or until the edges feel firm and dry. Set aside to cool to room temperature before filling.

5. To make the filling, place the cream cheese and vanilla extract in a large bowl, and beat with an electric mixer until smooth. Sprinkle the cornstarch over the cheese mixture, and beat until smooth. Add the sweetened condensed milk, and beat until smooth. Add the egg substitute, and beat until smooth. Finally, add the yogurt cheese, and beat until smooth.

6. Spread the batter evenly over the crust, and bake at 325°F for about 1 hour, or until the center is firm to the touch. (If you use a

---

## *Nutty Nutrition*

It's true—nuts are loaded with fat. In fact, one cup of nuts contains close to 800 calories and 70 grams of fat. Does this mean that you should never eat nuts again? Definitely not. Everyone needs some fat to maintain good health, and nuts provide the essential fats we need in their most wholesome and natural form. The fat in nuts is mostly unsaturated, and does not raise blood cholesterol levels. In fact, a number of studies have shown that people who eat nuts on a regular basis actually have a lower risk of heart disease. If you need another reason to eat nuts, keep in mind that they provide important minerals like magnesium, copper, zinc, and manganese, and are a good source of vitamin E. In addition, Brazil nuts, which grow in the selenium-rich soil of the Amazon rain forest, are the richest known source of selenium, a powerful antioxidant.

Like other plant foods, nuts also supply a variety of phytochemicals and other protective substances. For instance, all nuts contain flavonoids, which act as antioxidants to fight free radicals. Peanuts are rich in choline, a nutrient essential for the health of

the brain and nervous system, and in resveratrol, a compound that protects against heart disease and cancer. And walnuts and pecans contain ellagic acid, a compound that fights cancer.

Because of their nutritional value, their crunch, and their great taste, nuts are included in many of the recipes in this book, from salads to main dishes to breads to desserts. And, as you can see from the nutritional analysis of the recipes, when used moderately in low-fat recipes like the ones in this book, nuts will not blow your fat budget.

To bring out the flavor of nuts—and of seeds, too—try toasting them. Toasting intensifies the flavors of nuts so much that you can halve the amount used. Simply arrange the nuts in a single layer on a baking sheet, and bake at 350°F for 8 to 10 minutes, or until lightly browned with a toasted, nutty smell. (Watch the nuts closely during the last couple of minutes of baking, as they tend to brown quickly.) To save time, toast a large batch and store the extras in an airtight container in the refrigerator. That way, you'll always have a supply on hand.

dark pan instead of a shiny one, reduce the oven temperature to 300°F.) Turn the oven off, and allow the cake to cool in the oven with the door ajar for 1 hour. Remove the cake from the oven, cover, and chill for at least 4 hours.

7. To make the topping, drain the apricot halves well, reserving the juice and 1 of the halves. Cut each apricot half into 3 or 4 slices, and arrange the slices in concentric circles over the top of the cake.

8. Place $1/2$ cup of the reserved apricot juice, the reserved apricot half, the sugar, and the cornstarch in a blender, and process until smooth. Pour the mixture into a small saucepan, place over medium heat, and cook, stirring constantly, until the mixture is thickened and bubbly. Allow to cool for 5 minutes. Then stir the mixture and drizzle it over the cake, covering the apricots.

9. Cover the cake and chill for at least 3 additional hours, or until firm. Remove the collar of the pan just before slicing and serving.

## NUTRITIONAL FACTS
### (Per Serving)

| | | | |
|---|---|---|---|
| Cal: 223 | Carbs: 37 g | Chol: 5 mg | Fat: 2.4 g |
| Fiber: 0.8 g | Protein: 12.6 g | Sodium: 291 mg | |

# Simple Peach Sorbet

### Yield: 6 servings

2 cans (15 ounces each) sliced peaches in juice, undrained

$1/2$ cup plus 2 tablespoons frozen white grape juice concentrate, thawed

1. Place the peaches with their juice and the juice concentrate in a blender, and blend until smooth.

2. If using an ice cream maker, pour the mixture into a $1^{1}/_{2}$-quart ice cream maker, and proceed as directed by the manufacturer. If you do not own an ice cream maker, follow steps 3 through 5.

3. To make the sorbet in your freezer, pour the mixture into an 8-inch square pan. Cover the pan with aluminum foil, and place in the freezer for at least 8 hours, or until the mixture is frozen solid. (You can prepare the mixture a few days ahead of time, if you prefer.) Remove the frozen mixture from the freezer, and allow it to sit at room temperature for about 10 minutes, or until thawed enough to break into chunks.

4. Break the mixture into chunks, and place in the bowl of a food processor or electric mixer. Process or beat for several minutes, or until the mixture is light, creamy, and smooth. (Note that, depending on the capacity of your food processor, you may have to process the mixture in 2 batches.)

5. Return the mixture to the pan, cover, and return to the freezer. Freeze for at least 4 hours, or until firm.

6. Scoop the sorbet into individual serving dishes. (If it seems too solid, let it sit for 5 to 10 minutes at room temperature before scooping.) Serve immediately.

## NUTRITIONAL FACTS
### (Per $3/_4$-Cup Serving)

| | | | |
|---|---|---|---|
| Cal: 150 | Carbs: 37 g | Chol: 0 mg | Fat: 0 g |
| Fiber: 2.4 g | Protein: 1.1 g | Sodium: 6 mg | |

# Burst-of-Berries Sorbet

### Yield: 6 servings

5 cups sliced fresh strawberries, or 1½ pounds frozen (slightly thawed) unsweetened strawberries

½ cup plus 2 tablespoons sugar

½ cup cranberry juice cocktail

¼ cup Chambord raspberry liqueur

1. Place the strawberries, sugar, and cranberry juice cocktail in a 2½-quart pot, and stir to mix well. Cover and cook over medium heat, stirring occasionally, for about 5 minutes, or until the strawberries are soft and the liquid is syrupy. Allow the mixture to cool to room temperature.

2. Place the cooled strawberry mixture in a blender or food processor. Add the liqueur, and process until smooth.

3. If using an ice cream maker, pour the mixture into a 1½-quart ice cream maker, and proceed as directed by the manufacturer. If you do not own an ice cream maker, follow steps 4 through 6.

4. To make the sorbet in your freezer, pour the mixture into an 8-inch square pan. Cover the pan with aluminum foil, and place in the freezer for at least 8 hours, or until the mixture is frozen solid. (You can prepare the mixture a few days ahead of time, if you prefer.) Remove the frozen mixture from the freezer, and allow it to sit at room temperature for about 10 minutes, or until thawed enough to break into chunks.

5. Break the mixture into chunks, and place in the bowl of a food processor or electric mixer. Process or beat for several minutes, or until the mixture is light, creamy, and smooth. (Note that, depending on the capacity of your food processor, you may have to process the mixture in 2 batches.)

6. Return the mixture to the pan, cover, and return to the freezer. Freeze for at least 4 hours, or until firm.

7. Scoop the sorbet into individual serving dishes. (If it seems too solid, let it sit for 5 to 10 minutes at room temperature before scooping.) Serve immediately.

## NUTRITIONAL FACTS
### (Per ¾-Cup Serving)

Cal: 169     Carbs: 38 g     Chol: 0 mg     Fat: 0.6 g
Fiber: 3.2 g     Protein: 0.9 g     Sodium: 3 mg

# 14.

# Menus for a Long Life

In Chapter 1, you learned about the foundations of healthy eating, and you discovered how a few simple dietary guidelines can go a long way toward optimizing health and promoting greater longevity. Chapter 2 built upon these basic principles by showing you how to fine-tune your diet to target a number of common health problems. This chapter suggests sample menus that will help you do just that.

You will notice that although these menus were designed to prevent or treat different health disorders, they are more similar to one another than they are different. How are they alike? Each is built upon a foundation of wholesome whole grains; generous amounts of vegetables and fruits; lean meats, poultry, and seafood; vegetarian meat alternatives; and low-fat dairy products. Some health problems, though, do benefit from the inclusion of certain types of foods on a regular basis. For instance, calcium-rich foods are of special importance to people with osteoporosis, fish oils can be helpful to people with rheumatoid arthritis, and soy foods may benefit menopausal women. Thus, many menus provide greater amounts of specific foods, such as calcium-fortified soymilk, tofu, or fish.

Most of the menus presented in this chapter provide about 1,800 calories. The exceptions are the menus designed for weight loss, each of which provides about 1,500 calories. You will note that portion sizes have been specified for foods like fruit, yogurt, bread, and nuts. In the case of the dishes featured in this book, unless otherwise indicated, the recipe itself will guide you regarding portion size. Realize that you may have to either alter your portion size or add or subtract foods to make these menus meet your caloric needs. (See the table on page 11 for guidelines regarding the best calorie intake for your weight.)

Each of the following sections first reviews the key dietary strategies for targeting a specific condition. It then presents two sample daily menus that will help you put these principles into practice. I think you'll be pleased to discover that it is possible to follow a healthy diet without depriving yourself of the foods you love.

# CANCER

There is no doubt that smart food choices can dramatically reduce your risk of developing cancer. And though there are many kinds of cancer, the same general strategies target most types. These strategies are as follows:

❏ Eat a wide variety of vegetables, fruits, legumes, and whole grain products. These foods provide the nutrients, fiber, antioxidants, and phytochemicals that can help prevent and slow the growth of many cancers.

❏ Maintain a healthy body weight to prevent excessively high insulin and estrogen levels, which can promote the development of certain cancers.

❏ Keep your total fat intake low. High intakes of both saturated fat and omega-6 polyunsaturated fat have been shown to promote the development of various types of cancer. Keeping fat to a minimum will also help you control calories, and will leave more room in your diet for vegetables, fruits, whole grains, and other cancer-fighting foods.

❏ Purchase organic produce and meats whenever possible. This will help you avoid pesticides, hormones, and other additives that may promote the growth of cancer.

❏ Avoid highly processed foods, many of which contain additives that may promote the growth of cancer.

## Menu 1

### Breakfast

4 Multigrain Pancakes (page 69)
1/4 cup Warm Blueberry Topping (page 71)
Turkey Breakfast Sausage Patty (page 79)
1 cup skim milk or calcium-fortified soymilk

### Lunch

Roasted Onion Soup (page 100)
Vegetarian Roll-Up (page 176)
1 orange

### Afternoon Snack

1 ounce baked tortilla chips
1/4 cup bottled salsa

### Dinner

Greek Grilled Chicken Salad (page 124)
1 ounce warm whole wheat pita bread wedges
1/4 honeydew melon

### Evening Snack

Glazed Mocha Brownie (page 210)
1 cup skim milk or calcium-fortified soymilk

## Menu 2

### Breakfast

Cinnamon Apple-Raisin Granola (page 73)
1 cup skim milk or calcium-fortified soymilk
1 cup fresh mango slices

### Lunch

Tomato-Dill Soup (page 106)
Florentine Pasta Salad (page 114)
1 cup mixed fresh fruit

### Afternoon Snack

Cut fresh vegetables
3 tablespoons Honey-Mustard Dip (page 92)

### Dinner

Glazed Turkey Tenderloins (page 156)
Stuffed Acorn Squash (page 193)
Braised Cabbage With Bacon & Onions
  (page 192)
1 whole wheat roll

### Evening Snack

Apple Streusel Pie (page 203)
1 cup skim milk or calcium-fortified soymilk

# CARDIOVASCULAR DISEASE

The strategies presented in this section target both atherosclerosis and high blood pressure. These are two conditions that many people have simultaneously, and either one can lead to heart attacks and strokes. Your main goals are listed below.

❏ Maintain a healthy body weight to reduce the workload of the cardiovascular system and to help prevent the development of insulin resistance, which worsens cardiovascular disease.

❏ Using your fat budget as a guide to total fat intake, choose only heart-healthy fats, such as olive and canola oils, as well as foods like nuts, seeds, avocados, and olives. Avoid saturated and hydrogenated fats, which raise blood cholesterol levels.

❏ Eat fish at least twice a week, as the oils in fish protect against heart disease.

❏ Eat abundant vegetables, fruits, legumes, and whole grain products. These foods provide the nutrients, antioxidants, fiber, and phytochemicals that can control—and even begin to reverse—these conditions.

## Menu 1

### Breakfast

Ham and Pepper Omelette (page 77)
Honey Oat Bran Muffin (page 126)
1 cup mixed fresh fruit
1 cup skim milk or calcium-fortified soymilk

### Lunch

Mediterranean Chef's Salad (page 110)
9 reduced-fat Wheat Thins crackers
1/2 cantaloupe melon

### Afternoon Snack

1/4 cup mixed nuts

### Dinner

Capellini With Pesto Cheese Sauce (page 140)
Rocket Salad (page 112)
4 ounces steamed fresh asparagus
1 whole wheat roll

### Evening Snack

Black Forest Fudge Cake (page 211)

## Menu 2

### Breakfast

2 slices Banana French Toast (page 68) topped
  with 1/4 cup sliced bananas,
  2 tablespoons maple syrup, and
  1 tablespoon chopped pecans
Turkey Breakfast Sausage Patty (page 79)
1 cup skim milk or calcium-fortified soymilk

### Lunch

Unfried Falafel Pocket (page 174)
Golden Grains Soup (page 99)
1 cup grapes

### Afternoon Snack

1 ounce whole wheat pretzels

### Dinner

Grilled Lemon-Herb Fish (page 164)
2 cups fresh green salad with low-fat
  dressing
Southwestern Roasted Sweet Potatoes
  (page 189)
Celery Crunch Casserole (page 196)

### Evening Snack

Pumpkin-Orange Bread (page 132)
1 cup skim milk or calcium-fortified soymilk

# DIABETES

Diet can have a tremendous impact on both the prevention and the treatment of diabetes. And, as people who monitor their blood sugar can tell you, the body's response to diet can be rapid and rewarding. Indeed, you may see significant changes in your blood sugar from meal to meal, depending on your food choices. Here are some primary strategies for controlling blood sugar levels.

❐ Maintain a healthy body weight. When people are overweight, their cells become resistant to insulin, and the pancreas must work harder to keep blood sugar levels in check.

❐ When eating carbohydrates, choose foods that have a low to moderate glycemic index. (See page 36 for the glycemic index of some common foods.) These foods will require less insulin to be metabolized. Have some protein with each meal to help reduce the glycemic index of the meal as a whole.

❐ Eat plenty of vegetables, fruits, legumes, and whole grain products. These foods will provide the nutrients, fiber, antioxidants, and phytochemicals that can help prevent diabetic complications.

## Menu 1

### Breakfast
½ grapefruit
Cinnamon-Apple Oatmeal (page 75)
1 cup skim milk or calcium-fortified soymilk

### Lunch
2 cups Red Bean and Sausage Soup (page 98)
Berry Delicious Spinach Salad (page 111)
4 reduced-fat Triscuit whole wheat wafers

### Afternoon Snack
1 piece low-fat string cheese
1 pear

### Dinner
Cranberry-Apple Salad (page 120)
French Herb Chicken (page 152)
1 whole wheat roll

### Evening Snack
Deep, Dark, Delicious Chocolate Mousse
  (page 202)

## Menu 2

### Breakfast
½ cup scrambled fat-free egg substitute
2 strips extra-lean turkey bacon
2 Buttermilk Drop Biscuits (page 134)
1 cup sliced fresh strawberries
1 cup skim or 1% low-fat milk

### Lunch
Country Vegetable Soup (page 104)
Sandwich made with:
      6-inch whole wheat pita pocket
      2 ounces roasted turkey breast
      1 slice reduced-fat Swiss cheese
      Lettuce leaf, tomato slice, sprouts
      1 tablespoon low-fat mayonnaise

### Afternoon Snack
2 Ry-Krisp crackers
¼ cup Healthy Hummus (page 92)

### Dinner
Lasagna Siciliana (page 148)
2 cups mixed green salad with low-fat
  Italian Dressing
Italian Oven-Fried Eggplant (page 194)

### Evening Snack
Apricot-Pecan Bread (page 133)
1 cup skim or 1% low-fat milk

# MENOPAUSE

Diet has emerged as a powerful tool in the management of problems associated with menopause. By making smart food choices, you can not only help prevent the unwanted weight gain that often accompanies this time of life, but also keep your energy levels high and reduce many menopausal symptoms. Here are some strategies that can help smooth your transition through menopause.

❑ Aim for one to two servings of soy foods per day. These foods provide the phytoestrogens that can help reduce hot flashes and other symptoms of menopause. For additional phytoestrogens, include one to two tablespoons of flaxseeds in your daily diet.

❑ Eat generous amounts of vegetables, fruits, legumes, and whole grain products. These foods provide additional phytoestrogens, as well the nutrients, antioxidants, and phytochemicals you need to fight premature aging and disease.

❑ Include two to three servings of low-fat or nonfat dairy products or calcium-fortified soymilk in your diet every day to help protect your bones.

## Menu 1

### Breakfast

$^1/_2$ grapefruit
Marvelous Muesli (page 73) with
  1 tablespoon flaxseeds
1 cup skim milk or calcium-fortified soymilk
Zucchini-Spice Muffin (page 127)

### Lunch

Chunky Chicken Noodle Soup (page 107)
Sandwich made with:
  2 slices whole wheat bread
  $^1/_2$ cup Eggless Egg Salad (page 119)
  2 slices tomato
  1 leaf lettuce
  2 kiwi fruit

### Afternoon Snack

8 ounces nonfat or low-fat fruit yogurt

### Dinner

Roasted Eggplant Lasagna (page 160)
Gorgonzola Garden Salad (page 115)
1 whole wheat roll

### Evening Snack

Autumn Fruit Crisp (page 204)

## Menu 2

### Breakfast

4 Cottage-Apple Pancakes (page 70) with
  2 tablespoons maple syrup
Turkey Breakfast Sausage Patty (page 79)
1 cup skim milk or calcium-fortified soymilk

### Lunch

Crunchy Chicken and Rice Salad (page 123)
  over romaine lettuce
Tomato-Dill Soup (page 106)
9 reduced-fat Wheat Thins crackers

### Afternoon Snack

Whole Wheat Banana-Nut Bread (page 134)
1 cup skim milk or calcium-fortified soymilk

### Dinner

Tofu Lo Mein (page 140)
Sesame Slaw (page 113)
1 cup mixed fresh fruit

### Evening Snack

Deep, Dark, Delicious Chocolate Pudding
  (page 202)

# OSTEOARTHRITIS

As you learned in Chapter 2, proper diet is essential in the management of this "wear and tear" of the joints. The following strategies are especially important.

❑ Maintain a healthy body weight. This will take some of the stress off your joints, which will, in turn, help reduce pain and the progression of the disease.

❑ Eat generous amounts of vegetables, fruits, legumes, and whole grain products. These foods provide the nutrients, antioxidants, and phytochemicals you need to maintain healthy joints and slow the progression of arthritis.

❑ Include two to three servings of low-fat or nonfat dairy products or calcium-fortified soymilk in your diet every day to help maintain strong bones.

❑ Make sure you get enough vitamin D, which has been shown to slow the progression of osteoarthritis. A daily multivitamin can help insure adequate vitamin D intake.

## Menu 1

### Breakfast
Sausage and Potato Strata (page 78)
Blueberry Oat Muffin (page 126)
1 cup sliced fresh strawberries
1 cup skim milk or calcium-fortified soymilk

### Lunch
Country Vegetable Soup (page 104)
Skinny Sloppy Joes (page 185)
Carrot and celery sticks

### Afternoon Snack
1 ounce low-fat Cheddar cheese
1 apple

### Dinner
Honey Crunch Chicken (page 152)
Sweet Potato Salad (page 118)
Glorious Green Bean Casserole (page 195)
1 whole wheat roll

### Evening Snack
Cherry-Berry Cobbler (page 205)

## Menu 2

### Breakfast
Polenta Porridge (page 72)
$\frac{1}{2}$ grapefruit
1 cup skim milk or calcium-fortified soymilk

### Lunch
French Market Soup (page 101)
Roasted Vegetable Salad (page 112)
1 cup fresh cherries

### Afternoon Snack
Prune and Walnut Bread (page 135)
1 cup skim milk or calcium-fortified soymilk

### Dinner
Garden Meat Loaf (page 159)
Garlic Mashed Potatoes (page 190)
Dilled Zucchini and Carrots (page 193)
Moist Cornmeal Muffin (page 128)

### Evening Snack
Simple Peach Sorbet (page 215)

# OSTEOPOROSIS

As you learned in Chapter 2, lifestyle is one of the key factors that determine the degree of bone loss in later life. By focusing on the following points, you can make your diet work for you.

❏ Get plenty of calcium by eating two to three servings of low-fat and nonfat dairy products or calcium-fortified soy products daily. Also make sure that you get enough vitamin D, so that you can absorb the calcium you eat.

❏ Eat plenty of vegetables, fruits, legumes, and whole grain products. These foods provide nutrients like magnesium and boron, which are needed for building strong bones.

❏ Avoid excess animal protein, sodium, and caffeine, all of which can cause calcium to be lost from the body.

❏ Maintain a healthy body weight, as being underweight is a risk factor for osteoporosis.

## Menu 1

### Breakfast
2 slices Cinnamon-Vanilla French Toast
   (page 68)
$1/4$ cup Warm Apple Topping (page 71)
1 cup skim milk or calcium-fortified soymilk

### Lunch
Cauliflower-Cheese Soup (page 98)
Roasted Vegetable Sandwich (page 172)

### Afternoon Snack
1 ounce baked tortilla chips
Bueno Bean Dip (page 91)

### Dinner
Cabbage-Apple Salad (page 113)
2 cups Salsa and Spice Chili (page 158)
Buttermilk Cornbread (page 130)

### Evening Snack
Honey-Vanilla Custard (page 204)

## Menu 2

### Breakfast
California Crunch Granola (page 74)
8 ounces nonfat or low-fat vanilla yogurt
1 cup mixed fresh fruit

### Lunch
Sicilian Grilled Chicken and Pasta Salad
   (page 121)
2 plums

### Afternoon Snack
3 Ry-Krisp crackers
$1^1/_2$ ounces low-fat cheese

### Dinner
Savory Stuffed Fish (page 164)
Spinach-Noodle Casserole (page 199)
Glazed Rosemary Carrots (page 194)
1 whole wheat roll

### Evening Snack
Triple Berry Sundae (page 206)

# RHEUMATOID ARTHRITIS

Although important questions remain about the treatment of rheumatoid arthritis, research has shed some interesting light on this subject over the past few years. Key dietary strategies for controlling this disorder include the following:

❑ Maintain a healthy body weight. This will take some of the stress off your joints, which will, in turn, help reduce pain and the progression of the disease.

❑ Include one to two servings of fish in your daily diet. This is one case in which you *want* oily fish like salmon, sardines, mackerel, and herring, as these foods provide the omega-3 fatty acids that can reduce joint inflammation. For additional omega-3 fatty acids, include 1 to 2 tablespoons of flaxseeds in your daily diet.

❑ Limit your consumption of foods rich in omega-6 fatty acids, as these foods can interfere with the body's use of omega-3 fats. (See Chapter 1 to learn about the foods richest in omega-6 oils.)

❑ Eat generous amounts of vegetables, fruits, legumes, and whole grain products. These foods provide the nutrients, antioxidants, and phytochemicals you need to maintain healthy bones and joints.

## Menu 1

### Breakfast
½ cup scrambled fat-free egg substitute
Turkey Breakfast Sausage Patty (page 79)
Banana Oat Bran Muffin (page 127)
1 cup skim milk or calcium-fortified soymilk
½ cantaloupe melon

### Lunch
Cauliflower-Cheese Soup (page 98)
Dilled Salmon Burger (page 162)
Carrot and celery sticks

### Afternoon Snack
2 ounces sardines in mustard or tomato sauce
2 slices Wasa bread

### Dinner
Penne California (page 138)
1 cup steamed broccoli
1 whole wheat roll

### Evening Snack
Spiked Strawberries (page 212)

## Menu 2

### Breakfast
Breakfast Brown Rice Pudding (page 75) with
  1 tablespoon flaxseeds
1 cup mixed fresh fruit
1 cup skim milk or calcium-fortified soymilk

### Lunch
Cool Gazpacho (page 108)
Black Bean Burrito (page 173)

### Afternoon Snack
8 ounces nonfat or low-fat fruit yogurt

### Dinner
Mediterranean Foil-Baked Fish (page 167)
Greek Cottage Fries (page 188)
Asparagus With Honey Mustard Sauce
  (page 192)
1 whole wheat roll

### Evening Snack
Phyllo Apple Dumpling (page 209)

# WEIGHT PROBLEMS

A healthy calorie-controlled eating plan combined with a regular exercise program is the only effective means of keeping weight under control. And even small changes, when followed consistently, can make a big difference. The following tips will help you feel full and satisfied while enjoying weight loss success.

❑ Include plenty of vegetables and fruits in meals and snacks. Low in calories and high in fiber, these foods will fill you up, but not out.

❑ Have some protein at each meal. Protein-rich foods are very filling, and so will help keep you feeling satisfied until your next meal.

❑ Control portions of starchy foods like bread, rice, pasta, and potatoes. Though low in fat, when eaten in excess, these foods can quickly push you over your calorie budget.

❑ Keep fats and sugar to a minimum. This will help keep calories under control.

❑ Eat at least three meals per day, spacing them out evenly. This will keep your metabolism going strong throughout the day.

## Menu 1

*Breakfast*
Spring Vegetable Frittata (page 78)
$1/2$ grapefruit
Molasses Bran Muffin (page 129)

*Lunch*
Savory Vegetable-Beef Soup (page 105)
Portabella Mushroom Sandwich (page 173)

*Afternoon Snack*
1 nectarine

*Dinner*
Italian Baked Chicken (page 153)
$3/4$ cup brown rice
Rocket Salad (page 112)

*Evening Snack*
2 Maple Jumbles (page 210)
1 cup skim milk or calcium-fortified soymilk

## Menu 2

*Breakfast*
Cinnamon-Apple Oatmeal (page 75)
1 cup sliced fresh strawberries
1 cup skim milk or calcium-fortified soymilk

*Lunch*
Chutney Chicken Salad (page 122)
9 reduced-fat Wheat Thins crackers

*Afternoon Snack*
Apple Crunch Parfait (page 77)

*Dinner*
Crispy Oven-Fried Fish (page 166)
Country Corn Pudding (page 198)
1 cup steamed fresh green beans

*Evening Snack*
Blueberry Bread Pudding (page 202)

As you can see, it is not difficult to plan meals that are both delicious *and* good for you. Nor is it difficult to create meals that target problems ranging from cardiovascular disease to excess weight. I hope that the menus and strategies presented in this chapter will inspire you to plan your own healthful meals—meals that not only are in keeping with the Guidelines for Good Eating, but also combine slimmed-down versions of old favorites with delicious new dishes to satisfy each and every member of your family.

# Conclusion

There is no doubt that food is one of the most powerful tools you have to promote optimal health and longevity. If you've gotten this far, you've taken a major step toward achieving these goals. I hope that by now you've had a chance to incorporate the secrets of cooking for long life into your everyday diet. If so, you may already be reaping some of the benefits that many others have enjoyed—benefits like greater weight control; increased energy; a stronger immune system; a reduced risk of heart disease, diabetes, and cancer; and bolstered defenses against premature aging.

Both scientific studies and anecdotal experience have shown that the tips, guidelines, and strategies presented in this book *do* work. However, there are probably many more ways in which you can incorporate the preventive powers of nutrition into your life. Don't be afraid to devise your own secrets of cooking for long life. You may come up with great new techniques for improving your own favorite recipes and for including nutrient-packed foods in your diet. Then, if you'd like to share your ideas, please don't hesitate to write to me, care of Avery Publishing Group, 120 Old Broadway, Garden City Park, New York 11040.

I wish you the best of luck in all your healthy cooking adventures!

# Resource List

Most of the ingredients used in the recipes in this book are readily available in any supermarket, or can be found in your local health foods store or gourmet shop. But if you are unable to locate what you're looking for, the following list should guide you to a manufacturer who can sell the desired product to you directly or inform you of the nearest retail outlet.

## Whole Grains and Flours

Arrowhead Mills, Inc.
Box 2059
Hereford, TX 79045
(800) 749–0730

*Whole wheat pastry flour, oat flour, and other flours and whole grains.*

The Baker's Catalogue
PO Box 876
Norwich, VT 05055-0876
(800) 827–6836

*King Arthur white whole wheat flour, whole wheat pastry flour, unbleached pastry flour, and other flours, whole grains, and baking products.*

Mountain Ark Trading Company
PO Box 3170
Fayetteville, AR 72702
(800) 643–8909

*Whole grains and flours, unrefined sweeteners, dried fruits, fruit spreads, and a wide variety of other natural foods.*

Sovex Natural Foods, Inc.
PO Box 2178
Collegedale, TN 37315
(800) 227–2320

*Good Shepherd apple fiber, bulgur wheat, oat bran, wheat bran, and many other whole grain products.*

Walnut Acres Organic Farms
PO Box 8
Penns Creek, PA 17862-0800
(800) 433–3998

*Whole wheat pastry flour, unbleached pastry flour, unbleached flour, and other flours, whole grains, and baking products. Also unrefined sweeteners, dried fruits, and a wide variety of other organic and natural foods.*

## Sweeteners

Advanced Ingredients
331 Capitola Avenue, Suite F
Capitola, CA 95010
(408) 464–9891

*Fruit Source granulated and liquid sweeteners.*

Sucanat North America Corporation
/Wholesome Foods
525 Fentress Boulevard
Daytona Beach, FL 32114
(904) 258–4708

*Sucanat granulated sweetener.*

Vermont Country Maple, Inc.
76 Ethan Allen Drive
South Burlington, VT 05403
(800) 528–7021

*Maple sugar, maple syrup, and other maple products.*

## Dutch Processed Cocoa Powder

The Baker's Catalogue
PO Box 876
Norwich, VT 05055-0876
(800) 827-6836

Hershey's Chocolate World
(800) 544-1347

# Selected References

## Arthritis

Felson DT, Zhang Y, Anthony JM, Naimark A, Anderson JJ. Weight loss reduces the risk for symptomatic knee osteoarthritis in women. The Framingham Study. *Annals of Internal Medicine* 1992;116(7):535–539.

Fortin PR, Lew RA, Liang MH, Wright EA, Beckett LA, Chalmers TC, Sperling RI. Validation of a meta-analysis: the effects of fish oil in rheumatoid arthritis. *Journal of Clinical Epidemiology* 1995;48(11):1379–1390.

Geusens P, Wouters C, Nijs J, Jiang Y, Dequeker J. Long-term effect of omega-3 fatty acid supplementation in active rheumatoid arthritis. A 12-month, double-blind, controlled study. *Arthritis and Rheumatism* 1994;37(6):824–829.

Haugen MA, Kjeldsen-Kragh J, Bjerve KS, Hostmark AT, Forre O. Changes in plasma phospholipid fatty acids and their relationship to disease activity in rheumatoid arthritis patients treated with a vegetarian diet. *British Journal of Nutrition* 1994;72(4):555–566.

Kjeldsen J, Haugen M, Borchgrevink CF, Laerum E, Eek M, Mowinkel P, Hovi K, Forre O. Controlled trial of fasting and one-year vegetarian diet in rheumatoid arthritis. *Lancet* 1991;338:899–902.

Kremer JM. Effects of modulation of inflammatory and immune parameters in patients with rheumatic and inflammatory disease receiving dietary supplementation of n-3 and n-6 fatty acids. *Lipids* 1996;31(suppl):S243–S247.

Kremer JM, Lawrence DA, Petrillo GF, Litts LL, Mullaly PM, Rynes RI, Stocker RP, Parhami N, Greenstein NS, Fuchs BR, Mathur A, Robinson DR, Sperling RI, Bigaouette J. Effects of high-dose fish oil on rheumatoid arthritis after stopping nonsteroidal anti-inflammatory drugs. *Arthritis and Rheumatism* 1995;38(8):1107–1114.

McAlindon TE, Felson DT, Zhang Y, Hannan MT, Aliabadi P, Weissman B, Rush D, Wilson PW, Jacques P. Relation of dietary intake and serum levels of vitamin D to progression of osteoarthritis of the knee among participants in the Framingham Study. *Annals of Internal Medicine* 1996;125(5):353–359.

McAlindon TE, Jacques P, Zhang Y, Hannan MT, Aliabadi P, Weissman B, Rush D, Levy D, Felson DT. Do antioxidant micronutrients protect against the development and progression of knee osteoarthritis? *Arthritis and Rheumatism* 1996;39(4):648–656.

Schilke JM, Johnson GO, Housh TJ, O'Dell JR. Effects of muscle-strength training on the functional status of patients with osteoarthritis of the knee joint. *Nursing Research* 1996;45(2):68–72.

Sperling RI. Eicosanoids in rheumatoid arthritis. *Rheumatic Diseases Clinics of North America* 1995;21(3):741–758.

## Cancer

Adlercreutz H, Mazur W. Phyto-oestrogens and western diseases. *Annals of Medicine* 1997;29:95–120.

The American Cancer Society 1996 Advisory Committee on Diet, Nutrition, and Cancer Prevention. Guidelines on diet, nutrition, and cancer prevention: reducing the risk of cancer with healthy food choices and physical activity. *CA: A Cancer Journal for Clinicians* 1996;46(6)325–341.

Center for Science in the Public Interest. *Safe Food: Eating Wisely in a Risky World*. Venice CA: Living Planet Press, 1991.

Correa P. The role of antioxidants in gastric carcinogenesis. *Critical Reviews in Food Science and Nutrition* 1995;35(1&2);59–64.

Giovannucci E, Ascherio A, Rimm EB, Stampfer JM, Colditz GA, Willet WC. Intake of carotenoids and retinol in relation to risk of prostate cancer. *Journal of the National Cancer Institute* 1995;87(23):1767–1776.

Huang Z, Hankinson SE, Colditz GA, Stampfer MJ, Hunter DJ, Manson JE, Hennekens CH, Rosner B, Speizer FE, Willet WC. Dual effects of weight and weight gain on breast cancer risk. *Journal of the American Medical Association* 1997;278:1407–1411.

Kaaks R. Nutrition, hormones, and breast cancer: is insulin the missing link? *Cancer Causes and Control* 1976;7(6):605–625.

Rose, DP. Dietary fatty acids and cancer. *American Journal of Clinical Nutrition* 1997;66 (suppl):998S–1003S.

Steinmetz KA, Potter JD. Vegetables, fruit, and cancer prevention: a review. *Journal of the American Dietetic Association* 1996;96:1027–1039.

World Cancer Research Fund/American Institute for Cancer Research. *Food, Nutrition, and Cancer: A Global Perspective*. Menasha, WI: Banta Book Group, 1997.

## Cardiovascular Disease

Boushey CJ, Beresford SA, Omenn GS, Motulsky AG. A quantitative assessment of plasma homocysteine as a risk factor for vascular disease: probable benefits of increasing folic acid intakes. *Journal of the American Medical Association* 1995;274(13):1049–1057.

Daviglus ML, Stamler J, Orencia AJ, Dyer AR, Liu K, Greenland P, Walsk MK, Morris D, Shekelle RB. Fish consumption and the 30-year risk of fatal myocardial infarction. *New England Journal of Medicine* 1997;336(15):1046–1053.

Ernst ND, Obarzanek E, Clark MB, Briefel RR, Brown CD, Donato K. Cardiovascular health risks related to overweight. *Journal of the American Dietetic Association* 1997;97:S47–S51.

Gould KL, Ornish D, Kirkeeide R, Brown S, Stuart Y, Buchi M, Billings J, Armstrong W, Ports T, Scherwitz L. Improved stenosis geometry by quantitative coronary arteriography after vigorous risk factor modification. *American Journal of Cardiology* 1992;69(10):845–853.

Hodis HN, Mack WJ, LaBree L, Cashin-Hemphill L, Sevanian A, Johnson R, Stanley MA, Azen P. Serial coronary angiographic evidence that antioxidant vitamin intake reduced progression of coronary artery atherosclerosis. *Journal of the American Medical Association* 1995;273:1849–1854.

Kwitrovitch PO. The effect of dietary fat, antioxidants, and pro-oxidants on blood lipids, lipoproteins, and atherosclerosis. *Journal of the American Dietetic Association* 1997;97:S31–S41.

Losonczy KG, Harris TB, Havlik RJ. Vitamin E and vitamin C supplement use and risk of all-cause and coronary heart disease mortality in older persons: the established populations for epidemiologic studies of the elderly. *American Journal of Clinical Nutrition* 1996;64:190–196.

Ornish D, Brown SE, Scherwitz LW, Billings JH, Armstrong WT, Ports TA, McLanahan SM, Kirkeeide RL, Brand R, Gould KL. Can lifestyle changes reverse coronary heart disease? *Lancet* 1990;336:129–133.

Reaven GM. The role of insulin resistance and hyperinsulinemia in coronary heart disease. *Metabolism* 1992;41(5):16–19.

Reaven GM. Role of insulin resistance in human disease. *Diabetes* 1988;37:1595–1607.

Rimm EB, Ascherio A, Giovannucci E, Spiegelman D, Stampfer MJ, Willet WC. Vegetable, fruit, and cereal fiber intake and risk of coronary heart disease among men. *Journal of the American Medical Association* 1996; 275:447–451.

Rimm EB, Stampfer MJ. The role of antioxidants in preventive cardiology. *Current Opinion in Cardiology* 1997;12:188–194.

Rupp H. Insulin resistance, hyperinsulinemia, and cardiovascular disease. The need for novel dietary prevention strategies. *Basic Research in Cardiology* 1992;87:99–105.

Sacks FM, Obarzanek E, Windhauser MM, Svetkey LP, Vollmer WM, McCullough M, Karanja N, Lin P, Steele P, Proschan MA, Evans MA, Appel LA, Bray GA, Vogt TM, Moore TJ. Rationale and design of the dietary approaches to stop hypertension trial (DASH): a multicenter controlled-feeding study of dietary patterns to lower blood pressure. *Annals of Epidemiology* 1995;5:108–118.

## Diabetes

Foster-Powell K, Miller JB. International tables of glycemic index. *American Journal of Clinical Nutrition* 1995;62:871S–893S.

Jenkins DJA, Thomas DM, Wolever MS, Taylor RH, Barker H, Fielden H, Baldwin JM, Bowling AC, Newman HC, Jenkins AL, Goff DV. Glycemic index of foods: a physiological basis for carbohydrate exchange. *American Journal of Clinical Nutrition* 1981;34:362–366.

Salmeron J, Ascherio A, Rimm EB, Colditz GA, Spiegelman D, Jenkins DJ, Stampfer MJ, Wing AL, Willett WC. Dietary fiber, glycemic load, and risk of NIDDM in men. *Diabetes Care* 1997;20(4):545–550.

Salmeron J, Manson JE, Stampfer MJ, Colditz GA, Wing AL, Willett WC. Dietary fiber, glycemic load, and risk of non-insulin dependent diabetes mellitus in women. *Journal of the American Medical Association* 1997;277:472–477.

Wolever TMS, Jenkins DJA, Vuskan V, Jenkins AL, Buckley GC, Wong GS, Josse RG. Beneficial effect of a low glycaemic index diet in type 2 diabetes. *Diabetic Medicine* 1992;9:451–458.

## Fat

Blundell JE, Macdiarmid JI. Fat as a risk factor for overconsumption: satiation, satiety, and patterns of eating. *Journal of the American Dietetic Association* 1997;97:S63–S69.

Caughey GE, Mantzioris E, Gibson RA, Cleland LG, James MJ. The effect on human tumor necrosis factor and interleukin 1 production of diets enriched in n-3 fatty acids from vegetable oil or fish oil. *American Journal of Clinical Nutrition* 1996;63:116–122.

Dupont J, Holub BJ, Knapp HR, Meydani M. Fatty acid-related functions. *American Journal of Clinical Nutrition* 1996;63:991S–3S.

Hodgson JM, Wahlqvist ML, Boxall JA, Balazs ND. Can linoleic acid contribute to coronary artery disease? *American Journal of Clinical Nutrition* 1993;58:228–234.

Louheranta AM, Porkkala-Sarataho EK, Nyyssonen MK, Salonen RM, Salonen JT. Linoleic acid intake and susceptibility of very-low density and low-density lipoproteins to oxidation in men. *American Journal of Clinical Nutrition* 1996;63:698–703.

Simopoulos AP. Omega-3 fatty acids in health and disease and in growth and development. *American Journal of Clinical Nutrition* 1991;54:438–463.

Sugano M. Characteristics of fats in Japanese diets and current recommendations. *Lipids* 1996 Mar;31 (suppl):S283–286.

Troisi R, Willet WC, Weiss ST. Trans-fatty acid intake in relation to serum lipid concentrations in adult men. *American Journal of Clinical Nutrition* 1992;56:1019–1024.

Weisburger JH. Dietary fat and risk of chronic disease: mechanistic insights from experimental studies. *Journal of the American Dietetic Association* 1997;97:S16–S23.

Willet WC, Stampfer MJ, Manson JE, Colditz GA, Speizer FE, Rosner BA, Sampson LA, Hennekens CH. Intake of trans fatty acids and risk of coronary heart disease among women. *Lancet* 1993;341:581–585.

## Free Radicals and Antioxidants

Ames BN, Shigenaga MK, Hagen T. Oxidants, antioxidants, and the degenerative diseases of aging. *Proceedings of the National Academy of Sciences USA* 1993;90:7915–7922.

Jacob RA, Burri BJ. Oxidative damage and defense. *American Journal of Clinical Nutrition* 1996;63:985S–990S.

Rock CL, Jacob RA, Bowen PE. Update on the biological characteristics of the antioxidant micronutrients: vitamin C, vitamin E, and the carotenoids. *Journal of the American Dietetic Association* 1996;96(7):693–702.

## Healing Powers of Foods

De Oliveira e Silva ER, Seidman CE, Tian JJ, Hudgins LC, Sacks FM, Breslow JL. Effects of shrimp consumption on plasma lipoproteins. *American Journal of Clinical Nutrition* 1996; 64:712–717.

Dorant E, van den Brandt PA, Goldbohm RA, Sturmans F. Consumption of onions and a reduced risk of stomach carcinoma. *Gastroenterology* 1996;110(1):12–20.

Gartner C, Stahl W, Sies H. Lycopene is more available from tomato paste than from fresh tomatoes. *American Journal of Clinical Nutrition* 1997;66:116–122.

Jacobs DR, Meyer KA, Kushi LH, Folsom AR. Whole-grain intake may reduce the risk of ischemic heart disease death in post-menopausal women: the Iowa Women's Health Study. *American Journal of Clinical Nutrition* 1998; 68(2):248–257.

Knekt P, Jarvinen R, Seppanen R, Heliovarra M, Teppo L, Pukkala E, Aromaa A. Dietary flavonoids and the risk of lung cancer and other malignant neoplasms. *American Journal of Epidemiology* 1997;146(3):223–230.

Sivam GP, Lampe JW, Ulness B, Swanzy SR, Potter JD. Helicobacter pylori—in vitro susceptibility to garlic *(Allium sativum)* extract. *Nutrition and Cancer* 1997;27(2):118–121.

Smith BL. Organic foods vs supermarket foods: element levels. *Journal of Applied Nutrition* 1993;45:35–39.

Warshafsky S, Kamer RS, Sivak SL. Effect of garlic on total serum cholesterol: a meta-analysis. *Annals of Internal Medicine* 1993;119:599–605.

You WC, Blot WJ, Chang YS, Ershow A, Yang ZT, An Q, Henderson BE, Fraumeni JF, Wang TG. Allium vegetables and reduced risk of stomach cancer. *Journal of the National Cancer Institute* 1989;81(2):162–164.

## Menopause

Adlercreutz H, Mazur W. Phyto-oestrogens and western diseases. *Annals of Medicine* 1997; 29(2): 95–120.

Hammar M, Berg G, Lindgren R. Does physical exercise influence the frequency of post-menopausal hot flushes? *Acta Obstetricia Gynecologica Scandinavica* 1990;69:409–412.

Heymsfield SB, Gallagher D, Poehlman ET, Wolper C, Nonas K, Nelson D, Wang ZM. Menopausal changes in body composition and energy expenditure. *Experimental Gerontology* 1994;29(3-4):377–389.

Knight DC, Eden JA. A review of the clinical effects of phytoestrogens. *Obstetrics and Gynecology* 1996;87(5):897–904.

Murkies AL, Lombard C, Strauss BJ, Wilcox G, Burger HG, Morton MS. Dietary flour supplementation decreases post-menopausal hot flushes: effect of soy and wheat. *Maturitas* 1995;21(3):189–195.

Poehlman ET, Toth MJ, Gardner AW. Changes in energy balance and body composition at menopause: a controlled longitudinal study. *Annals of Internal Medicine* 1995;123(9):673–675.

Renli K, Block G. Phytoestrogen content of foods—a compendium of literature values. *Nutrition and Cancer* 1996;26(2):123–144.

## Osteoporosis

Abraham GE, Grewal H. A total dietary program emphasizing magnesium instead of calcium. *Journal of Reproductive Medicine* 1990; 35(5):503–507.

Devine A, Criddle RA, Dick IM, Kerr DA, Prince RL. A longitudinal study of the effect of sodium and calcium intakes on regional bone density in postmenopausal women. *American Journal of Clinical Nutrition* 1995;62:740–745.

Dreosti IE. Magnesium status and health. *Nutrition Reviews* 1995;53(9):S23–S27.

Heaney RP. Protein intake and the calcium economy. *Journal of the American Dietetic Association* 1993;93(11):1259–1260.

McBean LD, Forgac T, Calvert-Finn S. Osteo-porosis: visions for care and prevention—a conference report. *Journal of the American Dietetic Association* 1994;94(6):668–671.

Metz JA, Anderson JB, Gallagher PN. Intakes of calcium, phosphorus, and protein, and physical activity are related to radial bone mass in young adult women. *American Journal of Clinical Nutrition* 1993;58:537–542.

Naghii MR, Samman S. The role of boron in nutrition and metabolism. *Progress in Food and Nutrition Science* 1993;17:331–349.

Packard PT, Heaney RP. Medical nutrition therapy for patients with osteoporosis. *Journal of the American Dietetic Association* 1997;97(4): 414–417.

Sojka JE. Magnesium supplementation and osteoporosis. *Nutrition Reviews* 1995;53(3): 71–80.

Strause L, Saltman P, Smith KT, Bracker M, Andon MB. Spinal bone loss in postmenopausal women supplemented with calcium and trace minerals. *Journal of Nutrition* 1994; 124:1060–1064.

Volpe SL, Taper J, Meacham S. The relationship between boron and magnesium status and bone mineral density in the human: a review. *Magnesium Research* 1993;6(3):291–296.

## Protein

Campbell WC, Crim MC, Dallal GE, Young VR, Evans WJ. Increased protein requirements in elderly people: new data and retrospective reassessments. *American Journal of Clinical Nutrition* 1994;60:501–509.

Castaneda C, Charnley JM, Evans WJ, Crim MC. Elderly women accommodate to a low-protein diet with losses of body cell mass, muscle function, and immune response. *American Journal of Clinical Nutrition* 1995;62:30–39.

Evans WJ, Cyr-Campbell D. Nutrition, exercise, and healthy aging. *Journal of the American Dietetic Association* 1997;97(6):632–638.

## Vitamins and Minerals

Chandra RK. Effect of vitamin and trace element supplementation on immune responses and infection in elderly subjects. *Lancet* 1992; 340:1124–1127.

Connor JR, Beard JL. Dietary iron supplements in the elderly: to use or not to use? *Nutrition Today* 1997;32(3):102–109.

Kant AK, Schatzkin A. Consumption of energy-dense, nutrient-poor foods by the US population: effect on nutrient profiles. *Journal of the American College of Nutrition* 1994;13(3):285–291.

Krebs-Smith SM, Cleveland LE, Ballard-Barbash R, Cook DA, Kahle LL. Characterizing food intake patterns of American adults. *American Journal of Clinical Nutrition* 1997;65(4 suppl): 1264S–1268S.

Mertz W. A balanced approach to nutrition for health: the need for biologically essential minerals and vitamins. *Journal of the American Dietetic Association* 1994;94(11):1259–1262.

Russell RM. New views on the RDAs for older adults. *Journal of the American Dietetic Association* 1997;97(5):515–518.

"What we eat in America" survey. *Nutrition Today* 1997;32(1):37–40.

# Weight Problems and Obesity

American Health Foundation Roundtable on Healthy Weight. *American Journal of Clinical Nutrition* 1996;63(suppl):409S–477S.

Coleman E, Toth MJ, Katzel LI, Fonong T, Gardner AW, Poehlman ET. Body fatness and waist circumference are independent predictors of the age-associated increase in fasting insulin levels in healthy men and women. *International Journal of Obesity Related Metabolic Disorders* 1995;19(11):798–803.

Consumers Union. Weight: what have you got to lose? *Consumer Reports on Health* 1995;7(9): 97–100.

Manson JE, Willet WC, Stampfer MJ, Colditz GA, Hunter DJ, Hankinson SE, Hennekens CH, Speizer FE. Body weight and mortality among women. *New England Journal of Medicine* 1995; 333(11):677–685.

Miller WC, Niederpruem MG, Wallace JP, Lindeman AK. Dietary fat, sugar, and fiber predict body fat content. *Journal of the American Dietetic Association* 1994;94:612–615.

Nelson LH, Tucker LA. Diet composition related to body fat in a multivariate study of 203 men. *Journal of the American Dietetic Association* 1996;96:771–777.

Poehlman ET, Goran MI, Gardner AW, Ades PA, Arciero PJ, Katzman-Rooks SM, Montgomery SM, Toth MJ, Sutherland PT. Determinants of decline in resting metabolic rate in aging females. *American Journal of Physiology* 1993; 264(3 pt 1):E450–E455.

Poehlman ET, Toth MJ, Bunyard LB, Gardner AW, Donaldson KE, Colman E, Fonong T, Ades PA. Physiological predictors of increasing total and central adiposity in aging men and women. *Archives of Internal Medicine* 1995;155(22): 2443–2448.

Position of the American Dietetic Association: Weight management. *Journal of the American Dietetic Association* 1997;97:71–74.

Velthuis-te Wierik EJM, van de Berg H, Schaafsma G, Hendriks HFJ, Brouwer A. Energy restriction, a useful intervention to retard human aging? *European Journal of Clinical Nutrition* 1994;48:138–148.

Walford RL. The clinical promise of diet restriction. *Geriatrics* 1990;45:81–87.

# Metric Conversion Tables

## Common Liquid Conversions

| Measurement | = | Milliliters |
|---|---|---|
| $^1/_4$ teaspoon | = | 1.25 milliliters |
| $^1/_2$ teaspoon | = | 2.50 milliliters |
| $^3/_4$ teaspoon | = | 3.75 milliliters |
| 1 teaspoon | = | 5.00 milliliters |
| $1^1/_4$ teaspoons | = | 6.25 milliliters |
| $1^1/_2$ teaspoons | = | 7.50 milliliters |
| $1^3/_4$ teaspoons | = | 8.75 milliliters |
| 2 teaspoons | = | 10.0 milliliters |
| 1 tablespoon | = | 15.0 milliliters |
| 2 tablespoons | = | 30.0 milliliters |

| Measurement | = | Liters |
|---|---|---|
| $^1/_4$ cup | = | 0.06 liters |
| $^1/_2$ cup | = | 0.12 liters |
| $^3/_4$ cup | = | 0.18 liters |
| 1 cup | = | 0.24 liters |
| $1^1/_4$ cups | = | 0.30 liters |
| $1^1/_2$ cups | = | 0.36 liters |
| 2 cups | = | 0.48 liters |
| $2^1/_2$ cups | = | 0.60 liters |
| 3 cups | = | 0.72 liters |
| $3^1/_2$ cups | = | 0.84 liters |
| 4 cups | = | 0.96 liters |
| $4^1/_2$ cups | = | 1.08 liters |
| 5 cups | = | 1.20 liters |
| $5^1/_2$ cups | = | 1.32 liters |

## Converting Fahrenheit to Celsius

| Fahrenheit | = | Celsius |
|---|---|---|
| 200–205 | = | 95 |
| 220–225 | = | 105 |
| 245–250 | = | 120 |
| 275 | = | 135 |
| 300–305 | = | 150 |
| 325–330 | = | 165 |
| 345–350 | = | 175 |
| 370–375 | = | 190 |
| 400–405 | = | 205 |
| 425–430 | = | 220 |
| 445–450 | = | 230 |
| 470–475 | = | 245 |
| 500 | = | 260 |

## Conversion Formulas

| LIQUID | | |
|---|---|---|
| When You Know | Multiply By | To Determine |
| teaspoons | 5.0 | milliliters |
| tablespoons | 15.0 | milliliters |
| fluid ounces | 30.0 | milliliters |
| cups | 0.24 | liters |
| pints | 0.47 | liters |
| quarts | 0.95 | liters |

| WEIGHT | | |
|---|---|---|
| When You Know | Multiply By | To Determine |
| ounces | 28.0 | grams |
| pounds | 0.45 | kilograms |

239

# Index